D1736258

The Practice of Functional Analytic Psychotherapy

Jonathan W. Kanter · Mavis Tsai ·
Robert J. Kohlenberg
Editors

The Practice of Functional
Analytic Psychotherapy

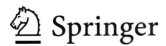 Springer

Editors
Jonathan W. Kanter
Department of Psychology
University of Wisconsin-Milwaukee
Milwaukee WI 53201
USA
jkanter@uwm.edu

Mavis Tsai
3245 Fairview Avenue East
Seattle WA 98102
USA
mavis@u.washington.edu

Robert J. Kohlenberg
Department of Psychology
University of Washington
Seattle WA 98195-1525
USA
fap@u.washington.edu

ISBN 978-1-4419-5829-7   e-ISBN 978-1-4419-5830-3
DOI 10.1007/978-1-4419-5830-3
Springer New York Dordrecht Heidelberg London

Library of Congress Control Number: 2010926926

Printed on acid-free paper

Springer is part of Springer Science+Business Media (www.springer.com)

To Zoe, Barbara, Andy, Paul and Jeremy, who taught us how wondrous and selfless parenthood can be.

Preface

Functional analytic psychotherapy (FAP) was born after a gestational period during which Kohlenberg and Tsai, as behavioral scientist practitioners, worked with clients who demonstrated profound changes far exceeding the specific stated goals of therapy through a highly emotional therapeutic process. Combining their clinical instincts, a genuine concern and therapeutic love for their clients, and precise behavioral analyses of the processes that seemed to be responsible for the profound changes observed, the full articulation of FAP appeared in 1991 with *Functional Analytic Psychotherapy: Creating Intense and Curative Therapeutic Relationships.*

FAP has evolved significantly since that first publication, with its many advances in research and clinical technique summarized in 2008 in *A Guide to FAP: Using Awareness, Courage, Love and Behaviorism* by Tsai, R. J. Kohlenberg, Kanter, B. Kohlenberg, Follette, and Callaghan. *A Guide to FAP* provides an update to the original FAP text, bringing together primary members of the community of FAP clinicians and researchers that has developed since the original book in a collaborative effort to refine and expand upon the initial framework.

The current volume originally was intended as Part II of *A Guide to FAP.* Through the process of writing and editing that book, we hoped to celebrate the larger FAP community and the compassion and intelligence that guide its work, by including chapters representing the contributions and ideas of FAP researchers and clinicians working with diverse populations and across a wide variety of settings. We realized, however, that this community is even larger and more vibrant than we thought, and thus this independent volume was born.

We gratefully acknowledge the diligent efforts of all 41 contributing authors. We would like to express our deep gratitude to these authors for their patience and respect of the editing process which resulted in multiple drafts of chapters being read at different times by different editors, such that authors received several rounds of feedback. It was truly a privilege to work with them. We hope the reader will be as inspired as we were in reading these chapters. We welcome you to join our worldwide FAP community, where we share an appreciation of the potential of individuals, where we work to weave a tapestry of behavior analytic precision and therapeutic love that is dedicated to ameliorating suffering and promoting transformation.

Milwaukee, WI   Jonathan W. Kanter
Seattle, WA   Mavis Tsai
Seattle, WA   Robert J. Kohlenberg

Contents

Contributors

Madelon Y. Bolling University of Washington, Seattle, WA, USA, mbolling@u.washington.edu

William M. Bowe University of Wisconsin-Milwaukee, Milwaukee, WI, USA, wmbowe@uwm.edu

Keri Brown University of Wisconsin, Milwaukee, WI, USA, keri_r_brown@hotmail.com

Andrew M. Busch The Warren Alpert Medical School of Brown University and The Miriam Hospital, Centers for Behavioral and Preventive Medicine, Providence, RI, USA, andrew_busch@brown.edu

Glenn M. Callaghan Department of Psychology, San Jose State University, San Jose, CA, USA, glennc@email.sjsu.edu

JoAnne Dahl Department of Psychology, University of Uppsala, Uppsala, Sweden, jo_anne.dahl@comhem.se

Thane A. Dykstra Behavioral Health Services, Trinity Services, Inc., Joliet, IL, USA, tdykstra@trinity-services.org

Rafael Ferro Centro CEDI (Educative and Development Childhood Center), Granada, Spain, rferro@cop.es

William C. Follette University of Nevada, Reno, NV, USA, follette@unr.edu

Alan S. Gurman University of Wisconsin School of Medicine and Public Health, Madison, WI, USA, asgurman@wisc.edu

Stig Helweg-Jørgensen Psychiatric Hospital Svendborg, Svendborg, Denmark, stighj@pc.dk

Renee Hoekstra Private Practice, Boston, MA, USA, renee_hoekstra@yahoo.com

Gareth I. Holman University of Washington, Seattle, WA, USA, gholman@u.washington.edu

Carl V. Indovina Autism and Family Resource Center, Trinity Services, Inc., Joliet, IL, USA, cindovina@trinity-services.org

Jonathan W. Kanter Department of Psychology, University of Wisconsin-Milwaukee, Milwaukee, WI, USA, jkanter@uwm.edu

Rachel R. Kerbauy Department of Psychology, University of São Paulo, São Paulo, Brazil, rachel.kerbauy@uol.com.br

Barbara S. Kohlenberg Department of Psychiatry and Behavioral Sciences, University of Nevada School of Medicine, Reno, NV, USA, bkohlenberg@medicine.nevada.edu

Robert J. Kohlenberg Department of Psychology, University of Washington, Seattle, WA, USA, fap@u.washington.edu

Sara J. Landes University of Washington at Harborview Medical Center, Seattle, WA, USA, sjlandes@u.washington.edu

Rachel C. Manos University of Wisconsin-Milwaukee, Milwaukee, WI, USA, rcmanos@uwm.edu

Akio Matsumoto School of Veterinary Medicine, Kitasato University, Japan, matsumot@vmas.kitasato-u.ac.jp

Daniel J. Moran Family Counseling Center, Trinity Services, Inc., Joliet, IL, USA, djmoran@trinity-services.org

Takashi Muto Department of Psychology, Doshisha University, Japan, taka610@mac.com

Reo W. Newring Children's Behavioral Health, Children's Hospital and Medical Center, Omaha, NE, USA, reo.newring@gmail.com

Kirk A.B. Newring Forensic Behavioral Health, Papillion, NE, USA; Nebraska Wesleyan University, Lincoln, NE, USA, newring@gmail.com

Hiroto Okouchi Department of Psychology, Osaka Kyoiku University, Japan, okouchi@cc.osaka-kyoiku.ac.jp

Chauncey R. Parker Independent Practice, Reno, NV, USA, chaunceyparker@gmail.com

Mary D. Plummer University of Washington, Seattle, WA, USA, maryplummer@gmail.com

Ethel Quayle Department of Applied Psychology, University College, Cork, Ireland, e.quayle@ucc.ie

Irwin S. Rosenfarb California School of Professional Psychology, Alliant International University, San Diego, CA, USA, irosenfa@alliant.edu

Maria R. Ruiz Rollins College, Winter Park, FL, USA, mruiz@rollins.edu

Laura C. Rusch University of Wisconsin-Milwaukee, Milwaukee, WI, USA, lrusch@uwm.edu

Benjamin Schoendorff University of Provence, Aix-Marseille, France, benjamin.schoendorff@gmail.com

Kimberly A. Shontz Behavioral Health Services, Trinity Services, Inc., Joliet, IL, USA, kshontz@trinity-services.org

Minoru Takahashi Department of Clinical Psychology, Mejiro University, Japan, m-takahashi@mejiro.ac.jp

Christeine Terry Psychosocial Rehabilitation Fellow, Palo Alto VA Healthcare System, Palo Alto, CA, USA, christeineterry@gmail.com

Mavis Tsai Psychological Services and Training Center, University of Washington, Seattle, WA, USA, mavis@u.washington.edu

Luis Valero School of Psychology, University of Malaga, Malaga, Spain, lvalero@uma.es

Luc Vandenberghe Pontifical Catholic University of Goiás, Goiânia, Brazil, luc.m.vandenberghe@gmail.com

Jennifer Waltz Department of Psychology, University of Montana, Missoula, MT, USA, jennifer.waltz@umontana.edu

Thomas J. Waltz University of Nevada, Reno, NV, USA, behavioralmystic@hotmail.com

Cristal E. Weeks University of Wisconsin-Milwaukee, Milwaukee, WI, USA, ceweeks@uwm.edu

Jennifer G. Wheeler Independent Practice, Seattle, WA, USA, dr.wheeler@yahoo.com

Regina C. Wielenska Instituto de Psicologia da Universidade de São Paulo, São Paulo, Brazil, wielensk@uol.com.br

About the Editors

Jonathan W. Kanter, Ph.D., is an Associate Professor of Psychology and Coordinator of the Psychology Clinic at the University of Wisconsin-Milwaukee (UWM). He directs the Depression Treatment Specialty Clinic which is collaboration between UWM and the Medical College of Wisconsin. His research focuses on behavioral and behavior analytic approaches to understanding and treating depression, with particular emphases on Functional Analytic Psychotherapy (FAP) and Behavioral Activation (BA), and an additional research interest in stigma related to depression. His research goal is to increase access to quality services for ethnic minorities and the underserved. He has written or co-edited five books on these topics, published over 50 articles and chapters, and currently is Principal Investigator and Co-Investigator on two National Institute of Health grants to study Behavioral Activation. He has presented numerous workshops on FAP and provides clinical supervision in both FAP and BA.

Robert J. Kohlenberg, Ph.D., ABPP, co-originator of FAP, is a Professor of Psychology at the University of Washington, where he held the position of Director of Clinical Training from 1997 to 2004. The Washington State Psychological Association honored him with a Distinguished Psychologist Award in 1999. He is on the Fulbright Senior Specialists Roster, and has presented "Master Clinician" and "World Round" sessions at the Association for Behavioral and Cognitive Therapies. He has presented FAP workshops both in the United States and internationally, and has published papers on migraine, obsessive-compulsive disorder, depression, intimacy of the therapeutic relationship, and a FAP approach to understanding the self. He has attained research grants for FAP treatment development, and his current interests are identifying the elements of effective psychotherapy, the integration of psychotherapies, and the treatment of co-morbidity.

Mavis Tsai, Ph.D., co-originator of FAP, is a clinical psychologist in independent practice. She is also Director of the FAP Specialty Clinic within the Psychological Services and Training Center at the University of Washington, where she is involved in teaching, supervision and research on treatment development. Her publications and presentations include work on healing posttraumatic stress disorder interpersonal trauma with FAP, disorders of the self, power issues in marital therapy, incorporating Eastern wisdom into psychotherapy, racism and minority groups, teaching youth to be peace activists, and women's empowerment via reclaiming purpose and passion. She is on the Fulbright Senior Specialists Roster, has presented "Master Clinician" sessions at the Association for Behavior and Cognitive Therapy, and has led numerous workshops nationally and internationally. She is interested in behaviorally informed multi-modal approaches to healing and growth that integrate mind, body, emotions, and spirit.

Chapter 1
Introduction to the Practice of Functional Analytic Psychotherapy

Jonathan W. Kanter, Mavis Tsai, and Robert J. Kohlenberg

The purpose of this book is to bring together, in a single volume, the diverse contributions and ideas of FAP researchers and clinicians working with a wide variety of populations, across a wide variety of settings, and using interventions associated with other therapeutic systems/orientations. As such, many chapters assume some familiarity with FAP and its theory. This introduction presents a brief history of FAP, summarizes its key principles and most recent research findings, and outlines the chapters to follow. Our intention is to provide a primer on FAP that may be helpful for those unfamiliar with it and an update for those more familiar.

The original text on FAP (Kohlenberg & Tsai, 1991) contained a basic explanation of the Skinnerian radical behavioral philosophy underlying FAP, a detailed description of the five rules that guide FAP therapists' behaviors, and behavioral analyses of clinical issues that traditionally were neglected or deemphasized by behavior analytic therapists such as emotion and memory, the self, and cognition. The book was not a treatment manual in any sense as it avoided telling the therapist what to do. The rules were not prescriptions for specific therapist actions but broad functional guidelines. Like the best of Skinner's writings on radical behaviorism (e.g., Skinner, 1953), the text started with established behavioral principles – reinforcement, stimulus control, and respondent conditioning – and composed a logical, theoretically precise functional analysis of important human behavior from them, in this case behavior that occurs in the psychotherapy relationship. The collective clinical wisdom, compassion, and behavioral precision of Kohlenberg and Tsai were woven into a framework upon which specific therapeutic techniques could be incorporated.

Understanding the original five rules of FAP first requires understanding *clinically relevant behaviors* (CRBs). Technically, CRBs are functionally defined behavioral response classes targeted by FAP. Less technically, they are instances of a client's interpersonal problems (CRB1s) and improvements in those problems

J.W. Kanter (✉)
Department of Psychology, University of Wisconsin-Milwaukee, Milwaukee, WI, USA
e-mail: jkanter@uwm.edu

J.W. Kanter et al. (eds.), *The Practice of Functional Analytic Psychotherapy*,
DOI 10.1007/978-1-4419-5830-3_1, © Springer Science+Business Media, LLC 2010

(CRB2s), as defined by the client's goals for therapy, as they occur in the live, here-and-now psychotherapy relationship.

Rule 1 is to *watch for CRBs*. Essentially this rule is a reminder to the FAP therapist that CRBs will occur in the therapy hour. A client who has trouble making friends may alienate the therapist. A client who is aggressive with others may be hostile with the therapist. A client who stutters, or yearns for affection, or avoids vulnerability, or experiences intense urges for cigarettes, will do so during the therapy hour, and so on. It is the therapist's job in FAP to observe and notice these behaviors as they occur.

Rule 2 is to *evoke CRBs*. In addition to observing CRBs (Rule 1), Rule 2 suggests structuring the therapy relationship to evoke them, which may include providing a detailed relationship-focused rationale (see Tsai et al., 2008) to the client before beginning or early in treatment, specifically prompting the client to engage in CRB2 in the moment, focusing on client emotional experiencing and expression, or co-opting techniques from other therapeutic approaches with an explicit awareness that these might functionally evoke key client behaviors.

Rule 3 in the original FAP text was to *naturally reinforce CRB2s*, which has been broadened in Tsai et al. (2008) to include contingent responding to any CRBs that occur in session. This is the essential rule that defines FAP's mechanism of action, and many of the chapters in this volume detail what is meant by it for different settings and populations. The key moments in FAP are when CRB2s (client improvements) occur and the therapist is naturally affected by this improved behavior. The therapist expresses or amplifies his or her natural response to the client in an attempt to reinforce the improved behavior. The emphasis in FAP is on *natural* reinforcement, thus FAP therapists develop genuine and caring relationships with clients and allow their natural reactions to clients in the moment to guide their expressed responses to CRBs.

Rule 4 is to *observe the potentially reinforcing effects of therapist behavior in relation to client CRBs*. To understand Rule 4, readers may be reminded that behaviorists define reinforcement functionally, as any event that leads to an increase in behavior, not topographically, as any specific kind or form of event. Thus, for a FAP therapist to know if Rule 3 is effectively occurring, Rule 4 encourages the therapist to observe client behavioral changes over time with respect to attempts at reinforcement.

Finally, Rule 5 has evolved over time. Originally in Kohlenberg and Tsai (1991) it was to *provide functional interpretations of client behavior* and was meant to highlight that any therapeutic talk in FAP should be as functional as possible, identifying antecedents and consequences to client target behavior. Such talk, theoretically, should enhance generalization of gains made in session to out-of-session settings. More recently (Tsai et al., 2008), Rule 5 has been expanded to encourage additional generalization strategies, specifically the provision of homework assignments. From a FAP perspective, the best homework assignments are those that flow from a successful in-session interaction in which CRB2s occurred and were positively reinforced by the therapist.

The five rules offer a framework for responding to CRBs during the psychotherapy session in which the therapist first notices the occurrence of CRB (Rule 1) or evokes a specific CRB (Rule 2), responds to it appropriately (Rule 3), checks that the response was reinforcing (Rule 4), and then talks about what just happened between the client and therapist, potentially including provision of a related homework assignment (Rule 5). A key is that CRBs are not defined in advance by FAP or the FAP therapist but are defined and redefined collaboratively by the client and therapist during therapy, depending on the client's goals. Thus, while a cognitive therapist may define a target in advance (e.g., depressogenic cognitions about the self, the world, and the future), the FAP therapist will not. Instead, whatever the targets brought to therapy and identified by the client, the FAP therapist will define collaboratively with the client CRB manifestations of those targets, and the therapist's behavior with respect to CRBs will be guided by the five rules.

Although FAP has been criticized for producing a preponderance of theoretical over empirical articles (Corrigan, 2001), and this volume adds to that imbalance, it is important to note that FAP can claim some unique empirical strengths. First, FAP's five rules are based on thoroughly accepted and time-tested behavioral principles: stimulus control (Rules 1 and 2), reinforcement (Rules 3 and 4), and generalization (Rule 5). Second, several compelling and converging lines of evidence supporting FAP exist from behavioral and other literatures (Baruch et al., 2008).

Third, in 1997, a pivotal event in the history of FAP occurred when Kohlenberg attained an NIMH treatment development grant to develop and evaluate FAP-Enhanced Cognitive Therapy (FECT). Based on the behavioral analysis of Cognitive Therapy (CT) first outlined in the original FAP book (Kohlenberg & Tsai, 1991), FECT included a package of enhancements designed to intensify the therapeutic relationship and focus the therapist on cognitive and other interpersonal CRBs that occurred in the context of the standard structure, case conceptualization, and treatment strategies of CT. Results of this study were encouraging, suggesting that the enhancements had measurable benefits in terms of improved interpersonal functional of clients and potentially decreased depression (Kohlenberg, Kanter, Bolling, Parker, & Tsai, 2002). In addition, process analyses found that the central enhancement provided by FAP to CT, focusing the therapist on cognitive CRBs (e.g., clients believing they are unlikable by the therapist), led to improvements in relational and overall functioning (Kanter, Schildcrout, & Kohlenberg, 2005).

Fourth, an intriguing line of research on FAP processes is promising. The intention of this line of research is to isolate FAP's mechanism of change – appropriate contingent responding by the therapist to client CRBs in the therapy session – and provide evidence that this mechanism occurs in successful FAP cases by observer coding of videotapes of the psychotherapy sessions. The impetus for this research was the development of the FAP Rating Scale (FAPRS; Callaghan, Ruckstuhl, & Busch, 2005), which first was demonstrated as a reliable and valid measure of the successful moment-to-moment FAP process by Callaghan, Summers, and Weidman (2003). Next, Busch, Callaghan, Kanter, Baruch, and Weeks (2010) replicated these results with a new client and provided evidence that an independent research team could produce reliable and valid FAPRS data. Then Busch et al. (2009) extended these results to a third client.

The client coded by Busch et al. (2009) was one of two FAP clients presented by Kanter et al. (2006), both diagnosed with major depression and a personality disorder, treated using a unique design in which treatment started with CT, and FAP techniques were withheld until a stable baseline on target problems was shown during the CT phase. Then, FAP techniques were applied. Results indicated immediate improvements in target problems for one client but not the other. The sessions from the successful client were submitted to FAPRS coding which identified the occurrence of contingent responding only after the phase shift to FAP techniques.

These results have been replicated by Landes, Kanter, Busch, Juskiewicz, and Mistele (2007) and Weeks, Baruch, Rusch, and Kanter (2009). In Landes et al., six clients with major depression and personality disorders were treated in a design similar to Kanter et al. (2006). In this study, the initial phase no longer included CT but instead focused simply on the formation of a FAP relationship, without contingent responding. When stable baselines on target problems were identified, contingent responding was initiated. Results indicated that four of the six clients showed improvements after the phase shift, while two did not. Weeks et al. (2009) then submitted the immediate post-phase-shift sessions of these clients to FAPRS coding. They found evidence for appropriate contingent responding to CRB2s for the successful cases, but a high frequency of responding to CRB1s, not CRB2s, in the unsuccessful cases.

Collectively, these results do not speak to FAP as a treatment package but rather to FAP process based on the five rules and the correspondence between application of this process and changes in target variables. The findings suggest several conclusions.

First, four separate process analyses now provide evidence for FAP's mechanism of action in successful but not unsuccessful cases. Second, the application of FAP techniques seems to be related directly to improvements in specific idiographically defined target variables in these clients, not molar variables such as depression (i.e., depression did improve for some of these clients but improvements were not directly associated with the phase shift to FAP techniques). Third, the results highlight the importance of responding to CRB2s for successful cases. In cases in which the therapist had difficulty evoking CRB2s and focused only on CRB1s, therapy seemed to become aversive for the client, leading to problems. Broadly stated, FAP needs to be constructive and focused on compassionately building new repertoires of behavior.

This research highlights how FAP's rules, because they are functionally defined, allow for considerable flexibility in what is defined as a CRB. This flexible framework can stand alone or be imported into other therapeutic approaches, potentially enhancing them. The general logic behind FAP as an enhancement to other approaches is that FAP's focus on CRBs in the therapeutic relationship could be used to enhance a variety of treatment techniques, all by helping the therapist focus on application of the technique to live instances of the problems occurring in the therapeutic relationship, and providing specific guidelines for what to do when the problems occur in session. So, cognitive therapy, which focuses on maladaptive cognitions, could be enhanced by focusing the therapist on instances of maladaptive cognition about the therapist, therapy relationship, or therapy process.

The integration of FAP with CT highlights how FAP provides a framework for psychotherapy integration and enhancement, and several FAP authors have proposed and refined integrations with other related treatment approaches. In Part I of this volume, on *FAP and Psychotherapy Integration,* several of these integrations are presented. First, Kohlenberg, Kanter, Tsai, and Weeks provide the latest conceptualization of FECT in Chapter 2 on *FAP and Cognitive Behavior Therapy.* Chapter 3 presents *FAP and Acceptance and Commitment Therapy* by Barbara Kohlenberg and Glenn Callaghan; Chapter 4 focuses on *FAP and Dialectical Behavior Therapy* by Jennifer Waltz, Sara Landes, and Gareth Holman; and Chapter 5 covers *FAP and Behavioral Activation* by Andrew Busch, Rachel Manos, Laura Rusch, William Bowe, and Jonathan Kanter. These treatments, ACT, DBT, and BA, often have been grouped with FAP because of shared behavioral sensibilities and an emphasis on acceptance (Hayes, Follette, & Linehan, 2004). The chapters demonstrate the potential power that integrations of these approaches, considered at the level of function and process rather than simple technique, have to offer. In Chapter 6, Irwin Rosenfarb capitalizes on the shared focus on the therapeutic relationship between *FAP and Psychodynamic Therapies,* clarifies their distinctive features, and discusses how FAP and psychodynamic approaches may learn from each other. Finally, in Chapter 7, Christeine Terry, Madelon Bolling, Maria Ruiz, and Keri Brown present an integration of *FAP and Feminist Therapies,* capitalizing on a shared contextual worldview, belief in an egalitarian therapeutic relationship, and use of self-disclosure between the two approaches.

As the chapters in this volume suggest, FAP as an enhancement may have additional indirect effects. Specifically, training in and practicing FAP requires a sensitivity to the nuances of the interpersonal interaction that occurs between the client and therapist, and the ability to sustain for extended periods intense, emotional interactions with clear articulation of one's own emotional reactions in a therapeutic manner. Thus, in FAP the therapy relationship comes alive for both parties, creating intimacy and love and deepening the relational quality of the larger therapeutic context. Acceptance and mindfulness, compassion, love, and courage become key repertoires for the FAP therapist.

Other indirect effects of FAP may stem from its radical behavioral philosophy, which focuses on environmental influences over behavior. FAP is committed to the notion that the ultimate source of a client's presenting problems is the context in which that client lives, and the history of that client in that context. Understanding the client's particular context in detail is key to identifying and responding to CRBs appropriately and ensuring that one's responses will generalize to the *appropriate* outside settings. With this attention to context comes humility, because we are ALL shaped by our contexts, and fully understanding a client's history and context reduces blame and judgment about the client's problematic behavior.

The importance of context and flexibility of the FAP framework, and the humility and compassion inherent in its application, is on full display in Part II of this volume on *FAP Across Settings and Populations.* Chapter 8, *FAP-Enhanced Couple*

Therapy: Perspectives and Possibilities by Alan Gurman, Thomas Waltz, and William Follette, presents informative guidelines and strategies for applying FAP with couples. Chapter 9 on *FAP with Sexual Minorities* by Mary Plummer provides useful insights into the context of sexual minorities, strategies to help FAP therapists increase their sensitivity to this context, and guidelines for the application of FAP with sexual minorities. Chapter 10 on *Transcultural FAP* by Luc Vandenberghe and his 13 co-authors, from countries spanning North and South America, Europe, and Asia, demonstrates how FAP can be applied with sensitivity across many ethnicities and cultures. Chapter 11, *FAP Strategies and Ideas for Working with Adolescents*, by Reo Newring, Chauncey Parker, and Kirk Newring, provides modifications and guidelines for working with adolescents and their families based on the authors' extensive experience in treating this population. Chapter 12, *The Application of FAP to Persons with Serious Mental Illness*, by Thane Dykstra, Kimberly Shontz, Carl Indovina, and Daniel J. Moran, presents FAP strategies for working with individuals at the level of an institutional milieu, developed by these authors from the nationally recognized program, Trinity Services, Illinois. Chapter 13, *FAP with People Convicted of Sexual Offenses*, by Kirk Newring and Jennifer Wheeler, outlines a strategy for assessing and intervening on CRBs related to sexual offending. Their chapter provides an excellent example of how CRBs are defined functionally, not topographically, such that actual sexual offense behavior is most often not the target of treatment, but rather the functions that give rise to that behavior are targeted. Finally, Chapter 14, *FAP for Interpersonal Process Groups,* by Renee Hoekstra and Mavis Tsai, discusses FAP in group settings. This chapter, like Chapter 8 on FAP with couples, shows how treatment can be enhanced because key aspects of the outside world are brought into the treatment setting, facilitating generalization of gains and clarifying the role of FAP's five rules in treatment.

FAP calls for behavior analytic precision; open-hearted generosity, vulnerability, expressiveness, and humility; and the continued pursuit of intellectual and emotional growth from its practitioners. We hope that this volume offers guidance and inspiration to a new generation of researchers and clinicians, who are stimulated by these ideas to further evaluate, develop, and refine these efforts.

References

Baruch, D. E., Kanter, J. W., Busch, A. M., Plummer, M. D., Tsai, M., Rusch, L. C., Landes, S. J., & Holman, G. I. (2008). Lines of evidence in support of FAP. In M. Tsai, R. J. Kohlenberg, J. W. Kanter, B. Kohlenberg, W. C. Follette, & G. M. Callaghan (Eds.), *A guide to FAP: Using awareness, courage, love and behaviorism*. New York: Springer.

Busch, A. M., Callaghan, G. C., Kanter, J. W., Baruch, D. E., & Weeks, C. E. (2010). The functional analytic psychotherapy rating scale: A replication and extension. *Contemporary Psychotherapy, 40,* 11–19.

Busch, A. M., Kanter, J. W., Callaghan, G. M., Baruch, D. E., Weeks, C. E., & Berlin, K. S. 2009. A micro-process analysis of Functional Analytic Psychotherapy's mechanism of change. *Behavior Therapy, 40,* 280–290.

Callaghan, G. M., Ruckstuhl, L. E., & Busch, A. M. (2005). *Manual for the functional analytic psychotherapy rating scale, Version 3*. Unpublished manual.

Callaghan, G. M., Summers, C. J., & Weidman, M. (2003). The treatment of histrionic and narcissistic personality disorder behaviors: A single-subject demonstration of clinical effectiveness using Functional Analytic Psychotherapy. *Journal of Contemporary Psychotherapy*, *33*, 321–339.

Corrigan, P. W. (2001). Getting ahead of the data: A threat to some behavior therapies. *the Behavior Therapist*, *24*, 189–193.

Hayes, S. C., Follette, V. M., & Linehan, M. (Eds.). (2004). *Mindfulness and acceptance: Expanding the cognitive-behavioral tradition*. New York, NY: Guilford Press.

Kanter, J. W., Landes, S. J., Busch, A. M., Rusch, L. C., Brown, K. R., Baruch, D. E., et al. (2006). The effect of contingent reinforcement on target variables in outpatient psychotherapy for depression: A successful and unsuccessful case using Functional Analytic Psychotherapy. *Journal of Applied Behavior Analysis*, *39*, 463–467.

Kanter, J. W., Schildcrout, J. S., & Kohlenberg, R. J. (2005). In-vivo processes in Cognitive Therapy for depression: Frequency and benefits. *Psychotherapy Research*, *15*, 366–373.

Kohlenberg, R. J., Kanter, J. W., Bolling, M. Y., Parker, C. R., & Tsai, M. (2002). Enhancing Cognitive Therapy for depression with Functional Analytic Psychotherapy: Treatment guidelines and empirical findings. *Cognitive and Behavioral Practice*, *9*, 213–229.

Kohlenberg, R. J., & Tsai, M. (1991). *Functional analytic psychotherapy: A guide for creating intense and curative therapeutic relationships*. New York: Plenum.

Landes, S. J., Kanter, J. W., Busch, A. M., Juskiewicz, K., & Mistele, E. (2007, November). *Functional analytic psychotherapy for depression and personality disorders: Investigating the application of basic behavioral principles to the therapeutic relationship*. Poster presented at the annual meeting of the Association of Behavioral and Cognitive Therapies, Philadelphia.

Skinner, B. F. (1953). *Science and human behavior*. New York: Macmillan.

Tsai, M., Kohlenberg, R. J., Kanter, J. W., Kohlenberg, B., Follette, W. C., & Callaghan, G. M. (Eds.). (2008). *A guide to FAP: Using awareness, courage, love and behaviourism*. New York: Springer.

Weeks, C. E., Baruch, D. E., Rusch, L. C., & Kanter, J. W. (2009, May). A process analysis of Functional Analytic Psychotherapy's mechanism of change. In J. W. Kanter (Chair), *A behavior analytic methodology for studying psychotherapy: New data on functional analytic psychotherapy*. Symposium presented at the annual meeting of the Association for Behavior Analysis, Phoenix, AZ.

Part I
FAP and Psychotherapy Integration

Chapter 2
FAP and Cognitive Behavior Therapy

Robert J. Kohlenberg, Jonathan W. Kanter, Mavis Tsai, and Cristal E. Weeks

The most accurate identification of cognitions is accomplished right after they occur.

(Beck, Rush, Shaw, & Emery, 1979, p. 180)

We have found it essential that schemas be challenged when they are triggered (in-session).

(Young, 1990, p. 39)

This chapter is intended to help practicing cognitive behavior therapists make their treatment more intense, interpersonal, and impactful for both therapists and clients by incorporating the methods of Functional Analytic Psychotherapy (FAP; Kohlenberg & Tsai, 1991; Tsai et al., 2008). Our approach is user friendly in that it builds on existing cognitive behavior therapy (CBT) methods and skills with which practicing therapists are already familiar. Since we use a behavioral rationale to explain how CBT works, this chapter also can help behavior analysts who might have shied away from using CBT because it is not "behavioral."

Before turning our attention to how FAP builds on and adds to CBT, we want to point out that there are compelling reasons for therapists to include cognitive techniques as part of their therapeutic armamentarium. First, the personal experience of most therapists, regardless of their theoretical orientation, corresponds to the cognitive approach when they deal with their own personal problems. That is, when we ask our colleagues what is the first approach they use when dealing with a problematic personal situation, most (but not all) say they try to use rationality and reason to counteract their initial reactions. They ask themselves something akin to "am I jumping to conclusions?" or "am I overreacting (catastrophizing)?" or "did I get the facts right?" or perhaps "what is the evidence for and against my conclusion?" After

R.J. Kohlenberg (✉)
Department of Psychology, University of Washington, Seattle, WA, USA
e-mail: fap@u.washington.edu

With permission of the publisher, portions of this chapter are based on Kohlenberg, Kanter, Bolling, Parker, and Tsai (2002).

J.W. Kanter et al. (eds.), *The Practice of Functional Analytic Psychotherapy*,
DOI 10.1007/978-1-4419-5830-3_2, © Springer Science+Business Media, LLC 2010

all, using intellect and reason and evaluating the facts were fundamental to their graduate training and successfully attaining an academic degree. To be sure, the approach does not always work but apparently it works well enough (i.e., has been sufficiently reinforced) to be a top choice. Incidentally, the idea that the cognitive approach may work in some instances but not others is important and is accommodated in our behavioral approach to CBT. Second, the cognitive approach has more empirical support than any other method for a wide range of specific disorders (DeRubeis & Crits-Christoph, 1998). Third, CBT has been disseminated widely, with a vast array of resources such as books, workshops, and videos that help therapists learn how to implement the treatment. Fourth, there is a wide range of supplemental pamphlets, books, forms, and other materials that have been created for the client and that facilitates treatment.

On the other hand, CBT is not perfect and there are a few problems. First, as is the case for all manualized treatments, it does not work for everyone or all situations. For example, although CBT usually does better than other treatments, 40–60% of depressed or anxious clients (Hollon, Stewart, & Strunk, 2006) are symptomatic at 1-year follow-up. Second, some clients reject the cognitive rationale, which posits that the client's faulty beliefs and attitudes are responsible for their problematic feelings and ineffective actions. Some clients insist their feelings occur no matter what thoughts they have. Third, a client's rejection of the CBT rationale is an indication of a counter-therapeutic client–therapy mismatch, and CBT has limited options for dealing with such mismatches. Our approach addresses these problems while at the same time does not make the mistake of "throwing out the baby with the bathwater" by wholly rejecting CBT.

The two quotes at the beginning of this chapter convey how CBT includes elements that are emphasized in FAP. The identification of cognitions "right after they occur" and schemas being challenged "when they are triggered" point to a focus on events happening here and now during the therapy session as they are evoked by the therapeutic relationship. This type of in vivo CBT work is consistent with the FAP proposition that in-session problematic behaviors provide exceptional opportunities for significant behavior change. On the other hand, the quotes point to a CBT–FAP schism that in that they refer to non-behavioral mental entities, "cognitions," and "schema," instead of here-and-now interpersonal behaviors. This schism might lead a CBT therapist to miss occurrences of here-and-now behaviors and associated therapeutic opportunities.

Our approach to CBT involves a behavioral interpretation of cognitions (the target of CBT interventions) and an increased emphasis on behavior occurring in the here-and-now. This approach leads to a version of CBT that we have termed "FAP-enhanced cognitive therapy" or FECT.

The comments of Mr. G., a 44-year-old client who experienced both standard CBT and FECT, illustrate a qualitative difference between the two approaches. Mr. G. was a subject in a treatment development study (Kohlenberg, Kanter, Bolling, Parker, & Tsai, 2002) involving 20 sessions of either CBT or FECT. He differed from the other clients in this study in that his treatment started with standard CBT until his therapist had a medical problem that necessitated a shift to another therapist after the eighth session. The second therapist (using FECT) continued the CBT focus on thoughts and feeling for the remaining 12 sessions and also followed the FAP rules. Obviously there is considerable confounding, but Mr. G. was in the unique position of being able to describe and compare his experience of both treatments. He had a long-standing history of major depression that had been unresponsive to a variety of prior medications and psychosocial treatments. Among his presenting problems was a deep dissatisfaction in his interpersonal relationships. He felt people rejected him and he was unable to achieve closeness with others. According to Beck Depression Inventory (BDI) scores, he was no longer depressed at the end of treatment and reported making progress in being more intimate with his wife and children. In this excerpt from the last session, Mr. G. describes how he experienced the difference between FECT and CBT:

> There's a lot of stuff going on in my personal life that we've been working on in here, depression and so on, and that has led to maybe the cognitive therapy way of handling things and looking at, ah, you know, the daily activity log and then doing the thought records and analyzing thoughts and how they lead to things. So that's over here [with the first 8 sessions of CBT]. And then on this other part, which I definitely got into with you [the second 12 sessions of FECT] was in my personal relationships and how that works, on both sides, myself and the other person. And then it became how that occurred for you and me as an example of that, [my appearing to others as] ominous. It's something I learned with you so that it would not persist in unintentionally coloring my relationships.

Here is our interpretation of Mr. G.'s comments. First, he acknowledged the utility of the standard CBT focus on thoughts during the first eight sessions. Second, he stated that during FECT, the second phase, he became aware of his problematic interpersonal behavior (not a cognition) that led others to see him as "ominous." Third, he recognized that this same interpersonal problem that occurred in his daily life also occurred in the therapy session between him and his therapist. Finally, he suggested that learning how to act differently and not be perceived as ominous by his therapist would help him in his relationships with others.

FAP-Enhanced Cognitive Therapy (FECT)

The methods and procedures of FECT are designed to produce the type of therapy experience that this client had, capitalizing both on the strengths of CBT and on use of the therapeutic relationship as a tool for improving interpersonal relationships while implementing CBT interventions. The two major FECT enhancements to standard CBT are (1) an expanded rationale for the causes and treatment of depression and (2) a greater use of the client–therapist relationship as an in vivo teaching opportunity.

Enhancement I: The Expanded Rationale

As suggested earlier, the rationale is a statement made by the therapist to the client that describes the therapist's view about the causes and cure of the problem. The rationale enters into treatment in two ways. First, it sets the stage for the kinds of changes expected from the client and the nature of the work to be done in therapy. Equally important, the rationale structures the nature and selection of interventions to be used by the therapist.

Clients who respond favorably to a treatment rationale are more likely to improve (Addis & Carpenter, 1999; Fennell & Teasdale, 1987; Teasdale, 1985). A "match" between the therapy and client rationale is hypothesized to promote more favorable outcomes due to factors such as increased rapport, therapeutic alliance, and willingness to do homework. On the other hand, a mismatch can have deleterious effects. For example, in comparative outcome studies it is not uncommon for a percentage of clients to drop out because they feel mismatched to the assigned treatment (Addis & Carpenter, 2000). Researchers have found that inflexible persistence with the cognitive rationale when the client claims it does not fit can be counter-therapeutic (Castonguay, Goldfried, Wiser, Raue, & Hayes, 1996); others have found that cognitive therapists do in fact persist in their approach even when the client is not progressing (Kendall, Kipnis, & Otto-Salaj, 1992).

The Cognitive Rationale

The core of CBT is the cognitive hypothesis, represented by the ABC paradigm illustrated in Fig. 2.1a. In that figure, A represents external environmental events, B represents cognition, and C is the resulting emotion or action. This paradigm contends that a person's irrational or inaccurate beliefs, assumptions, and attitudes about external events lead to problematic feelings. Our experience is that although the ABC paradigm fits the experience of many clients and leads to effective therapeutic interventions in many situations, it does not for others. For example, clients may not experience any thoughts that intervene between the environmental event and their subsequent feeling and/or action, as illustrated in Fig. 2.1b. In this case, the simple ABC rationale does not match the client's experience.[1]

Figure 2.1c represents a paradigm for the client who says, "I truly believe that I do not have to be perfect, but I still feel and act like I have to be." In this case, the cognitive hypothesis erroneously could lead the therapist to doubt that the client "truly believes" and persist in using cognitive interventions aimed at changing his/her beliefs. This potentially counter-therapeutic stance is consistent with Beck et al.'s (1979, p. 302) suggestion that clients who say they intellectually "know" they are not worthless, but who do not accept this on an emotional level, need more cognitive therapy because the dysfunctional feelings only can occur when they do not "truly believe" the rational thought. The prescription of "more cognitive therapy" is an indirect way of challenging the client's rejection of the CBT model. From a FAP perspective, these ABC-guided interventions do not allow for the possibility that a client's objecting to cognitive interventions or the CBT rationale could

---

[1] This problem has been addressed on a theoretical level by cognitive therapists (Hollon & Kriss, 1984). For a more complete discussion of their position as well as a behaviorally based critique and account of cognitive concepts such as cognitive products and structures, see Kohlenberg and Tsai (1991), pp. 101–120.

be desirable. For example, if a client's depression could be helped by increased assertiveness and willingness to express one's own opinions, then objecting to the therapist's rationale would be an improvement. That is, the client is being assertive and expressing opinions within the context of the therapy relationship. An expanded rationale facilitates the therapist's recognition of such client behavior as a within-session improvement that should be reinforced by acceptance and not punished by dogmatically implementing further CBT techniques.

Thus, there is a dilemma inherent in using the cognitive rationale. On the one hand, it sets the stage for using cognitive interventions that are often effective. On the other hand, at times its use can lead to counter-therapeutic mismatching of therapists and clients with different convictions, therapist perseveration, and punishment of assertive client behavior. This dilemma is resolved when using an expanded hypothesis based on a behavioral view of cognition.

The Behavioral View of Cognition

The expanded rationale used in FECT is based on the behavioral view of cognition and the importance given to a client's learning history in explaining current behavior. Cognition is defined as the activity of thinking, planning, believing, and/or categorizing. Thus cognitions, although covert, are simply behavior. This casts the often made distinction between thoughts, feelings and behavior, and the primacy of the cognition–behavior relationship in a new light. The relationship between these two becomes a behavior X–behavior Y relationship, e.g., a sequence of two behaviors. Here, behavior X is cognition (e.g., thinking, believing, saying things to oneself) and behavior Y is external behavior or emotional response (a bodily response). This view accommodates a variety of possibilities as to the causal connection between cognition (behavior X) and subsequent behavior (behavior Y), placing the degree of control exerted by cognitions on a continuum, varying depending on a particular client's history.

The expanded FECT rationale includes the cognitive rationale as well as the other two possibilities shown in Fig. 2.1. For example, Fig. 2.1b represents an AC sequence and matches the experience of the client who says, "I just reacted, I didn't

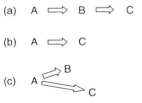

Fig. 2.1 Some cognition–behavior relationships according to the FECT-expanded rationale. A = antecedent event; B = belief/cognition; C = consequence (emotional reaction). (**a**) represents the standard cognitive model. (**b**) represents a situation in which there is no cognition. (**c**) represents a situation in which cognition precedes but is not causally related to the reaction

have any preceding thoughts or beliefs." In this case, although CBT would invoke an unconscious core belief that the client has not verbalized, the FECT view is that there is no intervening cognition and instead the client has a history in which AC was directly learned. To illustrate, consider the direct learning that took place in the famous case of little Albert, the infant who was classically conditioned to be fearful of white fury objects (Church, 1980). The fear was based entirely on the temporal pairing of a white rabbit and a very loud clanging noise. Similarly, Russell and Brandsma (1974) suggested that with enough repetitions of an ABC sequence (in which initially one's thoughts, beliefs, self-statements, or assumptions actually do have an influence), it will eventually transform into an AC sequence in which cognition no longer plays a role via the principles of classical conditioning. In such cases, although cognitive therapists have solutions to such problems (e.g., a core belief still may be identified in the absence of automatic thoughts), behavioral activation (Martell, Addis, & Jacobson, 2001) and acceptance-based interventions (Hayes, Strosahl, & Wilson, 1999) may be more appropriate candidates for treatment.

The behavioral view of cognition also includes ABC variations not shown in Fig. 2.1. For example, ACB would represent a client who reacts first before having a thought. In this case, since the thought has no influence on the occurrence of C, CBT is contraindicated. For clients whose experience matches ABC shown in Fig. 2.1a, FECT proposes that the methods of cognitive therapy would be maximally effective. However, for clients whose experience corresponds to one of the other two paradigms shown in Fig. 2.1, standard cognitive therapy might result in a client–therapy mismatch and a less effective treatment. It is also possible that multiple paradigms exist for a given client or that paradigms change from situation to situation.

An example of the expanded rationale presented to depressed clients includes the following:

> ...the way you think affects how you feel and what you do. CBT has been shown by research to be effective in treating depression. In our treatment, however, we also believe that sometimes feelings can lead to thoughts and actions, or that something else altogether can cause depressed thoughts, depressed feelings, and ineffective actions.

The use of the expanded rationale is illustrated in the case of a client, Mr. D., who had a problem of becoming angry too easily. He brought up an example of getting angry at other drivers at a four-way stop while driving to his appointment. He explained how the driver in front of him could have moved forward a little and allowed him to make a right turn. In this case, the therapist's use of the expanded rationale accommodated the client's experience and avoided a potential ABC mismatch:

Mr. D.:   I thought, "You idiot!"
Therapist: You remember during our discussion of the [FECT] brochure (rationale) that thought sometimes precedes feelings but can also occur after. At the four-way stop, you thought, "You idiot!" Were you aware as to

whether you had that thought first and then got angry, or did you get angry first and then have the thought?

Mr. D.:   I got angry first.

The FECT-expanded rationale also allows for using history to account for the client's reactions to the world either along with or as an alternative to the ABC hypothesis. This is consistent with a behavioral analysis of problems, tracing causality to external sources occurring in the reinforcement history of the individual. Although changing cognitions may be a useful therapeutic tool, cognition is never seen as the ultimate cause for problems according to a behavioral analysis. Recognizing historical antecedents for clients' problems and negative cognitions gives them a way to explain their behavior to themselves that can be less blaming than strict cognitive explanations. For example, a client might feel even more depressed after learning the cognitive hypothesis because he/she interprets it as "one more thing I'm doing wrong." Emphasizing historical antecedents exposes the function of self-blaming as understandable given the context of the client's prior experiences. In general, the expanded rationale allows for varying relationships between cognition and the client's problems and also facilitates discussions of the role that historical factors may have played in their development.

The FECT treatment development study described above (Kohlenberg et al., 2002) provides some preliminary support for the use of the expanded rationale. In that study, clients showed a significantly more positive response to the FECT-expanded rationale than to the standard CBT version. Further, there was a significantly more positive reaction to the ABC conceptualization when it was included in an expanded rationale than when it was presented in isolation as part of the standard CBT rationale. Though these results are promising in support of the expanded rationale, more research in this area is needed.

Enhancement 2: A Greater Use of the Client–Therapist Relationship

The underlying hypothesis of FAP is that the client–therapist relationship is a social environment with the potential to evoke and change actual instances of the client's clinically relevant behavior in the here-and-now. According to our behavioral analysis, there are times when this clinically relevant behavior corresponds to the focus of conventional CBT. Examples include in vivo automatic thinking about the therapist or therapy, doing the self-observation needed to complete a thinking record (discussed later in this chapter) during the session, or hypothesis testing with the therapist. For example, a client who does not express anger in his daily life because he assumes terrible things will happen if he does might get angry at the therapist but not express this anger. Such occurrences are opportunities for significant therapeutic change if and when these CBT-related behaviors occur and are recognized by the therapist. The therapist who evokes and notices these behaviors will be more likely to immediately shape, encourage, and nurture in vivo improvements.

Problematic Cognitive and Interpersonal Behaviors as Clinically Relevant Behaviors (CRBs)

CRB1s (in vivo problems) and CRB2s (in vivo improvements) (see Kohlenberg & Tsai, 1991) can be cognitive behavior and/or interpersonal behavior. Cognitive CRBs are in-session, actual occurrences of problematic or improved cognitions (e.g., thinking, assuming, believing, perceiving). In the above example, the angry client may assume that "the therapist will reject me if I express my anger," which would be a problematic in-session cognition. The occurrence of a problematic cognitive CRB provides a special opportunity for the therapist to do in vivo CBT. For example, the therapist could use a thought log or empirical hypothesis testing pertaining to the client–therapist interaction. Cognitive CRBs also are identified as having special significance in the CBT variants of Young (1990); Safran and Segal (1990), and several others (reviewed in Kanter et al., 2009).

The angry client example involves both cognitive and interpersonal CRBs. Interpersonal CRBs are actual in-session problematic interpersonal behaviors. A possible CRB1 could be that the client will not express his angry feelings toward the therapist. The therapist could encourage or prompt the client to express his anger instead of employing the in vivo cognitive intervention (e.g., the thought log) if such expression is conceptualized as a CRB2. This illustrates the importance of generating a clear case conceptualization (outlined below) from the outset and updating it as treatment progresses.

Generalization from Treatment to Daily Life

As therapy progresses, clients display more CRB2s (improvements in-session), and generalization of improvements from the client–therapist interaction to daily life is expected to occur. Generalization may occur naturally but can also be augmented by offering interpretations that compare within-session interactions to daily life. For example, the therapist might say, "Your belief that I will reject you if you criticize therapy seems to resemble the belief you have about others in your life." Successful within-session hypothesis testing and consequent mood improvement similarly could be related to uses in daily life. Standard CBT homework assignments can be built from this in vivo work. For instance, the therapist might say, "Now that you have found that your belief – that I will respond poorly if you express your feelings directly to me – is inaccurate, do you think a good homework assignment would be to check out that belief with your wife?"

Putting the Enhancements into Practice: Eight Specific Techniques

FECT treatment occurs simultaneously on two levels. At the first level, FECT therapists follow a CBT manual, for example, Beck and colleagues' (1979) CBT for depression. Beck's CBT consists of a 20-session structure with specific procedures such as (1) defining and setting goals, (2) structuring the session (setting and following an agenda; eliciting feedback from the client at the end of the session), (3) presenting a rationale, and (4) using cognitive-behavioral strategies and techniques. The FECT therapist, however, uses the expanded rationale rather than the standard CBT rationale. This requires the flexibility to drop the ABC hypothesis if it does not match the client's experience and/or if the client is not progressing.

The second level of therapy is perhaps the most important. At the same time that the above technical procedures are used, FECT therapists are observing intensely the client–therapist interaction and looking for the client's daily life problems and dysfunctional thoughts that actually are occurring in the moment, within the context of the client–therapist relationship. The following eight additions to CBT highlight the FECT approach and help therapists to work on both levels.

1. Set the Scene Early

The FECT interest in the client's history and observation of in vivo client behavior is established early. Either before treatment begins or during the first session FECT clients are given the following assignment: "Write an outline, a time chart, or an autobiography of the main events, enduring circumstances, highlights, turning points, and relationships that have shaped who you are as a person, from your birth to the present time." The assignment indicates to the client that the therapist is interested in history. At another level, it gives the therapist an opportunity to observe how the client deals with this task (e.g., procrastinates, gives sparse information, completes volumes of writings, assertively refuses to do it), which is used to generate hypotheses about potential CRBs that might appear in therapy. Both the historical information and the hypothesized CRBs enter into the formulation of an initial case conceptualization as described later.

2. Present the Expanded Rationale and Ask for Feedback

Underscoring FECT's inclusion of CBT, the therapist presents a treatment rationale to the client in the form of two brochures, the Beck Institute's "Coping with Depression" (Beck & Greenberg, 1995) and the FECT brochure. "Coping with Depression" presents the cognitive hypothesis, a preliminary outline of types of thinking errors depressed people commonly make, and a brief overview of the direction of treatment. The FECT brochure acknowledges the ABC hypothesis and the value of learning new ways to think. It also allows for the possibility that the ABC paradigm might not always match the particular client's experiences and discusses alternative paradigms. For example, the brochure states,

> The focus of your therapy will depend on the causes of your problems. Thus, along with cognitive therapy, your treatment might also include: exploring your strengths and seeing the best of who you are; grieving your losses, contacting your feelings, especially those that are difficult for you to experience; developing relationship skills; developing mindfulness, acceptance and an observing self; gaining a sense of mastery in your life.

The FECT brochure also emphasizes focusing on the here-and-now and using the client–therapist relationship to learn new patterns of behavior.

Presenting the rationale is a critical juncture in therapy and must be accompanied by observation of how the rationale is received by the client, what parts of it evoke particular enthusiasm, or what parts evoke disagreement. Because the FECT-expanded rationale is flexible, client feedback is important to help determine the course of therapy or the particular type of interventions to be used. At the same time, all client reactions should be viewed as potential CRBs. For example, a female client may say, "That's fine, whatever," in reaction to the brochures. What is going on in this case? Is this the way the client deals with others as well – accepting whatever is dished out? Is she afraid to express her real reaction to the therapist, just as she is with others? Or is this particular response not an instance of the client's daily life problems? This process of noticing potential CRBs is essential to FECT and is sharpened by the use of the case conceptualization form as discussed below.

3. Use Case Conceptualization as an Aid to Detecting CRBs

In FECT, case conceptualization is the sine qua non of therapeutic work. It is, in fact, a functional analysis of relevant client behaviors (thinking and feeling in addition to physical and verbal events). The FECT case conceptualization serves three purposes. First, it generates an account of how the client's history resulted in the current daily life problems. This account provides an explanation of how current problem behaviors were adaptive at the time they were acquired, and sets the stage for the client to learn new ways of behaving. Second, it identifies possible cognitive phenomena that may be related to current problems. Third and most important, FECT case conceptualization identifies and predicts how CRBs may occur during the session within the client–therapist relationship. Hence, the case conceptualization helps therapists notice CRBs as they occur and to use these opportunities to shape and reinforce improvements in vivo.

The FECT case conceptualization form is a working document to help maintain a focus on the goals of therapy as well as increase therapist detection of in-session problematic thinking and behavior and their improvements. The form is filled out as soon as there is enough information. Sometimes it is filled out jointly with the client – at the very least, it is presented to the client for feedback – and modified throughout the course of therapy as more information is gathered. The primary categories on the form are described here. Portions of Mr. G.'s (case presented earlier in this chapter) case conceptualization are used for examples.

Relevant history. History can go as far back as childhood and consists of significant events across the life span, including more recent experiences, that account for the thoughts, actions, and meaning that may be implicated in daily life problems. The purpose of this category is to generate an explanation of how the current problems were learned initially and how they were adaptive at the time they were acquired. Historical interpretations set the stage for the client to learn new ways of behaving. For example, Mr. G. reported growing up in a family environment that severely punished warmth and vulnerability.

Daily life problems. These are the client's complaints. For example, Mr. G. complained of a lack of close relationships and rejection by others.

Problematic beliefs. Mr. G. had the core belief that he was defective, incapable of ever forming a close relationship or being liked by others.

Assets and strengths. Mr. G. is a competent professional and overcame many obstacles to advance in his career through sheer persistence. He is responsible and ethical in his dealings with others and works at being a good husband and father.

CRB1s (in-session problematic behaviors and thoughts). It was hypothesized that Mr. G. would act in ways that would interfere with forming a close relationship with the therapist. It was in this context that Mr. G.'s "ominous" style of interacting was identified as a CRB1 by the therapist. This style most often emerged when the therapist was open and expressed warmth toward Mr. G. Mr. G. also believed his core unlikability occurred in the session with the therapist and that the therapist did not and could not like him.

CRB2s (in-session target behaviors and improvements). In-session behaviors can be observed as improvements in the client–therapist relationship. In Mr. G.'s case, his remaining vulnerable by saying, "I don't want to appear ominous now," when the therapist told him that he cared about and liked Mr. G., was identified as an improvement. The therapist acknowledged the improvement and confirmed that their relationship had been strengthened because of Mr. G.'s CRB2.

Daily life goals. Mr. G.'s goals were to be less depressed and to have more intimacy and closeness in his relationships.

T1s (therapist in-session problems). The therapist was aware of his discomfort with Mr. G. but was reluctant to bring this up since he was not sure whose problem this was and did not want to take a risk of being embarrassed. Since Mr. G. became ominous whenever the therapist expressed caring, the therapist was reluctant to do so even though he was very concerned about his client's well-being.

T2s (therapist in-session target behaviors). The therapist took a risk in expressing his caring for Mr. G. as well as describing his reactions to his client when he presented an "ominous" façade.

4. Notice CRBs: Both Problems and Improvements

Based on the case conceptualization, FECT therapists hypothesize about and look for specific CRBs. A few of the most common domains are the following:

Cognitive CRBs. Important cognitive CRBs can be pinpointed by examining the client's core beliefs, which are identified in the course of standard CBT. Core beliefs can be translated into cognitive CRBs, which will facilitate the therapist's being vigilant for their occurrence. Table 2.1 presents several core beliefs identified by Beck (1995) along with possible corresponding CRBs that can be anticipated in-session.

Intimacy CRBs. At the beginning of therapy, FECT therapists tell their clients that when they express their thoughts, feelings, and desires in an authentic, caring, and assertive way, they will be more likely to find joy in life and to be less depressed. The therapy relationship is an opportunity to build these skills because the therapist

Table 2.1 Potential core beliefs and corresponding anticipated CRBs

Core issue	Anticipated CRB
Alone	Feels this way, even with therapist
Defective	As seen by therapist
Different	As seen by therapist or in reactions to therapy
Doesn't measure up	As seen by therapist
Failure	In therapy, with therapy tasks, homework
Helpless	In relation to therapist, can't influence therapist
Inadequate	To understand the therapy, to get better with this treatment
Incompetent	In therapy
Ineffective	In therapy
Inferior	To therapist, to other clients
Loser	In relation to therapist, as seen by therapist, to be in therapy
Loser (in relationships)	In therapy relationship

can offer the client something that no one else can in the same way: perceptions of who the client is, the ways he or she is special, and the ways that he or she impacts the therapist. Throughout therapy, emphasis is placed on the client being able to express what is difficult for him/her to express to the therapist. Questionnaires given to the client at the beginning, middle, and end of therapy (see appendices in Tsai et al., 2008) encourage the client to say what is generally difficult to say, whether it be criticisms, fears, longings, or appreciation. FECT therapists model intimacy skills for their clients by expressing caring and other feelings, telling clients their perceived strengths, talking about concerns in a way that validates them, and making requests (I want, I need, I would like). FECT therapists also model self-disclosure when it is in the client's best interests (i.e., when relevant to the client's issues, offering support, understanding, encouragement, hope, and the sense that he or she is not alone) (Tsai, Plummer, Kanter, Newring, & Kohlenberg, 2010).

Avoidance CRBs. From a behavioral viewpoint, avoidance is one of the major factors in the etiology and maintenance of clinical depression, and avoidance CRBs are often a target in FECT. For many clients, therapeutic change is facilitated when avoidance is gently blocked and clients are encouraged to take risks outside of their usual comfort zone both in the session and in their daily life. For example, a client remains silent for a moment and looks troubled in response to a question. When the therapist inquires further, the client says, "Oh, I don't know, nothing important." This may be a CRB1. That is, in daily life, the client may avoid talking and feeling about troubling topics by using such dismissive phrases. This type of CRB1 precludes the possibility of the client's resolving the issue that is being avoided and interferes with forming more satisfying relationships. Gentle inquiry into "nothing important" may prompt CRB2s, which in this case may be the client identifying and expressing feelings of discomfort. The therapist should take care that his or her response to the CRB2 will naturally reinforce the new behavior. This may involve risk-taking and real emotional involvement, so the therapist should also be aware of his or her own avoidance CRBs.

5. Ask Questions to Evoke CRBs

FECT therapists ask questions that bring the clients' attention to what they are think-ing and feeling in the moment about the therapy or therapeutic relationship. Some common questions include the following: What are you thinking or feeling right now? What's your reaction to what I just said? What were you thinking or feeling on your way to therapy today/while in the waiting room? What are your hope and concerns as you start this therapy relationship with me? What are your behaviors that tend to bring closeness in your relationships – how would you feel about us watching for your behaviors in here which increase or decrease closeness? What are your feelings/reactions to our session today? What's hard for you to say to me? Are your reactions to me similar to your reactions to X?

6. Increase Therapist Self-Awareness as an Aid to Detecting and Being Aware of CRBs

FECT therapists use their personal reactions to alert them to client CRBs. The more therapists are aware of and understand their own reactions to their clients, the easier it will be for them to detect CRBs and respond appropriately. For example, the third author (MT) noticed in supervision while watching a tape of a session that when the client expressed warmth and appreciation toward the student therapist, he changed the subject without acknowledging what the client had said. MT also noticed that this therapist tended to be uncomfortable when she complimented him. When this was pointed out, he became more aware of this discomfort and focused on being more receptive and reinforcing when complimented. Subsequently he was better able to detect and naturally reinforce positive interpersonal behaviors of his clients. Tsai, Callaghan, Kohlenberg, Follette, and Darrow (2008) present questions that can be used during supervision of FECT therapists to increase self-awareness related to provision of FECT. These questions include the following: What feelings/thoughts does your client bring up in you? What feelings do you tend to avoid letting yourself get in contact with toward your client? What do you identify with in your client? What are you avoiding addressing with your client? An additional question specific to FECT that is added to the list is "What concerns and apprehensions do you have as you begin seeing FECT clients?"

7. Use the Modified Thought Record

We modified the thought record used during cognitive therapy (Beck et al., 1979, p. 403) in the following ways. First, the instructions were modified to include the expanded rationale: The client is asked to consider whether the ABC, AC, or ACB paradigms fit his/her particular experiences. The instructions read as follows:

> Begin filling out this record with the problematic situation, what you did, or what you felt. If possible, denote whether the thinking, feeling, or doing came first, second, or third (which did you experience first, second, and third?).

Second, a new column, "In Vivo," was added to the form to facilitate the therapist–client focus. After denoting the thoughts, feelings, and actions that occurred in response to the particular event in daily life, the client is asked, "How might similar problematic thoughts, feelings, and/or actions come up in-session, about the therapy, or between you and your therapist?"

8. Emphasize Opportunities for Improving Acceptance and Mindfulness Implicit to Doing CBT

Clients who are being treated with CBT are requested to observe and rate their thoughts and feelings. The therapist's encouragement and shaping of the behaviors of self-observing and objective rating pulls for the mindful experience of thoughts: seeing thoughts as thoughts and obtaining enough distance from them to label and provide intensity ratings of them (as requested on the thinking record). Similarly, the thinking record asks for a "believability rating" of automatic thoughts. Such a rating (1) conveys the idea that it is possible to have a thought and "not believe it," that is, not take it literally, and (2) sets the stage for not having to change the content of the thought or to "get rid of it" in order to act in more productive ways. This sentiment is also conveyed by the new column added to the thinking record: "Alternative More Productive Ways of Acting" which asks clients to come up with other ways of acting that would help them achieve their goals. The client is also asked to rate his or her "Commitment to Act More Effectively" using the following scale:

0% None. I can't act better while I have negative thoughts and/or feelings.
50% Some. I am willing to give it a try.
100% Very much. I will act effectively and have my negative thoughts and feelings at the same time.

Based on acceptance (Hayes, Strosahl, & Wilson, 1999; Linehan, 1993) and behavioral activation (Jacobson et al., 1996; Martell, Addis, & Jacobson, 2001) approaches, this column can be used to raise the possibility that one can act effectively even if one has negative thoughts and feelings. This approach is particularly useful for helping clients who have persistent negative thoughts, who do not improve with standard cognitive therapy interventions, and/or who reject the cognitive hypothesis.

Case Example: Bruce

Bruce, 27, was a very bright young man who presented with major depressive disorder and high Beck Depression Inventory scores ranging from 36 to 42 during the 3 weeks prior to beginning treatment. He had been depressed for the past 3 years and had little hope. He had been unable to get the kind of work that he wanted (work that was interesting and held promise for advancement), was in danger of losing his less satisfying job due to poor attendance and performance, and was thinking about quitting. Although he desired relationships, he admitted to having poor social skills and few social contacts and to doing little to improve his social life. He believed his problematic family background doomed him to isolation, and he avoided establishing relationships and being open with others, particularly "normal people," since he assumed they would have little in common with him. He had never checked this thought out, even though his therapist had urged the CBT "hypothesis testing" as a homework assignment. He told the therapist his life "sucks," is "shit," and he hadn't got out of the house for 3 days. From the case conceptualization, anticipated CRB1s included in vivo "all or nothing" thinking about the therapist being able to "understand him" and reluctance to directly check out his assumptions. An anticipated CRB2 was in vivo hypothesis testing with the therapist. The following is a transcript segment from one of his sessions:

T: I guess I wonder sometimes if you – I mean, we've talked about all or nothing thinking. I don't know if there is really a corollary, but I'm going to suggest there is with all or nothing behaving. [C: Um hmm] And I'm wondering if you have a tendency to do that. That either the job is exactly what you want or it has some good long-term possibilities or you don't do it at all. 'Cause, even though last week you were working on a job that you weren't very satisfied with and really couldn't possibly see yourself doing long term, you still felt a little better. You felt a little better about yourself. [C: um hmm] And now, you're staying in bed for three sunny days in a row and not even showering. So, just like if this was like you're thinking that things are all good/all bad, [C: um hmm] you know, you are not trying to find a middle somewhere or a continuum. (Therapist points out daily life black-and-white thinking, points out the relationship between working and feeling better, and is urging behavioral activation).

C: I guess it's hard for me to get across to you, who has a car, how it feels to not have a car, you know? I don't have a car. I don't have any motivation to do anything that doesn't require a car on the weekends, you know? So, I mean, I can explain until I'm blue in the face but you just don't understand, you know? (CRB1: an in-session belief about the therapist that he does not check out; that is, he does not ask therapist directly whether he understands what it's like not to own a car).

T: How can you test that out? Do you have any evidence that I don't understand? (Prompting & evoking CRB2s via in vivo hypothesis testing and in vivo gathering evidence for and against his belief).

C: No, but the scientific evidence is, just from looking outside, the majority of America has a car. (CRB1: ignores therapist prompt to attend to relationship).

T: Okay, has the majority of America always had a car, do you think?

C: Yeah, I think so.

T: Here's one other thought. Do you think I've always had a car. (Therapist brings global daily life belief about America and the world into an in vivo belief about the therapist).

C: Well, I'm assuming that since you're from New England, that's pretty rural, and you can't really do much without a car except play with cows or whatever you do up there. So, I'm going to assume that you've always had a car since you were sixteen. So, and that's, you know, that's assuming a lot but the odds are with me. You know what I mean?

T: How are the odds with you?

C: Well, because that's how it is with most Americans. Most Americans grow up in the 2.2 kid family, they get a car when they're sixteen, you know, they get the hand-me-down car or whatever like that and most people in America, I mean, it's a car culture.

T: Sure, okay, but let's not get confused. What I'm asking you to test out is a specific belief that I don't understand you because I have a car now, and granted, I have a car sitting in the back lot. But your belief is that I probably came from a 2.2 kid family and had a car when I was sixteen. (Therapist bringing discussion back to the here-and-now in the therapist–client relationship and prompting in vivo hypothesis testing).

C: Okay, I don't believe that specifically about you, but I believe that chances are that you did. You know, I'm not saying that you did. I'm not saying, you know, I'm saying that the odds are that you won't understand me. That's why I say you probably won't understand what I'm talking about. So, I don't mean to say you don't. (A CRB1 in that client is not directly asking therapist for information).

T: And I'm not trying to be argumentative here, but what I am saying is that right now you have the opportunity to test it out. [C: um hmm] And that this happens out in the real world. [C: um hmm] I think you make a lot of assumptions about people. That hurts you. It makes you feel crappy about yourself. And, what could you do to find out if someone understands you? (Again, prompting hypothesis testing and the important social skill of asking others about their beliefs and experiences).

C: Let me ask you something first. Did you ever talk to people who didn't have a car for a week. Do you ever see the trauma that they go through? The big bitch whine, you know, like somebody's cut off their legs. Then I tell them that I don't have a car and they look at me like I'm some little refugee boy, like, "Poor you. I don't know what I'd do without my car." I mean, how would that make you feel? That pisses me off so bad. I feel like saying, "You know, fuck you. Live my life for a couple of months without a car." You know. (A CRB2, an improvement in that a direct question about the therapist's experience was asked, although not as direct as it could be).

T: I understand that, but you almost have the answer to my question of how can you test if someone understands you. (Rule 3, reinforces CRB2). And then you said, "Can I ask you something?" That's the answer. You can ask someone if they understand you. [C: um hmm] You're making an assumption. Right now you're making an assumption that I don't understand you, that I don't understand what it's like to go without a car. But, you're not checking out whether or not I do. (Rule 2, more explicit CRB2 prompting to hypothesis test).

C: That's a good point.

T: Do you think sometimes that you might find that you have more in common with people than you think you do? Even the people you would think you don't have much in common with? [C: Yeah, probably.] (Rule 5, relating in-session experience to daily life). So, then...

C: Somewhere along the line, some switch flipped in me, you know what I mean? It's like a dog. You beat it with a stick or something. After about the tenth time, the dog doesn't care. Anyone he sees with a stick, he's not going to, like, want to sit there and you know? (CRB1 – Avoiding being interpersonally direct and testing hypothesis).

T: When did that switch flip?

C: I don't know. I don't know. Somewhere along the line, I just stopped, especially when I stopped drinking, you know?

T: So, what we're trying to do here, some of the things in terms of focusing on some of the behaviors right now, is trying to get that switch turned. [C: Um hmm] But one of the things is that this is a thought, not a behavior. This is a thinking pattern – you make assumptions. That's the thought. You assume about someone. And then, that leads to a certain behavioral pattern of not ever checking things out. You assume that either someone's an asshole because they're driving a certain car or they have a certain house or whatever. [C: Um hmm] You assume that people don't understand you, that they haven't been in the same spot. And that assumption prevents you from then going one step further and checking out to see that maybe there are some people in the world that kinda' know what you're feeling. They may not feel the exact same thing. They may never have but may have felt something similar. So, what I'm trying to push you to do right now is to actually change the behavior and test the assumption that I don't understand how you feel about the car.

C: So, you want me to ask you if you've ever not had a car? Is that what you're saying? (An indication of how difficult it is for this client to ask a direct question and view his assumption as an hypothesis that needs to be tested).

T: Well, that would be a way of testing that assumption.

C: Yeah. Do you know how it feels to not have a car from the age of sixteen to the age of 27?

T: Not to the age of 27, no I don't. But, I don't remember how old I was when I got my first car, but I was well into my twenties. I spent many years without one. [C: Hmm] And even though I grew up tipping cows for a living, I didn't have a car. And so I do have some understanding of the hardships that you can go through without a car. And, I understand what it's like to live in a world, a place with no buses and not have a car, and have to rely on the kindness of friends and family if they have that to get places. So, I know, I do know that it can be very frustrating. Um, that was many years ago. Granted, there is some truth in that I don't understand right now (self disclosure – a possible natural reinforcement, Rule 3, for client's direct question).

C: But still, I would never have guessed that at all. I mean, you seem pretty well adjusted so I automatically assumed that you had decent parents and, you know, who would, like, help you out and stuff. I mean, that's a big assumption, too, I guess, 'cause you could've had schizo parents like mine. I mean, I can fool a lot of people when I first meet them as well. They think, "Oh, you're so together."

T: Well, be careful with the assumptions you're making now: that I didn't have decent parents or that I'm fooling you or a number of things. There are some other assumptions that I don't – I don't want this to be a "you ask me about my life" session. [C: Yeah.] But, I just want to point out that even in this thing, and this was a good example because I do know what it's like to not have a car. There are probably other experiences that you've had that I don't share and probably some that I share.

C: Or some that you do and I don't. (In cognitive terms, a more balanced view).

Conclusion

We believe the selective use of CBT interventions is compatible with FAP. Our data (Kohlenberg et al., 2002) indicate that adding FAP to CBT does not compromise CBT adherence or competence. Further, using FAP has the potential to increase the potency of CBT while at the same time avoiding some of its weaknesses. This is supported by promising findings indicating that FECT improves interpersonal functioning, acceptance of the therapeutic rationale, and therapist–client matching. The FAP approach to CBT consists of the following: (1) be flexible and be ready to give up the cognitive rationale if it is not productive and (2) do *it* in vivo. The *it* we are referring to includes observing and evoking in-session thinking and believing about the therapist, as well as in-session use of cognitive techniques such as hypothesis testing, developing balanced thinking, and using a thinking record about the therapeutic relationship. It is of interest to note that comparisons across studies show that master cognitive therapists do *it* in vivo to a much greater extent than competent cognitive therapists that typically participate in research studies (Castonguay, Hayes, Goldfried, & DeRubeis, 1995; Goldfried, Raue, & Castonguay, 1998).

In conclusion, we wish to leave you with a final clarification – that we are suggesting the application of CBT techniques from a FAP perspective, and not FAP from a CBT perspective. This clarification simply means that, deep down, whether or not clients have dysfunctional cognitions, our primary concern is how they act interpersonally both in vivo with their therapist as well as in their daily lives. This primary concern, coupled with CBT techniques, will ultimately lead to a change in thoughts as well as behavior, which is the FECT therapist's ultimate goal. At times it can be difficult to conceptualize, as a therapist, what the reinforcing response to a client should be when you are discussing dysfunctional cognitions or doing in vivo cognitive restructuring. The greater concern, however, is how to elicit the client's cognitions in vivo or to encourage the client to test hypotheses directly with the therapist. Homework is then assigned that gives clients practice in acting differently outside of therapy, much in the manner that they did in-session with the therapist. The result is an intense therapeutic relationship that leads to changes both in client thoughts and in the way they act in their daily lives.

References

Addis, M. E., & Carpenter, K. M. (1999). Why, why, why? Reason-giving and rumination as predictors of response to activation- and insight-oriented treatment rationales. *Journal of Clinical Psychology, 55*(7), 881–894.

Addis, M., & Carpenter, K. (2000). The treatment rationale in cognitive behavioral therapy: Psychological mechanisms and clinical guidelines. *Cognitive and Behavioral Practice, 7*(2), 147–156.

Beck, J. S. (1995). *Cognitive therapy: Basics and beyond.* New York: Guilford.

Beck, A. T., & Greenberg, R. (1995). *Coping with depression* (Rev. ed.). Bala Cynwyd, PA: Beck Institute for Cognitive Therapy and Research.

Beck, A. T., Rush, A. J., Shaw, B. F., & Emery, G. (1979). *Cognitive therapy of depression.* New York: Guilford.

Castonguay, L., Goldfried, M., Wiser, S., Raue, P., & Hayes, A. (1996). Predicting the effect of cognitive therapy for depression: A study of unique and common factors. *Journal of Consulting and Clinical Psychology, 64*(3), 497–504.

Castonguay, L. G., Hayes, A. M., Goldfried, M. R., & DeRubeis, R. J. (1995). The focus of therapist interventions in cognitive therapy for depression. *Cognitive Therapy and Research, 19*(5), 485–503.

Church, R. (1980). The Albert study: Illustration vs. evidence. *American Psychologist, 35*(2), 215–216.

DeRubeis, R., & Crits-Christoph, P. (1998). Empirically supported individual and group psychological treatments for adult mental disorders. *Journal of Consulting and Clinical Psychology, 66*(1), 37–52.

Fennell, M. J., & Teasdale, J. D. (1987). Cognitive therapy for depression: Individual differences and the process of change. *Cognitive Therapy and Research, 11*(2), 253–271.

Goldfried, M. R., Raue, P. J., & Castonguay, L. G. (1998). The therapeutic focus in significant sessions of master therapists: A comparison of cognitive-behavioral and psychodynamic-interpersonal interventions. *Journal of Consulting and Clinical Psychology, 66*(5), 803–810.

Hayes, S. C., Strosahl, K. D., & Wilson, K. G. (1999). *Acceptance and commitment therapy: An experiential approach to behavior change.* New York: Guilford Press.

Hollon, S. D., & Kriss, M. R. (1984). Cognitive factors in clinical research and practice. *Clinical Psychology Review, 4*(1), 35–76.

Hollon, S. D., Stewart, M. O., & Strunk, D. (2006). Enduring effects for cognitive behavior therapy in the treatment of depression and anxiety. *Annual Review of Psychology, 57*, 285–315.

Jacobson, N., Dobson, K., Truax, P., Addis, M., Koerner, K., Gollan, J., et al. (1996). A component analysis of cognitive-behavioral treatment for depression. *Journal of Consulting and Clinical Psychology, 64*(2), 295–304.

Kanter, J. W., Rusch, L. C., Landes, S. L., Holman, G. I., Whiteside, U., & Sedivy, S. K. (2009). The use and nature of present-focused interventions in cognitive and behavioral therapies for depression. *Psychotherapy: Research, Theory, Practice, Training, 46*, 220–232.

Kanter, J. W., Schildcrout, J. S., & Kohlenberg, R. J. (2005). In vivo processes in cognitive therapy for depression: Frequency and benefits. *Psychotherapy Research, 15*(4), 366–373.

Kendall, P. C., Kipnis, D., & Otto-Salaj, J. (1992). When Clients Do Not Progress: Influences On and Explanations for Lack of Progress. *Cognitive Therapy and Research, 16*, 269–281.

Kohlenberg, R. J., Kanter, J. W., Bolling, M. Y., Parker, C., & Tsai, M. (2002). Enhancing cognitive therapy for depression with functional analytic psychotherapy: Treatment guidelines and empirical findings. *Cognitive and Behavioral Practice, 9*(3), 213–229.

Kohlenberg, R. J., & Tsai, M. (1991). *Functional analytic psychotherapy: A guide for creating intense and curative therapeutic relationships*. New York: Plenum.

Linehan, M. M. (1993). *Cognitive-behavioral treatment of borderline personality disorder*. New York: Guilford.

Martell, C. R., Addis, M. E., & Jacobson, N. S. (2001). *Depression in context: Strategies for guided action*. New York: W.W. Norton and Co Inc.

Russell, P., & Brandsma, J. (1974). A theoretical and empirical integration of the rational-emotive and classical conditioning theories. *Journal of Consulting and Clinical Psychology, 42*(3), 389–397.

Safran, J., & Segal, Z. (1990). *Interpersonal process in cognitive therapy*. Lanham, MD: Jason Aronson.

Teasdale, J. D. (1985). Psychological treatments for depression: How do they work?. *Behavioral Research and Therapy, 23*(2), 157–165.

Tsai, M., Callaghan, G. M., Kohlenberg, R. J., Follette, W. C., & Darrow, S. M. (2008). Supervision and therapist self-development. In M. Tsai, R. J. Kohlenberg, J. W. Kanter, B. Kohlenberg, W. C. Follette, & G. M. Callaghan (Eds.), *A guide to functional analytic psychotherapy: Using awareness, courage, love and behaviorism*. New York: Springer.

Tsai, M., Kohlenberg, R. J., Kanter, J. W., Kohlenberg, B., Follette, W. C., & Callaghan, G. M. (2008). *A guide to functional analytic psychotherapy: Awareness, courage, love and behaviorism*. New York: Springer.

Young, J. E. (1990). Schema focused cognitive therapy for personality disorders. In A. Beck & A. Freeman (Eds.), *Cognitive therapy for personality disorders*. New York: Guilford Press.

Tsai, M., Plummer, M. D., Kanter, J. W., Newring, R. W., & Kohlenberg, R. J. (2010). Therapist grief and functional analytic psychotherapy: Strategic self-disclosure of personal loss. *Journal of Contemporary Psychotherapy, 40*, 1–10.

Chapter 3
FAP and Acceptance Commitment Therapy (ACT): Similarities, Divergence, and Integration

Barbara S. Kohlenberg and Glenn M. Callaghan

When our clients seek psychotherapy, it is usually because they are suffering and want to feel better. They often wish for more in life ... more love or more satisfying love, better relationships, a sense of meaning and values, and deeper understandings and connections to what is held dear. In short, clients want a better connection with both their own intrapersonal experiences and their experiences with others. Therapists are in the privileged position of hearing the story of a client's suffering and longings, and in so hearing, to offer help. We believe it is common across all therapists and psychotherapies to want our clients to feel at the end of therapy that it was important and meaningful, and as a measure of successful treatment, that their lives are better with respect to strategies for working toward their needs and values.

We also believe that it would be an unusual therapist who would not draw upon all of her learning history in the service of trying to help clients. That is, a therapist would draw upon her own life experience, her science-based academic and intellectual training, and her specific training in various psychotherapeutic modalities in attempting to help her clients. Therapists who have received behavioral training may draw explicitly upon Functional Analytic Psychotherapy (FAP; Kohlenberg & Tsai, 1991; Tsai et al., 2008) and Acceptance and Commitment Therapy (ACT; Hayes, Strohsal, & Wilson, 1999), rather than other behavioral treatments such as Dialectical Behavior Therapy, Mindfulness Based Cognitive Therapy, or Integrative Couples Therapy, as these two treatments are studied frequently in behaviorally oriented clinical graduate training programs. The use of these therapies (or aspects of each) may feel seamless to the person doing a thoughtful, conceptualization-based intervention. In fact, all of these treatments are consistent theoretically, and could offer a very coherent intervention if integrated.

An integration of FAP and ACT could occur in which the principles of behavior change are employed to alter contingencies of both overt and private events. Although using these therapies simultaneously, or even interchangeably, can be

B.S. Kohlenberg (✉)
Department of Psychiatry and Behavioral Sciences, University of Nevada School of Medicine, Reno, NV, USA
e-mail: bkohlenberg@medicine.nevada.edu

J.W. Kanter et al. (eds.), *The Practice of Functional Analytic Psychotherapy*,
DOI 10.1007/978-1-4419-5830-3_3, © Springer Science+Business Media, LLC 2010

incredibly helpful and feel very natural to the therapist, there are some important distinctions between each that merit discussion. The differences between ACT and FAP can at times pull the therapist in different directions, despite being consistent paradigmatically at the broadest level. It is the purpose of this chapter to focus, on the ways that FAP and ACT originated, to explore their similarities and differences, and to consider their use together.

Although much of the source material referred to in this chapter is academically referenced, some of the history that is recounted is influenced by the particular relationships that the chapter authors have with FAP, ACT, and their originators. Barbara Kohlenberg is both the daughter of Robert Kohlenberg and received her graduate training with Steve Hayes; thus, she was part of the intellectual climate in which ACT developed. Glenn Callaghan was a graduate student of William Follette, one of Dr. Kohlenberg's first FAP supervisees and was influenced intellectually and personally by Drs. Hayes, Kohlenberg, and Follette as well as by Dr. Tsai. Thus, the following account is consistent with published scientific writings, and is also influenced by decades of personal, emotional, and intellectual relationships with the work and the people involved.

FAP Origins

FAP was developed by Robert J. Kohlenberg and Mavis Tsai. Their first published work on FAP occurred in *Psychotherapists in Clinical Practice* (Jacobson, 1987). In this work, they describe several events that stimulated the creation of FAP. These events came from intellectual sources, from experiences conducting behavior therapy over the years, and also from the interpersonal experiences of R. J. Kohlenberg and Tsai with each another and with others. Each of these sources of influence is discussed briefly.

Intellectual Underpinnings

FAP is a treatment firmly rooted in radical behavioral, functional analytic sensibilities. That is, R.J. Kohlenberg and Tsai had lengthy histories of behavior analytic training that defined their intellectual framework as psychologists.

R.J. Kohlenberg, however, had been noticing, in his clinical work as well as his personal life, some areas involving intimate relating for which he did not have a behavioral account. It was at this time that he came across the work of Steve Hayes, who served as an important intellectual stimulus in the development of FAP. Specifically, Kohlenberg attended a workshop presented at the Association of Behavior Analysis in the early 1980s by Hayes on Comprehensive Distancing (the name at that point for what is now considered ACT). Kohlenberg notes that at that time he had been a traditional behavior therapist for many years, and that Hayes introduced the possibility of applying radical behaviorism to adult outpatient psychotherapy in a way that was extremely exciting for him. From this introduction,

Kohlenberg began thinking about how to extend radical behavioral principles to adult outpatient psychotherapy.

Clinical Underpinnings

As experienced behavior therapists, Kohlenberg and Tsai state (1991) that over the course of their careers they noticed that some clients experienced change that far exceeded the specific stated goals of therapy. They noted that in these cases there was a feeling of emotional intensity in the therapeutic relationship. Tsai in particular was very interested in relationship-oriented psychotherapies, and was struck by the apparent power of relationship-focused approaches. Thus, they together began wondering how to account for this in terms of behavioral principles.

Personal Underpinnings

R. J. Kohlenberg and Tsai (personal communication) also noted that they both experienced and observed the tremendous behavior change that can occur when intimate, caring interpersonal relationships are in place. They experienced, both through their relationship with each another, and through awareness of the relationships of others, how powerful human relationships can be in terms of promoting satisfying lives. They observed that intimate human relationships that are rooted in compassion, the ability to be vulnerable, to take risks, and to give and receive love, are the kind of relationships that seem to go along with effective and meaningful lives.

Thus, R. J. Kohlenberg and Tsai developed therapeutic guidelines in response to the stimulus of an intellectual framework that allowed the extension of behavior analytic principles to help understand the general phenomenon of the powerful effects of intense, intimate human relationships. The clinical application of how the therapeutic relationship can promote effective psychotherapy became known as FAP.

ACT Origins

ACT was originally developed by Steve Hayes, and the first published description of this treatment (under the name "Comprehensive Distancing") was also published in *Psychotherapists in Clinical Practice* (Jacobson, 1987). In this chapter, Hayes described some of the origins of ACT, including a scholarly analysis of the progression of behavioral approaches to language and cognition. Hayes argued that a Skinnerian analysis does not explain adequately some important verbally based phenomena, and proposed a new account. He further described the kinds of problems that people seek therapy for as being in part due to the verbal context in which those problems occur; his therapeutic account focused on developing methods of altering the verbal contextual elements that give rise to human suffering. In part, this verbal context is problematic because language itself can be a barrier to fully contacting one's experience in the moment. The reader is referred to other resources for a more complete account of the underpinnings of ACT (e.g., Hayes, Strosahl, & Wilson, 1999).

Intellectual Underpinnings

Zettle (2005), in his overview of the evolution of ACT, divides the history of ACT into three phases, the first phase being an initial formative period in the late 1970s, when basic behavior analytic approaches to verbal and rule-governed behavior were applied to clinical phenomena. This was followed by a transitional period, beginning in the 1980s, in which relational frame theory (RFT) was developed as a post-Skinnerian account of language. In the last two decades, ACT has been developed and disseminated, and is described by Zettle as "a fully integrated functional contextualistic approach to psychotherapy grounded in RFT" (p. 78).

Clinical Underpinnings

ACT is also inspired by contact with the depth of human suffering seen in clinical situations, as well as more broadly. Hayes was not satisfied with the lack of depth seen in some behavioral approaches to human suffering, and looked toward other therapy approaches, such as experiential treatments, to learn more about methods of understanding and helping people. Being a thoughtful and rigorous scientist, he grappled with existing behavioral approaches and their application to both the depths of human suffering and to the compassion and seeming effectiveness of non-behavioral, experiential kinds of treatments. Concluding there were fundamental problems with behavioral accounts of language, he focused on the development of RFT as a behavioral approach to cognition that had more potential to understand and treat the kinds of suffering human beings endure. For a complete account of RFT see Hayes, Barnes-Holmes, and Roche (2001).

Personal Underpinnings

Hayes also has made clear that ACT is deeply sensitive to how much human suffering there is, and how extraordinarily painful it can be to be human. In an interview published in *Time* magazine (Cloud, 2006), Hayes disclosed his own intimate personal experiences with the debilitating effects of anxiety, and described how he learned to live a meaningful life, even with tremendous suffering.

Thus, ACT is a therapy that grew in response to Hayes' connection to the vast pervasiveness of human suffering. Hayes also felt that behavior analytic principles did not adequately account for some of the properties of language that he argues are crucial to the understanding of human suffering and human potential. So along with the growth and development of ACT, basic science has blossomed around RFT, a theory that has given rise to empirical data that can inform our understanding of suffering and its treatment (Hayes et al., 2001). Furthermore, ACT is also a therapy that is firmly committed to helping people discover what they value in life, and to help them lead lives that matter in a way that is consistent with an individual's deeply held values.

FAP and ACT: Historical Commonalities

FAP and ACT share a common background rooted in functional analysis and radical behavioral philosophy. In another sense, it is also the case that R. J. Kohlenberg and Hayes had interests that were similar prior to the development of FAP and ACT. Both considered themselves to be Skinnerians. Further, both utilized radical behaviorism and the principles of behavior analysis applied to various content areas of interest. Both Kohlenberg and Hayes published in the area of behavioral approaches to community psychology, specifically focused on energy conservation (e.g., Hayes & Cone, 1977; Kohlenberg, Phillips, & Proctor, 1976). Both published in the area of sexual dysfunction (Kohlenberg, 1974a; Brownell, Hayes, & Barlow, 1977) and both published in the general area of behavior therapy (Kohlenberg, 1974b; Hayes, 1976). Kohlenberg and Hayes both can be described as people who loved playing with concepts and technology to help make a difference in the lives of individuals and in our community. In these early works, both were focused on making a difference by focusing on overt behaviors that held meaning both for the community and clinical significance.

In addition, Kohlenberg and Hayes are both clinical psychologists, and were intrigued with the complexity of human suffering and the parsimony of behavioral philosophy and technology. It is also the case that both Kohlenberg and Hayes began to be interested in human struggles and problems that seemed to be characterized by different kinds of content than normally addressed by traditional behavioral and cognitive behavioral therapies. ACT and FAP arose from the same behavioral tradition, and thus at their core, understand and change behavior by examining contingent relationships (Kohlenberg, Hayes, & Tsai, 1993). Both FAP and ACT can be thought of as pioneering treatments as they pushed forward behavioral theoretical and technological innovation in the clinical arena.

FAP and ACT and the Behavioral and Cognitive Behavioral Therapies

FAP and ACT emerged at a time when traditional behavioral and cognitive behavioral therapies were doing very well, and yet had specific limitations. Traditional behavioral approaches to treatment typically were focused on specific behaviors that required changing, either increasing or decreasing, and these behaviors generally were studied and modified in restrictive settings where the behaviors could be observed and manipulated. For instance, behavioral therapies excelled with respect to phobias, classroom behaviors, and problematic behaviors seen in inpatient settings. Cognitive behavioral treatments also focused on instances of problematic behavior, including thoughts and feelings that occurred outside of the session, and discussions of which were recorded in session. The agenda that cut across both behavioral and cognitive behavioral therapies was focused on the importance of helping people try to *change* problematic behaviors, whether these behaviors were publicly observable or were more private in the domain of thoughts and feelings.

Taken together, the domains of interest to R. J. Kohlenberg and Tsai, intimacy and relationships, and Hayes, human suffering and meaning, were not typical realms for which behavioral treatments were well suited. However, in both FAP and ACT, there never has been a move to abandon behavioral philosophy and values in order to study these meaningful areas of human experience. Both FAP and ACT can be described as having extended the content areas of behavioral treatments. FAP stayed within existing behavioral principles, as these parsimonious accounts were completely adequate for the purposes of its authors. Hayes, however, did not feel that traditional behavioral principles were adequate for the understanding of cognition, and thus extended behavioral principles to include RFT. Furthermore, both FAP and ACT were more interested in helping people learn to *accept*, and thus *change their relationship with their thoughts and feelings*, rather than on helping change or eradicate specific thoughts or feelings. The agenda shared by both treatments, then, is constructivist rather than eliminative. FAP and ACT both seek to build on client histories to develop strategies to experience powerful emotions and to cultivate skills to interact in ways that better serve their needs and values. They are not therapies that seek to eliminate thoughts or feelings and replace them with more effective or accurate beliefs, thoughts, or feelings. This constructivist approach shared by both is paradigmatically consistent with behaviorism.

Unique Contributions of FAP to Behavioral and Cognitive Behavior Therapies

Impact and Meaning of the Therapy Relationship, and the Parsimony of Functional Analytic Behavioral Explanation

FAP has made many revolutionary contributions to contemporary behavior therapy. A particularly significant contribution is the notion that the therapy relationship is in itself a powerful force that can affect behavior change through the contingent reactions that occur in session, in the here-and-now. Though a focus on the healing power of the therapeutic relationship, and the therapeutic alliance, has been well articulated at a general level (e.g., Bordin, 1979; Safran & Muran, 2000), and there have been behavioral translations of psychodynamic psychotherapies[**], the importance of the therapeutic relationship had been underplayed in the behavioral therapies (see Kohlenberg, Yeater, & Kohlenberg, 1998 for a more complete discussion of these issues).

Thus, FAP has helped provide behavioral, parsimonious ways of understanding the way the client–therapist interaction can produce behavior change due to contingent responding in session (Follette, Naugle, & Callaghan, 1996). Because of FAP, there is now a way to conceptualize the contingencies present in the therapy relationship as being the primary agent of behavior change, rather than previous behavioral accounts suggesting that the therapy relationship is ancillary to other specified behavioral techniques (O'Donohue, 1995; Rimm & Masters, 1979). Said more plainly, FAP has helped behavior therapists move from an understanding of the therapeutic relationship as utilitarian, aiming to gain and further client adherence, to one that fully appreciates and addresses the complex interpersonal process that occurs between two people working toward healing and growth. Though FAP can be said to "use" the therapeutic relationship to affect clinical change, its use is in managing the rich contingencies that occur in session to help clients effectively and efficiently reach their goals in treatment (see also Callaghan, Naugle, & Follete, 1996).

Value of Intimacy in Human Interactions

FAP therapists also believe that much of human suffering is connected to problems involving interpersonal relationships. Many of the varied diagnoses listed in the Diagnostic and Statistical Manual of Mental Disorders (DSM IV) (APA, 1994; DSM IV-Revised, APA, 2000) entail problems with functioning interpersonally as part of the diagnostic criteria. FAP is an optimal treatment for increasing skill in the area of emotional intimacy, as the therapy is ideally suited to evoke and consequate emotionally intimate relating.

In FAP, the ability to create satisfying intimate human relationships is seen as an essential part of a meaningful life. In fact, one can argue that this is a logical starting point of FAP as an approach to psychotherapy. Working with people on developing and enhancing the repertoires involved in creating close, loving relationships is a particular area of sensitivity in FAP. In addition, it is well known that when intimacy is distorted, such as when a child is abused by a trusted caregiver, this can be highly predictive of later psychopathology (Kessler, Sonnega, Bromet, Hughes, & Nelson, 1995). With regard to these kinds of trauma histories, FAP offers many ideal opportunities for clients to work through the later interpersonal effects of such trauma (Kohlenberg, Tsai, & Kohlenberg., 2006).

A Focus on the Interpersonal as the Subject Matter of Interest

FAP primarily focuses on the contingent interpersonal relationship found in therapy as being the essential factor to bring about behavior change. Although both historical and current relationships are fundamental in bringing about some forms of human suffering, the therapeutic relationship is not seen as a metaphor for those past or other outside-the-room interactions. Instead, the client–therapist relationship is understood as one of many relationships the client has, one in which client behaviors that occur in the context of other human interactions also can occur. These are the "real deal" behaviors, not symbolic interactions. They are live or in vivo with the therapist, and are the primary focus of FAP.

The therapeutic relationship is the context for the mechanism of clinical change to occur via contingent responding by the therapist to in-session client problems and improvements. That is, the interactions that occur between the client and the therapist are the critical ingredients that occasion and shape clinically relevant behavior. Thus, when a client is working on trying to express a particular emotion, what is of interest is how that expression functions in the therapy relationship. The therapist works to contingently shape emotional expression that promotes effective interpersonal interactions.

Impact and Meaning of Clinical Supervision

FAP also has opened the door to the necessity of therapist awareness in the conduct of therapy. This is because the therapist must be aware and able to discriminate relevant aspects of both clinically relevant behaviors emitted by the client in session, and their own responses to that client behavior. Not only does the therapist need to observe and then determine which client behaviors are effective as they occur during treatment, the therapist must also be able to distinguish effectively between his or her private reactions that are pertinent to client change, and those reactions that are not representative of the social or verbal community. Thus, self-awareness skills are essential to the therapist and are a focus of supervision. This kind of clinical supervision invites the discussion of the personal emotional reactions of the therapist, both to the clients they are treating and to the supervision itself.

FAP supervision also is focused on expanding the abilities of the therapist to make discriminations about clinically relevant behavior, and to evoke and reinforce those in-session client behaviors. FAP supervision thus supports therapists in developing interpersonal courage in so far as the therapist must recognize and challenge emotional avoidance as it occurs for both their clients and for themselves. This involves interpersonal risk taking in the service of promoting emotional intimacy, a task that can be challenging for both the client and the clinician. Clinical supervision can be seen as a "learning laboratory" during which such skills are practiced and reinforced. Just as in FAP therapy, the skills of FAP therapists are evoked and contingently responded to during the supervision session. This "parallel process" as it is sometimes called creates opportunities for the supervisor to focus on the therapist's interpersonal repertoire as it occurs in the supervisory session in the service of creating a more effective FAP therapist. Though provocative and powerful, this experience by clinicians during FAP therapy can be very effective in modeling how to respond in difficult clinical situations, as well as creating a more compassionate and effective therapist response to client suffering. For a thorough discussion of FAP supervision, including ethical issues and other challenges, see Callaghan (2006a) and Tsai, Callaghan, Kohlenberg, Follette, and Darrow (2008).

Unique Contributions of ACT to Behavioral and Cognitive Behavior Therapies

Ubiquity of Human Suffering

ACT also has made many revolutionary contributions to contemporary behavior therapy. First and foremost, ACT has approached and embraced the subject matter of the depth and pervasiveness of human suffering. ACT has put forth the idea that suffering goes beyond particular problems, and is found instead in the very nature of language and cognition itself. ACT, in a meaningful way, joins many spiritual, religious, and psychotherapy traditions in trying to help human beings develop new relationship to their suffering, rather than adhering to the position of some cognitive behavioral therapies, which can be described as trying to help people change or regulate their suffering.

Relational Frame Theory, a Post-Skinnerian Account of Language and Cognition

ACT has brought along with it a basic science and theory of language and cognition that helps explain how language itself can create suffering. As briefly described above, Relational Frame Theory (RFT) explains how describing, categorizing, or evaluating aversive events can itself have aversive effects, and suggests that forming arbitrary relations between events is the core of human language. While RFT focuses on cognition, it is not in fact a cognitive therapy analysis. Briefly, cognitions, thoughts, feelings, and other human experiences are understood as behaviors occurring in context under the control of basic contingencies of reinforcement. According to RFT, some unique aspects of human language or cognition require a substantive extension of Skinner's (1957) seminal analysis of verbal behavior. This analysis is at the core of the principles of ACT.

A Focus on the Intrapersonal: Language, the Human Struggle, and a Vital, Valued Life

ACT's treatment model targets acceptance and mindfulness processes, along with commitment and behavior change processes, to produce psychological flexibility. This involves helping people acquire the skills to respond to their own experience in ways that promote engaging in behavior that is more effective for them, given their values. ACT is focused on using the processes of acceptance and mindfulness in the service of helping people respond differently to their thoughts and feelings. Again, the agenda of ACT, and its radical departure from eliminative approaches, is to help clients learn to experience a thought differently from the way many people have learned to deal with unwanted experiences, which is to get rid of them. Instead, ACT provides training that serves to help people learn to actively embrace emotion, to look mindfully and dispassionately at thoughts and feelings, to be more fully in the present moment, to be in contact with a transcendent sense of self, to make contact with their cherished life values, and to engage in behavioral patterns of committed action in the service of these values (Hayes, Luoma, Bond, Masuda, & Lillis, 2006). ACT, in many ways, offers a rich compendium of skills designed to help people respond more compassionately to their own thoughts and feelings, thus freeing them from the negative effects of entanglement with their own language, and promoting behavioral progress in life that is congruent with their values.

FAP and ACT: Mutual Influence and Integration

As noted in the introduction to this chapter, these two treatments often are options for clinical training in a variety of clinical psychology training programs. Thus, practitioners frequently may think about these treatments together when they are conceptualizing clinical problems and designing and implementing treatment strategies. In addition, as both FAP and ACT share a common behavioral philosophy, they fit together rather easily from a conceptual point of view, and given ACT's emphasis on the intrapersonal and FAP's focus on the interpersonal, they can operate in a complementary manner as well. We argue that it happens commonly that ACT therapists are guided by FAP's interpersonal sensibilities and techniques, and that FAP therapists are guided by ACT's intrapersonal sensibilities and techniques. However, how these two treatments co-exist both conceptually and practically is open for discussion.

The first conference presentation in which FAP and ACT were presented as treatments with mutual influence and integration was by Kohlenberg and Gifford (1998). This paper was an attempt to articulate a treatment that was theoretically consistent and true to the goals of each separate therapy. An outline describing integration strategies has been offered by Callaghan, Gregg, Marx, Kohlenberg, and Gifford (2004), and is described in some detail below.

Callaghan et al. (2004) describe three different approaches to using FAP and ACT together. The first is to use the therapeutic relationship in FAP, while doing ACT, to directly shape acceptance and mindfulness skills in the service of psychological flexibility and committed action. The goal here is to utilize the therapeutic relationship to achieve the intrapersonal outcomes set forth by ACT. The second approach is to use ACT, while doing FAP, to help clients respond differently to their thoughts and feelings so that they can engage in new behavior that impacts the therapy relationship and is amenable to contingent consequation. The goal in this approach is to attempt to use strategies of acceptance and mindfulness-based action to create more meaningful interpersonal relationships for clients both in and outside of therapy. The third approach is to have both ACT and FAP be equally present at any given moment, and to use the interpersonal processes of the therapeutic relationship to shape the intrapersonal processes of avoidance and acceptance as they are seen in the here-and-now of the therapy relationship.

One way that FAP therapists can utilize the strategies of ACT is with their own challenges in experiencing frustration, anguish, or even joy and happiness in the room with a client. The goal of the FAP therapist is to respond not only in the moment, contingent to how the client interacts with the therapist, but to do so genuinely, openly, and honestly. Given the rich histories that we all have as humans (both as clients and therapists), there may be certain emotions, needed for effective FAP, that are harder to feel and express to clients. These feelings may be essential to share with clients as they impact the therapist, but the therapist may not know how to experience or express that feeling. It would be far easier to avoid the experience and move on with therapy, but ACT gives the FAP therapist principle-based strategies to experience feelings and then share them with the client. Rather than change the subject, or even laugh off the awkwardness, we can learn to fully experience ourselves and the client, to embrace the moment of therapy even when it is exquisitely difficult to do so, and then move forward in the direction of our values as therapists, namely being effective in the service of the client's needs.

FAP and ACT: Empirical Investigations of Their Co-use

FAP and ACT have been used together in several single case designs and in one controlled clinical trial. These studies are reviewed below.

Baruch, Busch, Juskiewicz, and Kanter (2009) employed FAP and ACT consecutively to treat a client with major depression and paranoid behaviors. In this case study, they assessed and treated both the intra- and interpersonal aspects of the clinical presentation. During their 37 weeks of sessions, they employed ACT to focus on the intrapersonal behaviors of paranoia. During these first 7 sessions, they worked with the client on de-literalizing language, and on identifying values, mindfulness, and willingness. Specifically, they focused on helping the client accept his paranoid thoughts and symptoms of depression while acting in a value-consistent manner. Starting in Session 8, they continued with ACT, and started to implement FAP focused on his problematic behaviors of being reluctant to share personal information, social disengagement, and emotional expression deficits. This case was evaluated using both self-report and behavioral observations. Using self-report measures, the client showed improvement with depression, acceptance, and social relationships. The client's self-monitoring records showed that his paranoid thinking decreased and his mindful responses to his paranoid thoughts increased. One month after treatment ended, he reported a stable mood and an expanding social network. He still reported having paranoid thoughts but they interfered only mildly with interpersonal functioning.

Paul, Marx, and Orsillo (1999) used both ACT and FAP consecutively to treat a court referred exhibitionist. The treatment involved helping the client acquire the skills to accept undesired and intolerable affective states, as well as social anxiety, exhibitionism, and the use of marijuana. Urges to expose, acts of exhibitionism, and drug use were assessed throughout the 1 year of treatment, and at 6-month follow-up. Results suggested that urges to expose and public masturbation were reduced significantly from baseline. In addition, the client improved his social skills, and drug use decreased along with symptoms of depression and anxiety.

Gifford et al. (under review) developed a psychosocial treatment designed for smoking cessation that used ACT processes to help undermine experiential avoidance, while also making value-based behavioral choices. In this study, FAP processes were used to shape contingently these very behavior change processes as they occurred in the context of the therapy relationship. Three hundred and three smokers were randomly assigned to one of two conditions: bupropion, a smoking cessation medication; or bupropion plus the ACT-/FAP-based treatment. Subjects in the ACT-/FAP-based treatment received one 2-hour group and one individual session per week for 10 weeks. The group session involved a focus on ACT processes and techniques, while the individual session focused on contingently shaping FAP- and ACT-based skills. At 1-year follow-up, quit rates were 35.1% in the combined condition vs. 20% in the medication alone condition. Furthermore, the combined treatment was mediated by acceptance-based responding and the therapeutic relationship.

FAP and ACT: Differences

Treatment Delivery

One major place where FAP and ACT diverge is in the required methods of treatment delivery. To date, ACT has been delivered via individual therapy, group therapy, workshops, and self-help book materials. In other words, ACT can be delivered both in the context of an interpersonal relationship, as well as completely independent of an interpersonal relationship, such as by reading a self-help book. FAP, on the other hand, can only be delivered in the context of an interpersonal relationship. By definition, FAP requires contingent shaping, which requires the presence of an interpersonal relationship.

Evoking and Consequating Clinical Problems

In FAP, it is largely assumed that the client's clinically relevant behavior will be occasioned by the ongoing interaction between client and therapist that occurs in session. In other words, if a client tends to become passive and withdrawn when angry, and he becomes angry because the therapist forgot the name of his spouse, but fails to express his anger, this would be an opportunity to work with this particular clinically relevant behavior (CRB). The CRB would be evoked naturally as part of the ebb and flow of the therapy relationship. Generally in ACT, client problems can be illuminated via experiential exercises and metaphors that facilitate client exploration of their internal behavioral reactions. There is no need for the therapist–client interaction to elicit or occasion these behaviors.

In FAP, it is essential that clinically relevant problems and improvements be noted and consequated by the therapist. In ACT, this immediate, contingent response is not available, as there may not even be a therapist if the treatment is delivered by reading a book. This is a key difference between these two treatments.

Assessment

While both treatments value idiographic assessment, they do have different areas of emphasis. FAP focuses on functional analysis, and may utilize an assessment strategy developed called the Functional Idiographic Assessment Template (FIAT; Callaghan, 2006b). The FIAT promotes fine-grained assessment of clinically relevant behavior, with that assessment tied closely to clinical intervention and evaluation. In ACT, a focus is placed on the assessment of values, and outcomes are measured based on progress toward one's values. In addition, ACT processes are measured using self-report questionnaires, such as the Acceptance and Action Questionnaire (AAQ), and progress would be evaluated in part based on how this process measures changes.

Both treatments, naturally, also employ traditional measures of psychopathology, particularly when the purpose of treatment is research. However, both treatments are quite interested in assessments that are theoretically tied to their hypothesized mechanisms of action.

Values

Both FAP and ACT attach importance to incorporating client values into the treatment. In ACT, however, values may be assessed more systematically, via a self-report measure, than would be done in FAP. In ACT, values are defined primarily as related to categories that matter to the client in their lives; there is no focus on progress toward values also being evident for in-session behavior. In FAP, however, there is a clear dictate that values would be relevant both out-of-session as well as in-session. In this way, in-session improvements, or evidence of problems, would be directly shaped by the contingent reactions occurring in the therapy session. This would be expected to generalize to effective value-consistent behavior out of the session.

Conclusion

Clinical work with our suffering clients is extremely humbling. Though it is so meaningful to effectively help our clients, there are times in any therapist's experience when it is difficult to make a real difference. FAP is a system of therapy that promotes tender, compassionate growth, taking full advantage of interactions in the here-and-now of the therapy room. FAP therapists must acquire the skills to be excellent observers of their client's problems and their improvements. FAP therapists must also develop an ability to be very present with their clients, so as to not only notice problems and improvements, but also to respond effectively to these behaviors. And yet, even when all of this is working quite well, there are still times when one might be left with not knowing how to help, and what to do. In times like this, appealing to a different rich therapy system feels not only like conversing with an intellectual brother or sister, but also is new and interesting, and something about which one can be quite grateful. For many FAP therapists, ACT is just such a rich therapy system. ACT offers a wide variety of techniques and sensitivity to processes that can help clients compassionately hold their own emotional experiences so that they can then respond more effectively in the here-and-now of the therapy room. The therapist can then react in a reinforcing manner to such improvements.

Similarly, ACT therapists experience the same frustrations with the therapy working so well at times; yet there are always those clients who continue to struggle and to suffer. For these therapists, too, it is useful to extend to treatments that are intellectually close to ACT while having a very different technical emphasis. FAP is such a therapy.

Clinical work is rich, deep, and can be quite challenging. Just as we promote flexible thinking and behavior in our clients, it is important to promote this kind of thinking in ourselves. Both FAP and ACT are grounded in behavioral principles. Both FAP and ACT are compassionate treatments, rooted in helping people live meaningful, fertile lives. And FAP and ACT have different areas of conceptual and technical focus. This is why the mutual influence of FAP and ACT has helped both of us become more effectual, skillful therapists. And just as we value our clients taking their whole histories with them as they live meaningful lives, we as therapists also take our whole histories with us as we strive to provide the most compassionate, effective therapy that we can.

References

American Psychiatric Association. (1994). *Diagnostic and statistical manual of mental disorders* (4th ed., text revision). Washington, DC: Author.

American Psychiatric Association. (2000). *Diagnostic and statistical manual of mental disorders* (4th ed., text revision). Washington, DC: American Psychiatric Association.

Baruch, D. E., Kanter, J. W., Busch, A. B., & Juskiewicz, K. (2009). Enhancing the therapy relationship in Acceptance and Commitment Therapy for psychotic symptoms. *Clinical Case Studies, 8,* 241–257.

Bordin, E. (1979). The generalizability of the psychoanalytic concept of the working alliance. *Psychotherapy, 16,* 252–260.

Brownell, K. D., Hayes, S. C., & Barlow, D. H. (1977). Patterns of appropriate and deviant arousal: The behavioral treatment of multiple sexual deviations. *Journal of Consulting and Clinical Psychology, 45,* 1144–1155.

Callaghan, G. M. (2006a). Supervision in Functional Analytic Psychotherapy. *The International Journal of Behavioral Consultation and Therapy, 2,* 416–431.

Callaghan, G. M. (2006b). The Functional Idiographic Assessment Template (FIAT) System. *The Behavior Analyst Today, 7,* 357–398.

Callaghan, G. M., Gregg, J. A., Marx, B., Kohlenberg, B. S., & Gifford, E. (2004). FACT: The utility of an integration of Functional Analytic Psychotherapy and Acceptance and Commitment Therapy. *Psychotherapy: Theory, Research, Practice, Training, 41,* 195–207.

Callaghan, G. M., Naugle, A. E., & Follette, W. C. (1996). Useful constructions of the client–therapist relationship. *Psychotherapy: Theory, Research, Practice, Training, 33,* 381–390.

Cloud, S. (2006, February 5, Sunday). The third wave of therapy. *Time Magazine.*

Follette, W. C., Naugle, A. E., & Callaghan, G. M. (1996). A radical behavioral understanding of the therapeutic relationship in effecting change. *Behavior Therapy, 27,* 623–641.

Gifford, E. V., Kohlenberg, B. S., Hayes, S. C., Antonuccio, D. O., Piasecki, M. M., & Palm, K. Applying acceptance and the Therapeutic relationship to smoking cessation: A randomized controlled trial under review. *Behavior Therapy.*

Hayes, S. C. (1976). The role of approach contingencies in phobic behavior. *Behavior Therapy, 7,* 28–36.

Hayes, S. C., Barnes-Holmes, D., & Roche, B. (Eds.). (2001). *Relational Frame Theory: A Post-Skinnerian account of human language and cognition.* New York: Plenum Press.

Hayes, S. C., & Cone, J. D. (1977). Reducing residential electrical energy use: Payments, information, and feedback. *Journal of Applied Behavior Analysis, 10,* 425–435.

Hayes, S. C., Luoma, J., Bond, F., Masuda, A., & Lillis, J. (2006). Acceptance and Commitment Therapy: Model, processes, and outcomes. *Behaviour Research and Therapy, 44,* 1–25.

Hayes, S. C., Strosahl, K., & Wilson, K. G. (1999). *Acceptance and commitment therapy: An experiential approach behavior change.* New York: Guilford.

Jacobson, N. (1987). *Psychotherapists in clinical practice: Cognitive and behavioral perspectives.* New York: Guilford Press.

Kessler, R. C., Sonnega, A., Bromet, E., Hughes, M., & Nelson, C. B. (1995). Posttraumatic stress disorder in the National Comorbidity Survey. *Archives of General Psychiatry, 53,* 1048–1060.

Kohlenberg, R. J. (1974a). Directed masturbation and the treatment of primary orgasmic dysfunction. *Archives of Sexual Behavior, 3,* 349–356.

Kohlenberg, R. J. (1974b). In-vivo desensitization and aversive stimuli in the treatment of pedophilia. *Journal of Abnormal Psychology, 83,* 192–195.

Kohlenberg, B. S., & Gifford, E. (1998). *FACT (FAP and ACT): Clinical behavior analysts do it in-vivo.* Paper presented at the 24th Annual Meeting of the Association for Behavior Analysis, Orlando, FL.

Kohlenberg, R. J., Hayes, S. C., & Tsai, M. (1993). Radical behavioral psychotherapy: Two contemporary examples. *Clinical Psychology Review, 13,* 579–592.

Kohlenberg, R. J., Phillips, T., & Proctor, W. (1976). A behavioral analysis of peaking in electrical energy consumers. *Journal of Applied Behavior Analysis, 9,* 13–18.

Kohlenberg, R. J., & Tsai, M. (1991). *Functional analytic psychotherapy: Creating intense and curative therapeutic relationships.* New York: Plenum.

Kohlenberg, B. S., Tsai, M., & Kohlenberg, R. J. (2006). Functional analytic psychotherapy and the treatment of complex posttraumatic stress disorder. In V. Follette & J. Ruzek (Eds.), *Cognitive behavioral therapies for trauma* (pp. 173–197). New York: Guilford Press.

Kohlenberg, B. S., Yeater, E. A., & Kohlenberg, R. J. (1998). Functional analysis, therapeutic alliance, and brief psychotherapy. In J. D. Safran & J. C. Muran (Eds.), *The therapeutic alliance and brief psychotherapy* (pp. 39–62). Washington, DC: American Psychological Association Press.

O'Donohue, W. (1995). The scientist-practitioner: Time allocation in psychotherapy. *The Behavior Therapist, 18,* 117–119.

Paul, R. H., Marx, B. P., & Orsillo, S. M. (1999). Acceptance-based psychotherapy in the treatment of an adjudicated exhibitionist: A case example. *Behavior Therapy*, *30*, 149–162.

Rimm, D. C., & Masters, J. C. (1979). *Behavior therapy: Techniques and empirical findings* (2nd ed.). San Francisco: Academic Press.

Safran, J. D., & Muran, J. D. (2000). *Negotiating the therapeutic alliance: A relational treatment guide*. New York: The Guilford Press.

Skinner, B. F. (1957). *Verbal behavior*. Acton, MA: Copley.

Tsai, M., Callaghan, G. M., Kohlenberg, R. J., Follette, W. C., & Darrow, S. M. (2008). Supervision and therapist self-development. In M. Tsai, R. J. Kohlenberg, J. W. Kanter, B. Kohlenberg, W. C. Follette, & G. M. Callaghan (Eds.), *A guide to functional analytic psychotherapy: Awareness, courage, love and behaviorism*. New York: Springer.

Tsai, M., Kohlenberg, R. J., Kanter, J. W., Kohlenberg, B., Follette, W. C., & Callaghan, G. M. (2008). *A guide to functional analytic psychotherapy: Awareness, courage, love, and behaviorism*. New York: Springer.

Zettle, R. D. (2005). The evolution of a contextual approach to therapy: From Comprehensive Distancing to ACT. *International Journal of Behavioral and Consultation Therapy*, *1*, 77–89.

Chapter 4
FAP and Dialectical Behavior Therapy (DBT)

Jennifer Waltz, Sara J. Landes, and Gareth I. Holman

This chapter explores the intersections of Functional Analytic Psychotherapy (FAP; Kohlenberg & Tsai, 1991; Tsai et al., 2009) and Dialectical Behavior Therapy (DBT; Linehan, 1993a, 1993b) with a focus on how training and experience with each model can enhance work with the other. Both FAP and DBT understand behavior within its historical and current context, with DBT also adding the biological context. Seizing opportunities to address problem behaviors as they occur and actively reinforcing instances of more adaptive behavior are hallmarks of both treatments. Both emphasize forming a real relationship, characterized by compassion, awareness, and genuineness. Both treatments emphasize the importance of the therapist having experiential understanding of the behaviors or skills they are suggesting to clients, and a high level of self-awareness and ability to observe one's own reactions in the moment.

We believe that the experience of training in and practicing both treatments, as opposed to one or the other alone, enhances effectiveness doing DBT, and doing FAP-informed therapy. We have found that our work with both approaches has helped us to be more present to the current moment and open to whatever that moment presents. Both treatments have challenged us to synthesize scientific and theoretical rigor, with emotional depth and experiential understanding. We feel that doing FAP and DBT provides therapists with opportunities to deepen self-awareness and compassion. At this point, there is no empirical evidence available to address the question of whether training in either model enhances work with the other; such research would be quite difficult to conduct. Rather, the chapter is based on our experiences as therapists trained in both DBT and FAP, and our work training others. Those experiences have brought us to the conclusion that learning and doing each of these treatments can expand a therapist's awareness of, and ability to respond to, in-session behavior in a powerfully therapeutic way.

A crucial difference between FAP and DBT is that DBT is a comprehensive, stand-alone treatment model, whereas FAP is a set of rules that can be integrated

J. Waltz (✉)
Department of Psychology, University of Montana, Missoula, MT, USA
e-mail: jennifer.waltz@umontana.edu

J.W. Kanter et al. (eds.), *The Practice of Functional Analytic Psychotherapy*,
DOI 10.1007/978-1-4419-5830-3_4, © Springer Science+Business Media, LLC 2010

into many other treatment approaches. Although DBT utilizes a range of cognitive, behavioral, and mindfulness-based interventions, it is essentially a complete treatment in the sense that when clients are in DBT, they are just in DBT. In contrast, FAP may be implemented as an adjunct; thus, FAP-Enhanced CBT and FAP-Enhanced Behavioral Activation also are presented in this book. A second important difference is that DBT was developed for a specific client population, whereas FAP is theoretically applicable to any population whose problem behaviors can occur within the therapy setting. DBT was designed primarily as a treatment for people who have severe problems with emotion dysregulation and are chronically suicidal and/or engage in self-harm, many of whom meet criteria for Borderline Personality Disorder. DBT was designed to address specific problems experienced by this population, and consequently targets those problems very directly. DBT has subsequently been adapted for other populations for whom severe emotion dysregulation and behavioral dyscontrol are central difficulties (Dimeff & Koerner, 2007).

In terms of theory, FAP and DBT are both rooted in behaviorism, but DBT is additionally informed by a dialectical philosophy and by Zen. DBT has a specific model of etiology and a much broader, more specifically articulated set of strategies and interventions. The core of FAP is the process of contingent responding by the therapist to client clinically relevant behavior (CRB). Of all the currently available treatments that have empirical support for their efficacy, DBT is one of the few that specifically calls for the kind of interventions that are emphasized in FAP. Thus, we do not view FAP as an addition or change to DBT; rather, we believe that FAP training and experience are likely to increase a therapist's competence utilizing interventions and approaches that are already a part of DBT.

Our experience has been that training and experience with FAP increase a DBT therapist's ability to observe and describe in-session behaviors, both problematic and adaptive. We have found FAP to be helpful in expanding the therapist's comfort with, and repertoire available for, responding to relevant, in-the-moment behavior in an effective way. Similarly, DBT training and experience have enhanced our FAP-informed therapy work in a variety of ways, in particular around addressing more extreme CRB1s (i.e., clinically relevant behaviors that are problematic and occur in session), and providing a wider repertoire of CRB2s (e.g., clinically relevant behaviors that are improvements occurring in session) to encourage. Finally, we believe that both FAP and DBT training and experience can enhance a therapist's engagement in the therapeutic relationship in terms of his/her ability to be genuine, accepting, and engaged.

We begin this chapter with brief overviews of DBT and FAP. We then focus on ways that FAP and DBT training and experience can reinforce and augment each other. Given that DBT is a stand-alone treatment, and FAP may be an adjunct, this section of the chapter will be organized around the components of DBT to which FAP principles are most relevant. These include the acceptance-oriented elements of radical genuineness and reciprocal communication, and the change-oriented intervention strategies of targeting therapy-interfering behavior, observing limits, and promoting insight. Finally, we discuss how FAP training may help support DBT therapists in terms of their motivation to do the difficult work they do. It is important to note that we are not providing a full or complete explication of either approach. DBT includes many other important interventions and communication styles to which FAP is less relevant. For a complete description of DBT, the reader is directed to Linehan (1993a, 1993b). For a complete description of FAP, see Tsai et al. (2009).

Overview of Dialectical Behavior Therapy

The clients most typically served by DBT are individuals who meet criteria for Borderline Personality Disorder (BPD), or who struggle with other complex, multi-diagnostic problems that have not been responsive to more traditional types of treatment, and who share the common feature of emotion regulation deficits. Linehan (1993a) has proposed a way of understanding the diagnostic criteria for BPD centered around the notion of *dysregulation*. From this perspective, clients who meet BPD criteria are understood to experience some combination of emotional dysregulation (emotional lability, anger), behavioral dysregulation (impulsivity, suicidality/self-harm), interpersonal dysregulation (unstable relationships, fear of abandonment), cognitive dysregulation (dissociation/paranoia), and dysregulation in sense of self (identity disturbance, chronic emptiness). Typically, DBT clients meet criteria for one, or more than one, Axis I diagnosis, and often have serious problems in managing day-to-day life, relationships, work, and so on. Many clients come to DBT programs because other treatments (e.g., standard outpatient, inpatient) have not worked for them. Thus, DBT clients are often in intense emotional pain and have feelings of hopelessness, fear, shame, or frustration related to treatment.

Relevant to FAP, the presenting problems of DBT clients almost inevitably are very present in the therapy session and the therapeutic relationship. DBT clients often have interpersonal difficulties that are challenging for the therapist. They may be demanding, rejecting, desperate, lonely, critical, frightened, and/or dissociative. All of these client characteristics, and others, have shaped and influenced the development of DBT. Along with DBT's behavioral underpinnings, this influence has resulted in FAP-consistent strategies, with their focus on working on problems as they arise in the therapy session being integral to the delivery of DBT.

DBT (Linehan, 1993a) is a behavioral treatment based on a biosocial and transactional theory of BPD. The biosocial theory of the development and maintenance of BPD proposes that an on-going interplay of biologically based emotion dysregulation with a pervasively invalidating environment leads to BPD symptomatology. The theory hypothesizes that individuals who meet criteria for BPD have biologically based emotional sensitivity and reactivity. Their emotional reactions get set off more easily, are more intense and long-lasting than are those of others. Individuals meeting BPD criteria lack important abilities to modulate or regulate their intense emotional responses. This transacts with an environment that invalidates their emotional experiences and sense of self in a broad and persistent way. Invalidating environments communicate that the client is bad, wrong, pathological, unworthy, or unimportant (Linehan, 1993a). Over time this leads to extreme emotional dysregulation, inability to regulate emotions, and ultimately to the various kinds of dysregulation that are central to BPD.

In order to address the complexity and severity of the problems with which most DBT clients present, standard comprehensive DBT includes five components: (1) weekly individual therapy, (2) weekly skills training group, (3) phone coaching with the individual therapist, (4) team consultation for the therapist, and (5) ancillary treatments as needed (e.g., medication management). DBT is a team treatment, with the individual therapist, skills trainer, and other treatment team members working together and participating in regular consultation group meetings.

DBT utilizes a stage model of treatment; this chapter will focus on the Stage 1 interventions, as most of the treatment literature and research to date have been on this stage of DBT. The goal of Stage 1 is to move from a place of behavioral dyscontrol to behavioral control. The general idea is that DBT clients first need to develop the skills to manage painful emotions without resorting to intense suicidality, self-harm, or other highly destructive behaviors, and be able to engage effectively in treatment in a way that does not jeopardize the therapy relationship, before they move to work on Stage 2 topics, most typically trauma-related issues. DBT uses a hierarchy of treatment targets to organize individual therapy. This hierarchy is (1) life-threatening behavior (e.g., suicidal behavior, self-harm), (2) therapy-interfering behaviors (e.g., non-attendance, non-compliance, crossing therapist limits), (3) quality of life interfering behaviors (e.g., severe Axis I conditions, homelessness, severe work- or relationship-related behavioral deficits).

The primary intervention strategies in individual therapy are behavioral analysis and validation. Behavioral analysis (also referred to as "chain analysis") is used to identify the important contextual factors, skills deficits, and other behavioral "links" on the "chain" (series of events) to maladaptive behavior, as well as the consequences and other relevant features that contribute to the problem behavior. The therapist uses this information to inform interventions. For example, if the client engages in self-harm in the context of fear or anxiety, the therapist may use an exposure-based intervention to address the "dysfunctional link" of intense fear. If the client becomes highly suicidal in the context of dysfunctional thinking, the therapist may use cognitive interventions.

The other primary intervention strategy in DBT is validation. Validation involves communication to the client that his/her responses, emotions, thoughts, or behaviors make sense. The therapist communicates that the client's reactions or behaviors are normative, or normative given his/her history. The therapist takes the client's agenda seriously, and searches for the "kernel of truth" in the client's response. Validation is used to strengthen the therapeutic relationship; it also helps the client develop a clearer sense of normative responses, something many DBT clients lack due to their histories of invalidation. Validation counteracts the impact of the invalidating environment by communicating that the therapist understands, values, and respects the client (Linehan, 1997).

In DBT, skills are taught in a weekly skills training group (Linehan, 1993b). The skills are grouped into four modules: core mindfulness, interpersonal effectiveness, emotion regulation, and distress tolerance. The group is designed to teach the client skills information that the individual therapist will then draw on to help strengthen as more adaptive behaviors. Standard DBT also includes telephone coaching, in which the client calls the therapist for help in applying skills in difficult life situations, to increase generalization.

DBT has been shown to be effective in treating BPD and other multi-problem client populations. It has been evaluated in seven randomized controlled trials (RCTs) conducted across three independent research teams (Lynch, Trost, Salsman, & Linehan, 2007). In the first RCT of DBT, compared to treatment-as-usual, DBT resulted in less attrition, less parasuicidal behavior, and fewer days of hospitalization (Linehan, Armstrong, Suarez, Allmon, & Heard, 1991). Patients in this study treated with DBT reported less anger and demonstrated better social and overall adjustment (Linehan, Tutek, Heard, & Armstrong, 1994), and these gains were largely maintained at follow-up (Linehan, Heard, & Armstrong, 1993). DBT also has been shown to be effective in reducing symptoms from pre-treatment to post-treatment for clients completing a 3-month inpatient DBT program (Bohus et al., 2000). In another study, DBT reduced substance use and improved social and overall adjustment compared to treatment-as-usual in a population of drug-dependent women with BPD (Linehan et al., 1999). In a study of women veterans with BPD, those in DBT had significantly greater decreases in suicidal ideation, hopelessness, depression, and anger expression than those in treatment-as-usual (Koons et al., 2001).

To examine whether DBT's effectiveness was the result of clients receiving expert psychotherapy rather than specific DBT techniques, DBT with highly suicidal BPD clients was compared to a community treatment-by-experts condition. DBT was found to be superior, suggesting that the common factor of expert psychotherapy was not the critical factor in client outcome (Linehan et al., 2006). In addition to the empirical support for DBT being an efficacious treatment, it also has been shown to be effective in the community with women with BPD (Brassington & Krawitz, 2006), adolescents in a community residence (The Grove Street Adolescent Residence of the Bridge of Central Massachusetts, Inc, 2004), clients with BPD in a community-based outpatient program (The Mental Health Center of Greater Manchester NH, 1998), and clients with chronic self-injurious behavior in a community mental health setting (Comtois, Elwood, Holdcraft, Smith, & Simpson, 2007). In these studies, DBT was associated with reductions in number of days spent in the hospital and in number of instances of self-injury.

Overview of Functional Analytic Psychotherapy

Functional Analytic Psychotherapy (FAP; Kohlenberg & Tsai, 1991; Tsai et al., 2009) is a set of principles for conducting therapy based on a radical behavioral conceptualization of client problems and the therapeutic interaction. Following Skinner (1965) and Ferster (1972, 1979), FAP conceptualizes the psychotherapy interaction – the therapeutic "here-and-now" – as a context in which therapist and client influence each other according to the principles of operant and classical conditioning (i.e., as evoking, eliciting, and reinforcing stimuli).

The therapeutic interaction is an evocative interpersonal situation, and client behaviors in the here-and-now may be functionally related to the client's problems in everyday life. For example, an unassertive client who is deferential toward her boss (a behavior perhaps negatively reinforced by the boss ceasing to be critical) may become deferential with her therapist when the therapist offers a critical comment. Or, a client who is demanding of his wife in a way that damages his marriage (a behavior perhaps positively reinforced by his wife intermittently conceding to his demands) may be demanding of his therapist. Such behaviors are labeled, in FAP terminology, clinically relevant behaviors (CRBs). More specifically, CRB1s are behaviors that are representative of client problems, and CRB2s are improvements with respect to these problems. Accordingly, therapy aims to decrease the frequency of CRB1s and increase the frequency of CRB2s. In turn, changes in CRBs (e.g., increased strength of CRB2s) may generalize naturally to situations outside of therapy, although therapists and clients also may develop homework assignments to support generalization.

FAP therapists follow five deceptively simple rules related to CRBs. The first rule is to be aware of the occurrence of CRBs. This requires that therapists conduct an on-going functional assessment of client behaviors in the here-and-now. The second rule is that therapists evoke (i.e., provide discriminative stimuli for) CRBs. The natural processes of therapy, including the therapist's natural behavior as he or she conducts the therapy, often are sufficiently evocative. At times, however, a therapist may strategically evoke client CRBs. The third rule constitutes the heart of the theorized mechanism of change in FAP: the therapist responds contingently in order to naturally (rather than arbitrarily) reinforce and shape CRB2s and extinguish and/or punish CRB1s. Natural reinforcement is defined as reinforcement that resembles and functions similarly to reinforcement available in the client's everyday life, thus supporting generalization of behavior change. The fourth rule is that therapists must notice the impact of their response to CRBs, thus evaluating how effectively they are following Rule 3. Finally, the fifth rule is that therapists shape client's understanding of the functional relationships controlling their behavior. Readers familiar with applied behavior analysis or behavior therapy will recognize the above rules as an application of functional assessment and contingency management to the here-and-now therapy interaction.

It is clear from the above that FAP may be implemented only when relevant client problem behaviors (CRBs) actually occur in the therapeutic interaction. The technical aspects of FAP, developed considerably since publication of the original FAP book (Kohlenberg & Tsai, 1991), consist of a repertoire of instruments and techniques for assessing client interpersonal problems likely to be appropriate targets for FAP, evoking and shaping CRBs, and supporting generalization of improvements beyond the therapy relationship (see Tsai et al., 2009). However, the spirit of FAP lies in the creation of an evocative and naturally reinforcing therapeutic relationship.

Intersections of FAP and DBT

Jazz music is sometimes used as a metaphor for DBT as a treatment (Linehan, 2002; Swenson, 2006). The idea is that in jazz, one must learn all of the essential musical skills to a very high level, and then let go and improvise, responding to what arises in the moment with flexibility and creativity, while still adhering to basic principles. We would like to extend this metaphor to help elucidate the relationship between FAP and DBT. In a jazz ensemble, there are usually a number of different instruments, including a rhythm section. The rhythm section, the percussion and bass, is a constant presence in the music, the heartbeat of the ensemble. It is always present and holds the ensemble together; however, the rhythm section also at times solos, adding intensity and power to the music. We see FAP-supported interventions as the rhythm section of DBT. FAP encourages a constant presence of authentic relationship and mindful awareness of what is happening in the moment in the therapy interaction. FAP-supported interventions become a direct focus when the therapist brings attention to what is happening and uses that focus as a powerful opportunity for change. These are moments of intensity and movement.

DBT balances two general stances and styles. One is an acceptance-oriented stance characterized by warm engagement, attentiveness, attunement, validation, and genuineness. The other is a change-oriented stance involving pushing for behavior change, fully utilizing behavioral interventions, frankness about difficult topics, directness, and irreverence. We first explore in this section how FAP-supported interventions are relevant to the acceptance-oriented components of DBT, with particular focus on radical genuineness and reciprocal communication. We then focus on how FAP training might enhance the therapist's use of change-oriented interventions of targeting therapy-interfering behavior, observing limits and utilizing insight strategies.

Radical Genuineness

Therapists learning DBT and FAP who observe videotapes or roleplays of individual therapy sessions are often struck by the qualities of genuineness, honesty, and "realness" that the therapist brings to the interaction. They comment on the compassion, respectfulness, and directness of the therapist. In DBT, this orientation to the relationship is referred to as "radical genuineness." As the name implies, radical genuineness involves bringing one's true self into relationship with another person. Linehan (1993a) quotes Carl Rogers (Rogers & Truax, 1967) in her description of radical genuineness:

> He [sic] is without front or façade, openly being the feelings and attitudes which at the moment are flowing in him. It involves the element of self-awareness, meaning that the feelings the therapist is experiencing are available to him, available to his awareness, and also that he is able to live these feelings, to be them in the relationship, and able to communicate them if appropriate. It means that he comes into a direct personal encounter with his client, meeting him on a person-to-person basis. It means he is *being* himself, not denying himself. (p. 101)

In FAP, this theme is manifested in the principle that the therapist must behave naturally with respect to the client in order to evoke CRBs in the therapy relationship. CRBs are understood to occur more frequently in a genuine, real relationship; they are also more likely to be naturally reinforced in such a relationship, and ultimately to generalize beyond therapy. At a very basic level, FAP rules point the therapist consistently in the direction of authenticity: "... the client learns from being involved in a real relationship. A therapist who loves, struggles, and is fully involved with a client provides a therapeutic environment that evokes CRB1" (Kohlenberg & Tsai, 1991, p. 27).

Thus, in both DBT and FAP, the therapist is not only entering the therapy room with the knowledge and skills he/she has available, but also as a real person, willing to be affected by the client, experience and express his/her actual reactions to the client, and engage in a full way in the relationship. This "realness" communicates that the client is important enough for the therapist to be present with in an authentic way. We have experienced radical genuineness to be an extremely important aspect of DBT's therapeutic relationships, and being naturally reinforcing to be equally as important to FAP's. Of course there are times when a therapist's natural reactions may not be helpful to express, particularly in a raw form. Such candid expressions often can be extremely therapeutic, however, and we believe that for many clients, particularly DBT clients who may have had few chances for authentic relationships with a caring person, such a general stance is vital.

To be radically genuine (in DBT terms), or naturally reinforcing (in FAP terms), a therapist needs to develop a repertoire that includes expression of a broader range of reactions than may be typical in psychotherapy. Many approaches discourage the sharing of feelings such as a deep level of caring, annoyance/frustration, or vulnerability; however, we believe that something very crucial is lost when therapists cut off sharing these parts of themselves and their emotions and reactions. FAP therapists are encouraged to share these kinds of reactions to naturally punish CRB1s and evoke and reinforce CRB2s. DBT therapists, more specifically, are called on to share these kinds of reactions in the service of radical genuineness, to give the client feedback about how he/she is affecting the therapist (i.e., punishing CRB1s or reinforcing CRB2s), working on therapy-interfering behavior, and reinforcing target-relevant adaptive behavior (CRB2s). Our experience in practicing DBT and FAP-informed therapy has encouraged us to share a broader range of ourselves as therapists, in a way that has enhanced both our DBT and FAP work.

DBT encourages the therapist to express a balance of competence, knowledge, and strength, with open, matter-of-fact acknowledgment of relevant limits, limitations, and mistakes. The latter can be challenging. For example, many of us may find acknowledging therapeutic mistakes anxiety-provoking or irritating. We may have encountered rules or other experiences in the process of becoming therapists that suggest therapists should be consistently "right." DBT includes the assumption that in working with extremely difficult clients, mistakes are inevitable, and that direct acknowledgment of mistakes is often crucial. Linehan (1993a) notes that clients have commented that the most therapeutic thing they experienced in DBT was their therapist's willingness to acknowledge mistakes. A FAP perspective highlights that, to the extent that a therapist's acknowledging mistakes is reinforcing to the client, the acknowledgment should follow CRB2s. Such a CRB2 could be, for example, observing and/or bringing up a problem in the relationship or with the therapist's behavior. In this example, the therapist would be encouraged to reinforce the behavior in a natural way, by acknowledging the problem and apologizing. FAP helps us see the occasion of a therapeutic mistake as an opportunity to reinforce CRB2s, and to model and reinforce improved relationship-repair behavior (Kohlenberg & Tsai, 1991).

Our experience has been that a major impediment to radical genuineness is judgmental reactions by the therapist. When therapists are feeling judgmental of the client's behavior, they often fear hurting the client, and may withdraw, or respond in an artificial way. We believe that FAP augments and strengthens the non-judgmental stance toward client behavior that is a central part of DBT. FAP, also rooted in radical behavioral theory, helps us keep our focus on how client behaviors have been shaped by their learning histories and contexts. Consistently returning to that approach to understanding client behavior helps us "let go of judgment." It encourages empathic understanding and a sense of shared humanity – we are all shaped by our physiology and our experiences. This conceptualization makes it much easier to be radically genuine, firmly maintaining or returning to the stance that we are all products of our histories and shaped by our experiences.

We have found both FAP and DBT supervision and consultation extraordinarily helpful in expanding the capacity for radical genuineness/natural reinforcement. Our FAP and DBT supervisors, consultants, and colleagues have modeled radical genuineness in striking ways. They have reinforced our own self-generated behaviors and the emergence of our true selves in the process of supervision/consultation. FAP and DBT supervision/consultation have provided opportunities for exposure-based experiences that have helped us examine and work on our obstacles to radical genuineness.

Reciprocal Communication

DBT and FAP, at their best, both involve a kind of attentiveness and perceptive reading of the client's in-the-moment behavior that can be very powerful. In DBT, this kind of close observation is part of a "reciprocal communication style" which is "the usual mode in DBT" (Linehan, 1993a, p. 372). Linehan (1993a) uses the metaphor of "staying awake" during the session, and suggests that DBT therapists must be very careful observers of subtle client behaviors, including changes in facial expression and other non-verbal behaviors that may reflect changes in emotion.

Although this kind of attentiveness can sound straightforward or simple, it requires a strong commitment to being mindful of the client, relative freedom from preoccupation and strong emotion regulation skills. It also involves an ability to be aware of the client's behavior in the moment while working on other content material. This stance of alertness to what the client is doing or feeling in the current moment is similarly encouraged by FAP's Rule 1, to watch for CRBs, which are often subtle, non-verbal behaviors. Our experience has been that both DBT and FAP training help increase this kind of "awakeness" – FAP by providing Rule 1 as a central tenet, and DBT through its emphasis on the reciprocal communication style. Both models provide opportunities to practice and build our attentiveness to subtle, in-the-moment behavior.

Another aspect of reciprocal communication is the therapist expressing or sharing his/her reactions, thoughts, or experiences with the client; in other words, self-disclosure. Both FAP and DBT therapists talk about their reactions to their clients. This kind of self-disclosure is called "self-involving self-disclosure" in DBT. Self-involving self-disclosure involves noticing one's own reaction, noticing what the client's behavior was that triggered the reaction, sorting out whether describing and sharing that reaction would be helpful, and expressing the reaction in a way most likely to be therapeutic. Self-involving self-disclosure is encouraged in order to increase the sense of trust and equality in the relationship.

FAP emphasizes how therapist self-disclosures are often very reinforcing and thus may be used to shape CRB2s. Likewise, in DBT, self-involving self-disclosure is used to help give the client feedback about the impact of his/her behavior on the therapist, in the service of reinforcing target-relevant adaptive behavior, observing limits, or addressing therapy-interfering behavior. The therapist also will consider whether a target-relevant adaptive behavior (CRB2) has occurred where giving the feedback will be reinforcing. For example, a therapist might disclose "I'm so glad you have your diary card filled out completely. I'm appreciating the effort you put into that and it makes me feel motivated for our session" or "when you told me you were irritated about something I said, I felt great that you let me know, even though you were probably nervous about bringing it up." With these self-disclosures, as per FAP, essentially the therapist amplifies his/her private reaction to the client, making the reaction more salient and thus more likely to affect the client. Our experience has been that both FAP and DBT help therapists to be observant of and attentive to their own reactions to clients, and help them develop their repertoire of communicating reactions to clients.

Addressing CRB1s and Therapy-Interfering Behavior in DBT

DBT emphasizes "movement, speed and flow" in the therapy process (Linehan, 2002). Consistent with FAP, one aspect of this style is flexibly shifting focus from other therapy activities to CRB1s that arise during a session. In DBT, the decision to shift focus from other topics to the here-and-now when CRB1s occur is largely driven by the DBT target hierarchy. As described earlier, the top treatment target in DBT is any "life-threatening behavior." The therapist develops a conceptualization, based on multiple behavioral analyses of these behaviors, of what events and other behaviors seem to be most highly related to life-threatening behavior. When one of these "target-relevant" CRB1s, that is, CRB1 that is functionally related to life-threatening behavior, occurs during the session, DBT, like FAP, would recommend that the therapist seize the opportunity to work on the behavior in the moment as it is occurring. For example, if the client's self-harm behavior frequently occurs in the context of self-hatred, the occurrence of self-hatred in the session would likely become the focus. Thus FAP and DBT both direct the therapist to shift focus to CRB1s when they occur, with DBT providing additional direction regarding which CRB1s are highest priority, based on the target hierarchy.

Most clients entering DBT programs, having pervasive emotion regulation deficits and a variety of interpersonal difficulties, are likely to engage in behaviors (often CRB1s) that make benefiting from psychotherapy difficult. One of the hallmarks of DBT is a direct focus on these "therapy-interfering behaviors" as the second highest target in the hierarchy, following only life-threatening behaviors. For example, DBT clients may frequently miss or come late to sessions, experience intense emotions that lead to behavioral dysregulation in the session, come to sessions impaired by substances, lack skills to organize themselves to complete homework assignments, be compliant and unassertive with the therapist to a problematic extent, be overly critical or demanding with the therapist to a problematic extent, or a range of other difficulties. DBT recognizes the bind most DBT clients are in: they very much need help, but the problems that they are struggling with make it incredibly difficult for them to get that help. DBT attempts to respond to this dilemma by prioritizing assisting clients in developing behaviors that will do two very important things: preserve the therapy relationship and allow the client to get the most benefit from therapy. DBT therapists address therapy-interfering behaviors proactively and directly, from a non-judgmental, problem-solving stance.

Many times therapy-interfering behaviors are CRB1s, that is, they are behaviors that also occur outside of therapy and interfere in the client's daily life. In these situations, DBT strategies that target these behaviors are consistent with FAP strategies. FAP suggests the general principle that CRB1s should be ignored, blocked, or otherwise extinguished; these are interventions that a DBT therapist also would be likely to use. In addition, it is common for DBT clients to be relatively unaware of therapy-interfering behavior or its effect on others. It is also common that alternative, more adaptive behaviors are not in the client's repertoire; therefore, DBT therapists frequently intervene by describing the therapy-interfering behavior in a non-judgmental manner, doing a behavioral analysis on the behavior, assessing and intervening to increase the client's commitment to changing the behavior, and then teaching and reinforcing an alternative behavior, often a DBT skill. For example, a client who gets angry easily and yells at the therapist may be taught to use mindfulness skills to identify and describe his/her emotions and notice when anger is escalating, emotion regulation skills to reduce anger, and/or interpersonal effectiveness skills to address whatever problems are arising with the therapist.

In the service of insuring the preservation and health of the therapy relationship, DBT prioritizes those therapy-interfering behaviors that are most likely to have a strong, negative impact on the therapist. These are referred to as "limit relevant behaviors." DBT puts the onus on the therapist to know and observe his/her own limits, and to approach conversations about limits in a non-defensive, non-judgmental, and problem-solving manner. DBT encourages finding a balance between carefully monitoring and staying within one's limits, with extending limits temporarily as needed. DBT therapists are encouraged to be honest about their limits, and about when they are requesting a client change his/her behavior in the service of maintaining the strength of the therapy relationship and the therapist's motivation, rather than suggesting that the change is primarily for the client's direct benefit, if that is not the case. From a FAP perspective, the occasion of the therapist bringing up his/her own limits is a description of the conditions under which CRB1s will have a negative effect on the therapist. It is also an excellent opportunity to work on CRBs related to the client's reactions to the therapist's limits, the client's feelings about the therapist expressing those limits, and a whole range of reactions that might be evoked by that cue.

Some client behaviors may be difficult for the therapist and thus therapy interfering, but not have a negative impact on the client's life outside of therapy. From a DBT perspective, the therapist would still actively work to address this, most often by working with the client to change the behavior while in session. Thus, although the behavior may not be a CRB1, the DBT therapist would address the behavior in the service of preserving the quality of the relationship and the therapist's motivation. The therapist would acknowledge the rationale for the requested change being in the service of therapist's own limit or preference. For example, a therapist may feel frustrated by a client whose communication style involves giving lengthy, drawn-out, detailed responses to all questions. Although the client may not feel this communication style is problematic in his/her life, the therapist may still ask him/her to work on being briefer in session. It is also important to note that both FAP and DBT therapists examine strong reactions to client behavior and assess whether their own problematic repertoires may somehow be implicated. In the case of DBT, the therapist would likely discuss such an issue with the consultation team.

A common inclination DBT therapists have is to focus too exclusively on getting content work done (e.g., doing behavioral analyses or reviewing diary cards). In our experience, when therapists do notice problematic in-session behavior they are sometimes hesitant to address it, because doing so feels uncomfortable, they are avoiding a negative reaction from the client, or they do not know how to discuss it in a manner that feels likely to be therapeutic. We believe FAP training increases the likelihood that a DBT therapist will shift focus to address therapy-interfering behavior. FAP increases awareness of relevant in-session behavior, both CRB1s and CRB2s. FAP also provides rules for therapists that direct attention to in-session behavior and its meaning. FAP training helps support the prioritization of focusing on these behaviors, since this is one of the central tenets of FAP. FAP training helps the therapist develop his/her repertoire of responses to therapy-interfering behaviors.

Reinforcing Target-Relevant Adaptive Behavior

Reinforcing CRB2s is of primary importance in FAP-informed treatment. It is designated as "Rule 3: Reinforce CRB" (Kohlenberg & Tsai, 1991). DBT likewise places a high priority on being aware of and reinforcing adaptive behavior (Linehan, 1993a):

A central principle of DBT is that therapists should reinforce target-relevant adaptive behaviors when they occur. The therapist must at all times pay attention to 1) what the patient is doing; 2) whether the patient's behavior is targeted for increase, is targeted for decrease, or is irrelevant to current aims (i.e., whether the behavior is target-relevant); and 3) how he or she responds to the patient behaviors. In Kohlenberg and Tsai's (1991) terms, the therapist must observe clinically relevant behaviors and reinforce those behaviors that represent progress. (p. 301)

Noticing CRB2s particularly can be difficult in DBT for a number of reasons. It is common for the therapist to feel overwhelmed by the large number of problems and crises with which multi-diagnostic, complex clients present. Just keeping track of content issues can be taxing. Tracking both content and process can be exceptionally challenging with a client who is particularly emotionally reactive, sensitive to subtle stimuli, masking or partially masking reactions, or responding to complicated historical associations triggered by the current interaction. DBT clients often have difficulty observing and describing their own private behaviors, and thus the therapist being astute to the cues present, the client's learning history and the nature of the cues the therapist is presenting are all extremely important. Our experience is that DBT clients face many obstacles to trying out new behaviors; they may fear that if they try, they might fail and disappoint the therapist, or if they succeed, feel that they will be overwhelmed by the expectation of having to consistently engage in the new behavior in the future. Consequently, some CRB2s may be subtle, and, simultaneously, very important to reinforce.

FAP training helps therapists overlearn the skill of observing and noticing the on-going flow of behavior in the session. Monitoring whether the current behavior represents a CRB2 becomes more ingrained and consistent. DBT clients usually have many enormous obstacles to overcome to make change in their lives. In this context, noticing and reinforcing even subtle or small changes is crucial. The art of shaping is central to the work. For example, picture a client who experiences chronic shame, sits hunched over in her chair and makes very little eye contact. This shame-related way of being in the world interferes with developing relationships, an important goal for this client. In addition, many typical reinforcers, such as praise or direct acknowledgment, may be punishing to this client. At moments in session when this client's shame-related behavior decreases, it will be extremely important for the therapist to notice this and respond in a way that is naturally reinforcing for this particular client. The therapist must monitor and track this shame-related behavior and his/her own reactions to it, while simultaneously doing a behavioral analysis or discussing homework.

In order to notice and identify CRB2s, the therapist must have a clear idea of what a given client's CRB1s and CRB2s are. Identifying CRBs as part of one's case conceptualization will likely increase the salience of target-relevant adaptive behavior for the therapist. For example, imagine a client who is consistently extremely unassertive, and this unassertiveness is linked to other relevant targets. In a given session, the client starts pushing the therapist to deviate from the DBT target hierarchy and not do a behavioral analysis on self-harm. At one level this behavior is therapy interfering and a CRB1, in that the client is avoiding difficult therapy material and attempting to divert the therapist from the treatment protocol. At another level it may be a CRB2, in that the client is engaging in an assertive behavior that is new and target-relevant. The therapist who has identified CRB1s and CRB2s in the case conceptualization is likely to recognize that this behavior has elements of both therapy-interfering and target-relevant adaptive behavior. FAP, however, does not specify in detail what to do when both CRB1s and CRB2s occur, other than emphasizing the importance of reinforcing CRB2s. DBT adds specificity. The DBT therapist is encouraged to observe and describe both aspects of the behavior, and work to respond in a way that reinforces the adaptive elements of the behavior, while not reinforcing the therapy-interfering aspects. The dialectical philosophy informing DBT promotes "both–and" rather than "either–or" thinking, encouraging the therapist to observe situations where there is truth in apparent opposites, for example, when a behavior may have elements of being both therapy interfering (CRB1) and improvement (CRB2).

Regarding the nature of CRB2s, FAP does not specify any particular topography, while DBT has specific behaviors it encourages. DBT therapists integrate and coach DBT skills as CRB2s whenever possible. At moments when a CRB2 may be prompted, the DBT therapist will likely think through which DBT skill is most likely to be effective in the current situation, and which skills the client has already learned, in choosing an alternative, more adaptive behavior to encourage. For example, if a client walks into a session and immediately begins demanding that the therapist complete a needed form for him/her in an angry, off-putting manner, the therapist is likely to recommend and coach the client on the use of interpersonal effectiveness skills to make the request, with particular emphasis on the "GIVE" (gentle, interested, validate, easy manner) skills designed to help maintain a relationship effectively (Linehan, 1993b). DBT, then, provides a broad range of very helpful and specific CRB2s to promote as alternatives to CRB1s.

Our experience has been that FAP training helps therapists become more aware of the reinforcing or punishing effects of their own behavior, and better observers of the impact of their behavior (Rule 4). We believe that FAP can help increase therapists' sensitivity to subtle changes in behavior that mark the presence of CRB2s, and thus become more likely to reinforce those changes. This is particularly relevant for DBT clients who are often extremely sensitive to therapists' reactions. Without careful observation, the therapist may inadvertently punish or fail to reinforce a CRB2 if it goes unnoticed. FAP also provides ideas for reinforcers available to the therapist, and explicates the importance of amplification of therapist responses to make reinforcers more salient.

Insight Strategies

In both FAP and DBT, therapists observe and discuss functional relationships they observe in their clients' repertoires. Both approaches provide rules for when and how to express these observations. Rule 5 in FAP suggests that therapists make interpretations that describe variables that affect the client's behavior

(Kohlenberg & Tsai, 1991), which is very consistent with DBT's recommendation to "observe and describe patterns of stimuli and their associative relationships that elicit (classical conditioning model) or reinforce/punish (operant conditioning model) P's [patient's] behavior" (Linehan, 1993a, p. 267). Both approaches focus on in-session behavior in identifying what behaviors to make interpretations about. For example, Linehan (1993a) suggests that the most useful interpretations focus on client behaviors that occur within the therapy relationship.

FAP makes the same recommendation, but adds an emphasis on interpretations that relate in-session to out-of-session behavior (Kohlenberg & Tsai, 1991). For example, imagine a client who has experienced long-term invalidation from family members who have communicated pervasively that the client is worthless and undeserving. The client now becomes emotionally dysregulated when people express feelings of respect or appreciation for him/her; in particular, he/she becomes extremely sad. In describing this association, the therapist may observe "I notice that when I express respect for you or compliment you, you feel very sad." The therapist may do a behavioral analysis in which he/she assesses other feelings or thoughts that occur when he/she expresses respect or admiration. The therapist may also draw a link to the client's learning history and/or the occurrence of the response outside of therapy and the impact of that response on others.

The point of this intervention in both FAP and DBT is increasing clients' awareness of the variables influencing their behavior. Interpretations change the context of the behavior because following the interpretation the context now includes the description of the behavior and its controlling variables. Both approaches encourage therapists to formulate hypotheses about controlling variables, rather than making assumptions. FAP may put more emphasis on exploring the ways in which the behavior happening in the session is similar to behaviors that occur in the client's day-to-day life. The extent to which such exploration would occur in DBT would depend on the relationship between the in-session behavior and other treatment targets; for example, if the behavior also occurs in the context of higher treatment targets such as self-harm, this connection would be more likely to be a focus. If the behavior is therapy interfering but does not seem to be related to higher targets, the DBT therapist would be more likely to move into working on teaching and having the client practice an alternative behavior (CRB2), especially early on in treatment.

Inspiration and Motivation for the Therapist

DBT therapists regularly enter into relationships with clients who are in intense emotional pain, many of whom are suicidal, hopeless, and emotionally dysregulated. What keeps therapists feeling motivated to continue this difficult work? In other words, what are the reinforcers for DBT therapists? Working with clients who have problems with emotion dysregulation and behavioral dyscontrol, especially suicidality and self-harm, can be extremely stressful. Recognizing this, DBT takes a strong stance that therapists working with difficult clients need support, regular consultation, and a solid connection to a team who provides contingencies that support doing effective treatment.

Our experience has been that FAP training has helped promote our sense of motivation and excitement for doing DBT. We believe that learning and engaging with FAP can help support DBT therapists by bringing them more into contact with the reinforcing aspects of their work. There are at least three ways that FAP has provided us with inspiration and motivation in doing DBT. These are (1) becoming more knowledgeable of basic behavior principles in ways that we believe contribute to our effectiveness with our clients; (2) experiencing a sense of personal growth that also benefits us as therapists; and (3) promoting the development of deeper and more meaningful relationships, both with clients and with colleagues.

Learning FAP provides additional grounding in behavioral theory and greater depth and facility to many therapists' ability to apply behavioral concepts. There are a variety of ways to increase understanding of basic behavioral concepts; FAP provides one way that is particularly focused on the application of those concepts to psychotherapy. Our experience has been that knowing more about behavioral theory can help DBT therapists feel more confident with and hopefully more skillful in their use of behavioral interventions.

Both FAP and DBT training and practice provide opportunities for personal growth in the service of becoming more effective therapists. For many, such opportunities are very reinforcing. DBT primarily provides such opportunities in the context of the consultation team. Consultation team members discuss their reactions to clients and their own therapy-interfering behaviors. The team provides opportunities for the therapist to practice alternative behaviors and reinforces them. For many DBT therapists, the reinforcers the team provides are extremely important in keeping them motivated, particularly when clients are in extended periods of crisis. Our experience has been that involvement in FAP work also contributes reinforcement in the form of personal growth related to therapist effectiveness. FAP therapists actively explore their own histories and T1s (therapist in-session problems) and T2s (therapist in-session target behaviors) in order to understand what they are bringing to their therapy relationships. They explore their reactions to their clients in depth. FAP therapists typically complete activities that they suggest to clients.

FAP work can increase a therapist's comfort and skill with focusing on the here-and-now. Facility with such a focus is integral to the effectiveness of DBT consultation teams. Team members need to be able to notice when dialectical tensions are arising and observe and describe those. They must be able to recognize when they are feeling defensive or polarized, and be able to examine their responses. DBT consultation teams are described as "therapy for the therapist," in the sense that identifying and practicing new behaviors in the moment, with the team, are central. Our experience has been that FAP experience contributes to active engagement in here-and-now work in the team.

Both FAP and DBT support the development of rich and meaningful relationships with both clients and colleagues. The idea of having such relationships as part of our life's work is one of the things that drew many of us to be therapists. What FAP does well is deepen that aspect of therapy, and of consultation, for the therapist. FAP helps us notice and address our ways of avoiding that interfere with making direct contact with others. Through exposure, FAP helps reduce the anxiety and fear that can block us from being truly present to ourselves and others.

References

Bohus, M., Haaf, B., Stiglmayr, C., Pohl, U., Bohme, R., & Linehan, M. M. (2000). Evaluation of inpatient dialectical-behavioral therapy for borderline personality disorder: A prospective study. *Behaviour Research and Therapy, 38*, 875–887.

Brassington, J., & Krawitz, R. (2006). Australasian dialectical behaviour therapy pilot outcome study: Effectiveness, utility and feasibility. *Australas Psychiatry, 14*, 313–319.

Comtois, K. A., Elwood, L. M., Holdcraft, L. C., Smith, W. R., & Simpson, T. L. (2007). Effectiveness of dialectical behavioral therapy in a community mental health center. *Cognitive and Behavioral Practice, 14*, 406–414.

Dimeff, L. A., & Koerner, K. (2007). *Dialectical behavior therapy in clinical practice: Applications across disorders and settings*. New York: Guilford.

Frester, C. B. (1972). An experimental analysis of clinical phenomena. *The Pschological Record, 22*, 1–16.

Frester, C. B. (1979). A laboratory model of psychotherapy. In P. Sjoden (Ed.), *Trends in behavior therapy*. New York, NY: Academic Press.

Kohlenberg, R. J., & Tsai, M. (1991). *Functional analytic psychotherapy: Creating intense and curative therapeutic relationships*. New York: Plenum Press.

Koons, C. R., Robins, C. J., Tweed, J. L., Lynch, T. R., Gonzalez, A. M., Morse, J. Q., et al. (2001). Efficacy of dialectical behavior therapy in women veterans with borderline personality disorder. *Behavior Therapy, 32*, 371–390.

Linehan, M. M. (1993a). *Cognitive-behavioral treatment of borderline personality disorder*. New York: Guilford.

Linehan, M. M. (1993b). *Skills training manual for treating borderline personality disorder*. New York: Guilford.

Linehan, M. M. (1997). Validation & psychotherapy. In A. Bohart & L. Greenberg (Eds.), *Empathy reconsidered: New directions in psychotherapy*. Washington, DC: APA.

Linehan, M. M. (2002). *Dialectical behavior therapy intensive training course*. Slide presentation licensed to Behavioral Tech, LLC.

Linehan, M. M., Armstrong, H. E., Suarez, A., Allmon, D. J., & Heard, H. L. (1991). Cognitive-behavioral treatment for chronically suicidal borderline patients. *Archives of General Psychiatry, 48*, 1060–1064.

Linehan, M. M., Comtois, K. A., Murray, A. M., Brown, M. Z., Gallop, R. J., Heard, H. L., et al. (2006). Two-year randomized trial + follow-up of dialectical behavior therapy vs. therapy by experts for suicidal behaviors and borderline personality disorder. *Archives of General Psychiatry, 63*, 757–766.

Linehan, M. M., Heard, H. L., & Armstrong, H. E. (1993). Naturalistic follow-up of a behavioral treatment for chronically parasuicidal borderline patients. *Archives of General Psychiatry, 48*, 1060–1064.

Linehan, M. M., Schmidt, H., Dimeff, L. A., Craft, C. C., Kanter, J. W., & Comtois, K. A. (1999). Dialectical Behavior Therapy for patients with Borderline Personality Disorder and drug-dependence. *The American Journal on Addictions, 8*, 279–292.

Linehan, M. M., Tutek, D. A., Heard, H. L., & Armstrong, H. E. (1994). Interpersonal outcome of cognitive behavioral treatment for chronically suicidal borderline patients. *American Journal of Psychiatry, 151*, 1771–1776.

Lynch, T. R., Trost, W. T., Salsman, N., & Linehan, M. M. (2007). Dialectical Behavior Therapy for borderline personality disorder. *Annual Review of Clinical Psychology, 3*, 181–205.

Rogers, C. R., & Truax, C. B. (1967). The therapeutic conditions antecedent to change: A theoretical view. In C. R. Rogers (Ed.), *The therapeutic relationship and its impact.* Madison, WI: University of Wisconsin Press.

Skinner, B. F. (1965). *Science and human behavior.* New York, NY: Free Press.

Swenson, C. R. (2006). Foreward. In A. L. Miller, J. H. Rathus, & M. M. Linehan (Eds.), *Dialectical behavior therapy with suicidal adolescents.* New York: Guilford.

The Mental Health Center of Greater Manchester NH. (1998). Integrating dialectical behavior therapy into a community mental health program. *Psychiatric Services, 49,* 1338–1340.

The Grove Street Adolescent Residence of the Bridge of Central Massachusetts Inc. (2004). Using dialectical behavior therapy to help troubled adolescents return safely to their families and communities. *Psychiatric Services, 55,* 1168–1170.

Tsai, M., Kohlenberg, R. J., Kanter, J. W., Kohlenberg, B., Follette, W. C., & Callaghan, G. M. (2009). *A guide to functional analytic psychotherapy: Awareness, courage, love, and behaviorism.* New York: Springer.

Chapter 5
FAP and Behavioral Activation

Andrew M. Busch, Rachel C. Manos, Laura C. Rusch, William M. Bowe, and Jonathan W. Kanter

Depression is at the same time extremely common and extremely serious. In fact, depression is one of the most frequent presenting problems in outpatient psychotherapy, was listed as the single most burdensome disease in the world by the World Health Organization (Murray & Lopez, 1996), creates significant economic costs at the societal level, and results in major functional impairment and distress for depressed persons and those close to them. Suicide, of course, is the ultimate cost. How may FAP be used specifically with clients who present with depression? On the one hand, Tsai et al. (2008) present a working FAP model for the clinician to use with clients exhibiting diverse diagnoses, including depression, and it is our hope and belief that such a model will be useful. On the other hand, FAP is currently not empirically supported for depression, and several other treatments are.

One of these empirically supported treatments is Behavioral Activation (BA; Martell, Addis, & Jacobson, 2001). As described by Kanter, Manos, Busch, and Rusch (2008), FAP and BA share many important elements, including an underlying radical behavioral philosophy and a focus on reinforcement contingencies. The theory of depression espoused by BA describes depression as a function of losses of, reductions in, or chronically low levels of positive reinforcement; BA treatment strategies are designed to reconnect the client with stable sources of positive reinforcement in the outside world. Interestingly, while BA thus focuses on reinforcement in the outside world, it does not provide a corresponding set of reinforcement-based techniques for in-session work. FAP, in contrast, provides a model for use of reinforcement in session but, other than Rule 5 on generalization of gains made in therapy to the outside world, does not provide guidance or techniques for talking to depressed clients about outside problems.

Thus, integration of these two treatments may address limitations in each, capitalize on each treatment's strengths, produce a more complete behavioral model of depression with linked treatment strategies, and ultimately result in a more effective treatment than either approach alone. Kanter et al. (2008) critically reviewed BA

A.M. Busch (✉)
The Warren Alpert Medical School of Brown University and The Miriam Hospital, Centers for Behavioral and Preventive Medicine, Providence, RI, USA
e-mail: andrew_busch@brown.edu

J.W. Kanter et al. (eds.), *The Practice of Functional Analytic Psychotherapy*,
DOI 10.1007/978-1-4419-5830-3_5, © Springer Science+Business Media, LLC 2010

from a functional perspective, concluded that BA lacked a model for application of reinforcement in session, and suggested integration with FAP to address this limitation. This chapter focuses on the potential utility of integrating these two behavioral treatments from a more clinical perspective.

History of Behavioral Activation

BA grew out of early behavioral accounts of depression provided by Ferster (1973) and Lewinsohn (1974). Both argued that the symptoms of depression are naturally elicited by environments characterized by low rates of positive reinforcement. Specifically, depression results from losses of, reductions in, or chronically low levels of positive reinforcement. This position is supported by findings indicating that major negative life events (e.g., job loss) predict the onset, maintenance, and relapse of depressive episodes (Billings & Moos, 1984; Kessler, 1997; Mazure, 1998; Monroe & Depue, 1991; Paykel, 1982). In addition, persistent mild stress (e.g., work-related stress, negative interpersonal interactions), which can be conceptualized as consistently limiting positive reinforcement, also predicts depression (Mirowsky & Ross, 1989; Pearlin, 1989).

Early behavioral treatments for depression focused on pleasant event scheduling and skills training in an effort to increase client contact with consistent sources of positive reinforcement (Zeiss, Lewinsohn, & Muñoz, 1979). These early treatments showed great promise in treatment outcome trials. A recent meta-analysis of outcome trials that included a behavioral treatment using activity scheduling as the primary intervention concluded that these treatments produced large effect sizes and were comparable to Cognitive Therapy (CT) conditions (Cuijpers, van Straten, & Warmerdam, 2007). Interestingly, 14 of the 16 trials included by Cuijpers et al. were conducted prior to the mid-1980s, indicating that interest in and research on these behavioral treatments waned during the "cognitive revolution" for reasons unrelated to their effectiveness.

Interest in activation strategies was renewed following the landmark component analysis of CT conducted by Jacobson et al. (1996). In this study, 150 depressed outpatients were randomly assigned to one of three treatment conditions that varied the CT treatment techniques available to the therapist. In one condition, therapists were allowed to use the full CT package. In a second condition, therapists were restricted from cognitive restructuring techniques aimed at influencing core beliefs and schemas but were allowed to focus on automatic thoughts. In a final condition, therapists were not permitted to use restructuring techniques at all and only allowed to use the relatively few activation techniques included in the CT package. Findings indicated no significant differences in outcome among conditions at post-treatment or 2-year follow-up (Gortner, Gollan, Dobson, & Jacobson, 1998), suggesting that directly addressing cognitive variables may not be necessary for the effective treatment of depression and that activity scheduling alone may be sufficient. These results shocked the CBT treatment world; however, considering the findings of early BA studies reviewed by Cuijpers et al. (2007), they should not have been surprising.

Modern Behavioral Activation

Modern BA (Martell et al., 2001) stemmed from an attempt to develop a comprehensive behavioral treatment for depression following the promising results of Jacobson et al. (1996). While modern BA retained the core of earlier behavioral treatments (i.e., activity scheduling) it has become more contextual, idiographic, and incorporated a broader range of behavioral theory and research (Kanter, Callaghan, Landes, Busch, & Brown, 2004).

Most importantly, modern BA recognizes that too much avoidance of unpleasant feelings or events (excessive control by negative reinforcement) is as important to the maintenance of depression as a lack of approaching positive feelings and events (lack of control by positive reinforcement). Ferster's (1973) behavioral account of depression specifically suggested that a high frequency of escape and avoidance behaviors leads to inactivity and a narrow range of behavior which limits opportunities for positive reinforcement. In recognition of the idiographic nature of depression, these avoidant behaviors can take the form of well-recognized, passive depressed responses (e.g., staying in bed to avoid work stress) or behaviors that may be anti-depressant in many situations (e.g., going to the movies to avoid having a difficult but important discussion with one's spouse). The role of escape and avoidance responses in depression has been supported by numerous research findings (Ottenbreit & Dobson, 2004). Tendencies toward avoidant responding have been linked to future depression (Blalock & Joiner, 2000; Londahl, Tverskoy, & D'Zurilla, 2005), concurrent depression (Kuyken & Brewin, 1994), and maintenance of depression (Holahan & Moos, 1986).

Another addition of modern BA is its treatment of rumination. BA purports that rumination should be directly addressed in treatment and that it often functions as avoidance. Essentially, BA theory posits that engaging in rumination in reaction to stress or life problems, although not necessarily objectively pleasant, functions to avoid actively addressing the problem situation. Although those who ruminate frequently may feel rumination provides insight into their problems (Luybomirsky & Nolen-Hoeksema, 1993), the importance of rumination to the development and maintenance of depression is well established (Nolen-Hoeksema, Parker, & Larson, 1994).

BA's TRAP and TRAC Models

In BA, the *TRAP* (*T*rigger, *R*esponse, and *A*voidance *P*attern) model is used with clients to facilitate understanding of the reinforcing short-term effects and problematic long-term effects of avoidance. In this model, *T*riggers may consist of major negative life events (e.g., loss of a loved one, being fired) or an accumulation of smaller chronic negative life events or stressors (e.g., conflict with a boss, financial strain). In addition to specific negative life events, stimuli related to these negative life events may also function as triggers. For example, the death of a spouse (negative life event), as well as reminders of one's spouse (e.g., seeing a picture, mementos, having to tell others about the death) may function as triggers. According to the *TRAP* model, individuals respond to these triggers. These *R*esponses may include some of the symptoms of depression, such as negative affect, crying, fatigue, and anhedonia. When clients are experiencing these symptoms, it is key that the BA therapist express to the client that given the context (i.e., given the triggers), the individual *should* feel the way he or she is feeling. In BA, instead of focusing on the depressive response in session (including negative cognitions), the BA therapist focuses on the *A*voidance *P*attern that may ensue in response to these symptoms (e.g., staying at home, calling into work sick, staying in bed, socially withdrawing). BA therapists work with clients to replace this avoidant coping with *A*lternate *C*oping. Clients are taught that whereas avoidant coping leads to increased triggers, alternate coping interrupts the depressive cycle by activating behaviors that directly address the trigger (i.e., active problem solving). By directly addressing the trigger, the individual is more likely to come into contact with diverse and stable sources of positive reinforcement, which should maintain these behaviors after therapy.

For example, consider a client who was recently fired and is consequently experiencing financial stressors (*T*rigger) and sadness, crying, and loss of interest (*R*esponse). Consequently, this client has stayed in bed all day, not answered his phone, and not looked for employment opportunities (*A*voidance *P*attern). In this scenario a BA therapist would activate the client to get out of bed and begin a job search (*A*lternate *C*oping), which would directly address the trigger of losing his job and bring him in contact with sources of positive reinforcement. It is important to note that this type of activation would occur even when the client is still reporting depressive symptoms; the BA therapist challenges the client to activate despite the presence of depressive symptoms.

Outcome Support for BA

The efficacy of modern BA for moderate to severe adult depression was recently established in a large randomized controlled trial that compared BA, CT, Paroxetine (Paxil), and placebo (Dimidjian et al., 2006). While all three active treatments produced similar outcomes for moderate depression, BA demonstrated comparable effects to Paroxetine and larger effects than CT for severe depression (Coffman, Martell, Dimidjian, Gallop, & Hollon, 2007). As CT is the most well-established psychosocial treatment for depression and many consider SSRIs (Selective Serotonin Reuptake Inhibitors) the treatment of choice for severe depression, this trial was an important step in empirical legitimization of BA for depression.

A Note on BATD

A second version of BA was independently and concurrently developed by Lejeuz, Hopko, and Hopko (2002) and is referred to as Brief Behavioral Activation Treatment for Depression (BATD). This treatment is similar to Martell and colleagues' BA in many ways. Most importantly, it relies on increasing contact with positive reinforcement through activity scheduling. BATD also recognizes the importance of aversive control in depression. BATD, however, conceptualizes these behaviors by evaluating reinforcement for depressed versus non-depressed behaviors (Lejeuz, Hopko, LePage, Hopko, & McNeil, 2001). BATD has shown empirical promise including positive results from a randomized controlled trial for inpatient depression (Hopko, Lejeuz, LePage, Hopko, & McNeil, 2003). Although the discussion below is framed in terms of Martell et al.'s (2001) version of BA, integrating FAP with BATD would be theoretically beneficial for the same reasons. For a detailed review of the theory behind BA and BATD, as well as an attempt at an integrated approach to BA consistent with the current account, see Kanter, Busch, and Rusch (2009).

Rationale for Integration

As pointed out by Kanter et al. (2008), both BA and FAP are built upon the most basic premise of behavior analysis, reinforcement. Specifically, the frequency of a behavior can be increased when followed by certain environmental changes. When these changes are no longer contingent upon the target behavior or the behavior is punished, the behavior will decrease in frequency. The application of these principles in humans is well established (Catania, 1998). Further, both FAP and BA are rooted in a radical behavioral philosophy that looks to the context in which a behavior occurs and a person's history for causal explanations of human behavior. Both FAP and BA also rely on the therapist's understanding and ability to identify functional response classes. Specifically, BA requires that therapists recognize varied topographies in different contexts as functioning as "avoidance patterns" or "alternative coping behaviors" while FAP requires the differential identification of CRB1s (problems) and CRB2s (improvements) occurring in session and the recognition of functionally similar behaviors occurring in the client's relationships outside of session.

What FAP Adds to BA

As described in Kanter et al. (2008), BA does not capitalize on some fundamental principles of shaping behavior: immediacy and certainty. Behavior is shaped most effectively when consequences immediately follow the target behavior, but often reinforcement for non-depressed behaviors occurring in client environments is not immediate. For example, if a depressed client assertively calls a friend and leaves an invitation for a social outing on a voicemail (which could be an important anti-depressant behavior), he or she may not receive a call back for several days. Here the outcome may be reinforcing, but would be temporally removed from the target behavior and therefore would not be as effective as a reinforcer.

A related issue involves the lack of control the therapist has over consequences or the certainty of the outcomes related to assignments to engage in activation outside of session. In the example mentioned above, the client may engage in a non-depressed behavior by making the call, but this behavior may be punished because the friend is busy and does not have time to respond. The certainty of consequences is especially important when the goals of therapy are to develop new anti-depressant behaviors "from the ground up." With these clients, therapist control over the immediate social consequences following a client's behavior allows for the reinforcement of successive approximations that may be punished in real world social contexts.

For example, imagine a client who engages in almost no emotional disclosure, which has caused strain with his wife and children. For this client, any attempt to disclose emotions to others could be considered a successive approximation to more effective behavior. This client may say something like, "I really *hate* talking about my feelings because it makes me feel so weak" during a therapy session. Here, the therapist is in a position to reinforce this behavior in the service of helping the client refine it over time. These same words spoken to the client's wife, however, may not be as well received (i.e., she inadvertently may punish a weak instance of the behavior she desires more of). Thus, FAP allows for the recognition of small improvements in behaviors that may not be recognized as progress outside of therapy and provides a system for reinforcing those improvements. By continuing to do this in a graded fashion, the therapist can shape the client's behavior until it reaches the level of sophistication that can be reinforced outside of session.

A final element that FAP adds to BA is an explicit focus on developing and maintaining genuine, intimate interpersonal relationships. Research has found that difficulties with intimacy are associated with depression (Hammen & Brennan, 2002; Zlotnick, Kohn, Keitner, & Della Grotta, 2000). These difficulties can be conceptualized as leading to decreased positive reinforcement due to either a lack of intimate relationships or unsatisfying relationships. Furthermore, avoidance of conflict in intimate relationships can result in decreased positive reinforcement, decreased relationship growth, and increased interpersonal problems. Thus, as FAP techniques explicitly target these issues through the client–therapist relationship, they have the potential to enhance BA's effectiveness in changing interpersonal behavior.

BA Targets and the Five Rules of FAP

As the five rules of FAP are reviewed in Chapter 1 of this volume, they are described below only in relation to the process and targets of BA.

Rule 1: Watch for Clinically Relevant Behaviors (CRBs)

The first rule of FAP instructs therapists to merely observe their client's CRBs during session. CRBs can take the form of in-session behavior that is functionally similar to BA's outside of treatment targets or relate to other specific client goals for change. Observation of CRBs requires the therapist to mindfully engage in the present moment with the client and remain vigilant of in vivo change opportunities. As CRBs (and the targets of BA) are defined by each individual client's case conceptualization, neither a list of behavioral topographies or even functional classes that should be addressed with clients can be generated. Below is a list of examples of BA targets that could become relevant CRBs.

Avoidance patterns. As described in the *TRAP* model above, BA views avoidance as effective in reducing negative affective responses in the short term, but not leading to a reduction in stressful life problems, thus limiting access to positive reinforcement in the long term. BA assignments using the *TRAP* model explicitly instruct clients to engage in approach behavior (i.e., *A*lternative *C*oping in the *TRAC* acronym) in contexts where they previously engaged in avoidance. As many aspects of therapy elicit powerful emotions (i.e., *R*esponses), the stage is set for opportunities to shape approach behaviors in session.

The most easily conceptualized avoidance CRB involves the client avoiding the therapeutic interaction by skipping or arriving late for sessions. Showing up for session on time can be naturally reinforced by the therapist in session and used as a model for other approach behaviors. In addition, clients may avoid discussing difficult topics. This avoidance may consist of restricting discussion to superficial topics, making sarcastic remarks when difficult topics arise, or explicitly stating that the topic is not of concern or importance. For example, consider a client who has difficulty giving negative feedback to her husband. Suppose she is prompted in session to give the therapist negative feedback (e.g., "Can you tell me something that you would like to see change about our interactions or coming to therapy in general?"). The client may respond, "I don't really know, everything has been fine." Depending on the case conceptualization and the history between the client and therapist, this response could be conceptualized as avoidance of giving negative feedback, thus constituting a CRB1. Compassionate query into her response may prompt a CRB2, which in this case may be the client giving negative feedback to the therapist.

Rumination. Although rumination typically is seen as an internal behavior, some forms of client talk during sessions may have similar functions as rumination. For example, it is not uncommon for depressed clients to spend considerable time in session on monologues about their misery and hopelessness. Although this is public talk, the function may be quite similar to private rumination. Ultimately, this expression of misery and hopelessness may function as avoidance of negative emotions associated with more active problem-solving attempts. Thus, an individual may consider rumination useful because of its superficial similarity to active problem solving; however, unlike problem solving, rumination does not elicit the same negative emotions as active problem solving. Thus rumination in session may be identified as a CRB1 and directly targeted. This can be done by compassionately bringing to the client's attention how the ruminative behavior negatively impacts the therapeutic relationship because it is an ineffective use of therapeutic time in that it precludes attempts at active problem solving.

Passivity. Avoidance patterns also often involve passivity or passive coping. BA directly targets passivity by identifying avoidance patterns and working collaboratively with the client to identify alternating coping strategies for daily life problems. Essential to FAP is the idea that passivity that occurs outside of session will almost inevitably translate into passivity that occurs in session with the therapist. For example, a client may agree with the therapist's proposed therapy goals and rely on the therapist to dictate the sessions and course of treatment. If passivity is not recognized as a CRB1, the client's lack of active responding may either (a) extinguish the therapist's active behavior, resulting in a progressively more passive therapist, or (b) prompt the therapist to become more active and take sole responsibility for the therapy. Both therapist responses (passivity or increased activity on part of the therapist) are problematic and may result if passivity is not identified and targeted as a CRB1.

Assertiveness. In addition to avoidance patterns, rumination, and passive coping, depressed clients often have difficulty engaging in assertive behaviors that are typically necessary for successful, active problem-solving and goal-directed action. If assertiveness is conceptualized as a CRB2 for a particular client, then any appropriate request to the therapist may be a CRB2, and avoidance of such a request may be a CRB1. A client request may be quite simple, and without a FAP conceptualization, may be overlooked as a CRB2. For example, a CRB2 could be as basic as a client asking a therapist to close the window blinds because the sun is in the client's eyes.

It is possible for a client to be assertive and ask for something that appears counter-therapeutic. For example, a client may call to reschedule a session because of another commitment. This behavior could constitute a CRB1 (avoidance of the therapist), a CRB2 (assertively expressing needs), both, or neither. As another example, in BA it is recommended that prior to each session the client complete the Beck Depression Inventory (Beck, Ward, Mock, & Erbaugh, 1961) or another depression symptom measure. Consider a client who asks, "I really hate filling out that measure – would it be okay if I did not complete it?" A typical BA therapist might discuss with the client the importance of completing the measure and how data are necessary to track progress when conducting an empirically supported intervention. A FAP therapist, however, would react differently in this situation by considering whether the client's request was a CRB1 (avoidance), a CRB2 (assertiveness), both, or neither.

Rule 2: Evoke CRBs

Evoking CRBs often happens naturally, since the therapy process, setting, and relationship tend to be highly evocative in their own rights. In addition to noticing when

CRBs occur naturally, when integrating FAP and BA techniques therapists also strategically evoke CRBs. Evocation of CRBs often takes courage on the part of both therapist and client. Depending on the case conceptualization, evoking CRBs may call for the therapist to go out of his or her comfort zone and engage in evocative behaviors such as personal self-disclosure. Furthermore, it takes courage for the client to be at the receiving end of Rule 2. The emotional challenge of continuing in therapy knowing that sessions will be real and evocative interactions should not be underestimated.

In-session prompts to engage in CRBs may be seen as in-session parallels to the activation homework assignments given to clients in standard BA. As mentioned above, the advantage of having access to these behaviors in session is that the therapist can control the consequences that follow relevant behavior and shape approximations to the goal behavior (e.g., a weak but still improved attempt by the client to change meeting times) that might not be reinforced or may even be punished outside of session. If the therapist can evoke the relevant behaviors in session, it would provide a practice ground for corresponding behavioral homework assignments.

As an example, one common CRB1 that is particularly relevant to the integration of BA and FAP for the treatment of depression is in-session passivity. Therapists should pay close attention to the division of the therapeutic workload between the therapist and client. For instance, is the therapist doing most of the work (e.g., trying to convince the client to be more active, taking responsibility for almost all of the in-session activities)? Therapists not attuned to the function of the client's behavior may at best miss opportunities to shape more effective behavior and at worst unknowingly reinforce problematic behavior by relieving the client of session responsibility. If the therapist notices himself or herself taking on the vast majority of in-session responsibility with a client who is also problematically passive in social relationships, the therapist might say something like, "I notice that I have been very active during this session, while you have had little to say. This sounds a lot like how you describe interactions with your spouse. I was wondering what we could do here to break the pattern between us and have you become more active in session." This type of response hopefully will function to evoke improved behavior (i.e., increased active engagement in session) that then can be reinforced (see Rule 3 below). Clients may experience this kind of evocative talk from therapists as aversive, so it is important to evoke sensitively. In this example the therapist could do so by saying something like "I know this is tough for you, but this is a safe place for you to try new behaviors."

Rule 3: Reinforce CRBs Naturally

As described above, one of the most important benefits of adding in vivo work to standard BA is that the therapist can control the provision of reinforcement for activation relevant behaviors that occur in session. By taking advantage of the therapy room as a setting where the therapist has increased control over the consequences of a client's behavior, the therapist should be able to build a repertoire that will produce more reinforcing outcomes to out-of-session activation assignments (see Rule 5). There are three relevant issues related to Rule 3 to consider when adding FAP techniques to BA: the therapist's threshold for what behaviors constitute CRBs, schedules upon which the therapist responds to CRBs, and the arbitrariness of therapist responses.

Given that clients begin therapy with problematic in-session behavior and after treatment should be engaging in more effective in-session behavior suggests that the threshold for therapist responding should shift during treatment. This means that at first even very unskillful attempts at the target behavior should be reinforced by the therapist. Over time, the therapist adjusts the threshold for a behavior to be reinforced (much like the graded homework assignments that are central to BA) until the client is reinforced only for very skillful demonstrations of the target behavior. This pattern should mirror the therapist's expectations and homework assignments regarding out-of-session behavior. It is also easier to shape a new behavior when reinforcement is applied initially after every target response (i.e., a continuous ratio schedule). To facilitate generalization, however, the reinforcement schedule eventually should be adjusted to a point where it approximates what may actually take place outside of the therapy environment. This means that near the end of treatment the therapist should slowly reduce the rate at which he or she responds to CRB2s.

A final related issue is the therapist's sensitivity to natural versus arbitrary reinforcement (Ferster, 1967; Kohlenberg & Tsai, 1991). This may entail a therapist behaving quite differently than the usual therapist in some situations. For instance, in daily life, assertiveness is naturally reinforced by compliance with the assertive request. Therefore, an assertive CRB2 is naturally reinforced by the therapist granting the client's request whenever possible. This may involve changing homework assignments, changing appointment times, or having a longer session. This type of natural reinforcement contrasts with more arbitrary responses, such as "Great job being assertive!" that may not involve compliance with the request. In order to respond in a naturally reinforcing manner, it is often useful for therapists to amplify their private reactions, which may include demonstrating caring, telling the client how the therapist is feeling in the moment toward him or her, and nonverbal displays of interpersonal connection. This natural reinforcement of CRB2s often requires that therapists are therapeutically loving, in that they are willing to take such risks (e.g., demonstrating caring, expressing feelings of closeness and connection) in the service of their clients.

Responding to ambiguous CRBs. In some instances, responding to assertiveness CRB2s may be complicated. Consider the case of an assertive request not to be assigned any homework. Although this may be a CRB2 in terms of assertiveness, it is also potentially a CRB1 in terms of avoidance of difficult activation assignments. Usually, reinforcing a CRB2 is given priority over responding to a CRB1, but the therapist should be careful to discriminate between the behaviors as much as possible. In this example, the therapist may explore what the client dislikes about the homework and work to make it more agreeable without avoiding it completely.

In addition to responding to CRB2s, Rule 3 addresses responding to in-session avoidance behaviors and other instances of CRB1s. Although not always the case, in general the therapist should block avoidance when it occurs and prompt CRB2s. Special care should be taken when blocking avoidance, since this is often experienced as punishing. Thus, responding to CRB1s also requires therapeutic love in that therapists are sensitive to their clients' needs and are able to gently block behaviors and prompt new ones without damaging the therapeutic alliance. For example, the therapist could say, "It seems like you're trying to avoid discussing this topic. I know it's hard, but could you try to do something more active right now?"

Rule 4: Observe the Potentially Reinforcing Effects of Therapist Behavior in Relation to Client CRBs

Rule 4 suggests that therapists observe their effect on clients. One can only say that an in-session target behavior has been reinforced if the client demonstrates the target behavior with increased frequency, intensity, or both. Thus, it is important to observe the effect of contingent responding on the client over time. However, often it is also helpful to seek immediate feedback from clients regarding their reactions to the therapist's attempt at shaping. For example, after attempting to reinforce a generally passive client's in-session assertion of needs, the therapist might ask the client, "What was it like for you to get what you wanted and to hear my reaction after expressing your needs?" Seeking this type of in vivo client feedback is significantly different from the BA (and general CBT) practice of seeking general feedback at the end of each session.

Rule 5: Provide Functional Analytically Informed Interpretations and Implement Generalization Strategies

Rule 5 in FAP consists of the therapist giving functional descriptions of the client's behavior in order to facilitate generalization of in-session client gains to daily life. Commonly this is done by the therapist explicitly drawing attention to parallels between the therapeutic relationship and the client's outside of therapy relationships. For example, consider a depressed client who has difficulty asserting his needs. Suppose this client is able to assert himself with the therapist and this translates into a richer therapeutic relationship. The therapist can then draw a parallel between this and the client's difficulty asserting himself with a loved one with whom he has a strained relationship. The therapist can highlight that being assertive with the therapist enhanced their relationship and parallel this with the need for the client to be assertive with the loved one. Specifically, the therapist can use the BA activity chart to aid in generalization by scheduling a homework assignment of being assertive with the loved one. When integrating FAP and BA, the scheduling of activation assignments should flow directly from collaboratively determined functional similarities between in-session and out-of-session contexts.

Treatment Recommendations

As BA is an empirically supported treatment for depression, we recommend that behaviorally minded clinicians begin treatment of depressed clients with BA techniques. As described above, however, FAP techniques may take advantage of fundamental behavioral findings in ways that would improve BA. Thus, we suggest that therapists wishing to integrate these two treatments provide a rationale and obtain informed consent for FAP techniques early in treatment, but begin with a focus on out-of-session activation. The therapist who remains vigilant to CRBs is then free to incorporate FAP as BA targets show up in session, the client engages in therapy-interfering behavior, or activation assignments fail due to interpersonal problems that appear amenable to FAP.

Although speculative, the addition of FAP techniques to the practice of BA theoretically should be particularly helpful for populations with problematic interpersonal relations. This may include subpopulations of depressed clients with co-morbid personality disorders or relationship discord. Regarding the treatment of personality disorders, the American Psychological Association Task Force recently released guidelines that call specifically for treatments that include the therapeutic relationship as a mechanism of behavior change (Critchfield & Benjamin, 2006), which supports our contention that FAP would be an important addition to BA in this situation.

A Case Example

To highlight the usefulness of integrating FAP and BA techniques, this chapter concludes with a case description in which BA was augmented with FAP techniques to address a client's non-passive avoidance repertoires (that still prevented him from contacting important sources of positive reinforcement) and interpersonal repertoires that were amenable to in-session shaping.

John, a 31-year-old single Caucasian male, diagnosed with Major Depressive Disorder and Narcissistic Personality Disorder, was treated using an integration of FAP and BA for 15 sessions. John complained of hypersomnia, weight loss, reduced ability to concentrate, and anhedonia. He reported an inability to connect intimately with others, a history of shallow interpersonal relationships and romantic infidelity. John was raised in an upper middle class family and had high-paying jobs in the past, but at the time of treatment was making little money, returning to school, and experiencing legal problems. He reported having many acquaintances – specifically he had a large network of friends for playing sports and socializing – but few close friends for support. When John did identify that he needed support, he often asked for it in an unclear manner and reported that these attempts to elicit support made him feel weak and incapable. He reported dating much younger women because they tended to be more casual and willing to be non-monogamous.

Initial sessions were spent clarifying John's goals for treatment, assessing BA and FAP target behaviors, providing a rationale, and obtaining informed consent for the treatment. Two major interpersonal problems were identified: (1) excessive, interpersonally aversive behaviors aimed at impressing others, which the therapist and John collaboratively labeled as "impressing statements and behaviors," and (2) an inability to identify and express needs clearly. Corresponding goals for treatment were (1) decreasing impression management in social situations and (2) increasing asking others for assistance and emotional support when needed.

In terms of BA's *TRAP* model, both of these broad classes of behavior were functionally seen by John and his therapist as attempts to avoid feeling anxious or vulnerable in situations that elicited social discomfort or feelings of inadequacy. Thus, both behaviors were well-suited targets for BA interventions as they successfully avoided aversive private events in the short term but prevented John from having meaningful interpersonal relationships in the long term. This lack of meaningful relationships was conceptualized as an important variable maintaining his depression.

Regarding impressing statements, the *T*rigger could have been any social situation, the *R*esponse was social discomfort, feelings of vulnerability or anxiety, and the *A*voidance *P*attern was making impressive statements. These statements functioned to maintain a strong social image that effectively, temporarily avoided discomfort but also prevented John from developing close and genuine interpersonal relationships. John reported that impressing was often a problem when he tried to "one-up" people in social situations or when he was so concerned with networking or what people could do for him that he did not feel connected to them. Another area where impression management was a problem in John's everyday life involved completion of schoolwork, where he was unable to turn in work that he did not feel "reflected his potential." This became a significant problem as John missed deadlines while trying to produce near perfect work.

Likewise, *T*riggers for problems with need assertion were situations in which John needed some kind of help, his emotional *R*esponse included feeling incapable, vulnerable, or inadequate, and his *A*voidance Pattern involved not asking for help (and experiencing negative consequences) or asking for help in very subtle ways that had a low probability of evoking assistance. Examples of *TRAP*s regarding need assertion included being unable to ask for money that was owed to him (because it would look like he needed it) and denying academic difficulties (e.g., how far behind he was on assignments) to an academic counselor in order to preserve his image.

Although BA alone may appear to be a sufficient treatment given that the specific *TRAP*s were identified, there were several reasons why the addition of FAP appeared necessary for this case. First, John had a hard time identifying when he was engaging in impressing behaviors or opportunities to assert his needs. Thus, it would have been ineffective to assign him homework to change his responses before he was aware of specific instances of his own problem behavior. Second, John's impressing behavior was highly aversive and his first attempts at need assertion were not of high enough quality that they would be reinforced at an adequate rate in the outside world. Thus, an in-session focus was needed to shape John's behavior through reinforcement of successive approximations. John's lack of awareness and behavioral repertoire deficits highlight the potential limitations of implementing BA alone and indicate the benefits of incorporating FAP with clients who have certain interpersonal problems.

Early in treatment the therapist noticed aversive impressing behaviors occurring in session as CRB1s. For example, John came to session over-dressed (he also pointed out to the therapist that he was wearing a $200 shirt), described his active sexual and dating life in detail, and often referred to wealthy or important friends or family. More broadly, John often sounded scripted and engaged in storytelling in such a way that the therapist felt like John was trying to sell him something. Finally, John's need to impress teachers with school assignments generalized to therapy in that his written therapy homework assignments were either completed in considerable detail and full of misplaced psychological jargon (John admitted to efforts to make them sound clinical) or not completed at all. A lack of need assertion also occurred in session in more subtle ways including denying difficulty and emotion, and avoiding talk about problematic situations where he needed assistance from the therapist in favor of more abstract discussions.

Impressing statements occurred readily without explicit attempts by the therapist to evoke them (Rule 2) and the therapist contingently responded (Rule 3) by sharing his personal reactions to John's in-session behavior including sensitively telling him that he sounded scripted, like a salesman, over-controlled, or that it made it hard for them to get work done in therapy. In addition, with each contingent response to a CRB1 the therapist attempted to prompt a more effective behavior. For example, the therapist once responded, "Is that a salesman answer? Could you try responding in a different way?" Regarding therapy homework, John was asked to finish assignments in a complete and practical manner but resist making them perfect (i.e., typing his responses, writing full paragraphs, and using psychological jargon).

Over time, John's in-session behavior improved and he began to engage in less impression management. For example, John eventually was able to let the therapist know when he was confused (as opposed to pretending he understood the therapist), came to sessions in regular clothing (John described his new outfits as "less studied" than those earlier in treatment), turned in homework that was complete but not perfect, engaged in less impressive story telling, and generally sounded less deliberate and scripted. Consistent with both FAP and BA, these improvements led to homework assignments to engage in functionally similar out-of-session *Alternative Coping* (Rule 5). For example, John was asked to specifically refrain from making impressive statements in high-risk situations (e.g., meeting new people at a party), go to social events dressed in ways that made him slightly uncomfortable (i.e., underdressed), and to turn in homework assignments to teachers that he did not feel were perfect.

In-session problems with need assertion were less apparent and more often were evoked directly by the therapist. This required that the therapist wait until he understood John well enough to discriminate interactions where he was having difficulty, but was failing to bring up the topic or ask for assistance directly. These attempts to evoke CRB often took the form of questions like, "What can I do to be most helpful to you right now?" or "What do you need from me at this moment?" These evocative questions often initially resulted in John denying difficulty or attempting to change the topic. The therapist responded by blocking his avoidance and prompting an alternative response. For example, when John had experienced a very painful interaction with an ex-partner between sessions, he joked about the interaction in session and described it as "amusing" and "curious" but was noticeably shaken. The therapist contingently responded by pointing out the incongruence between previous descriptions of the importance of this relationship, his in-session affect, and his verbal presentation, then prompted the client to express his needs and difficulties in the moment.

During treatment John began to admit difficulties and express his needs to the therapist. It is important to note that seeking therapy and continuing to come were functionally CRB2s for John as it implied needing help. This was discussed and explicitly reinforced throughout treatment. These improvements led to homework assignments to engage in out-of-session *Alternative Coping* (Rule 5), ranging from asserting very simple requests early in treatment, like needing help moving, to more emotional requests later in treatment (e.g., asking a friend to spend some time talking about a painful issue). BA's weekly activity chart was used to facilitate this graded improvement.

Symptoms of depression essentially were resolved by the 12th week of treatment and remained low until termination. Additional sessions were spent (1) solidifying gains made in impressing behaviors and need assertion and (2) discussing additional steps John could take toward closer interpersonal relations, including increased emotional expression and reduced reliance on rigid social rules. In addition, John reported engaging in several out-of-session behaviors demonstrating improvement, including making requests to friends that made him feel embarrassed about his current financial standing (e.g., asked friends for second hand furniture and for opportunities to do odd jobs for extra money), being more forthcoming with peers regarding his financial and social position, and asking peers for emotional support. John also reported being more mindful of engaging in overly impressive behavior and that it now made him feel "showy." In addition, he reported noticing how well his new behaviors were working at getting his needs met and feeling closer to people, suggesting that these behaviors eventually shifted from instructional to contextual control.

Conclusion

In summary, both BA and FAP are behavioral treatments that focus on reinforcement as the key mechanism of change. In BA, the goal is to activate new client behaviors in the natural environment to contact stable sources of positive reinforcement. In FAP, the goal is to naturally and differentially reinforce in-session behavior that is functionally similar to out-of-session targets. BA relies on instructing and encouraging clients to seek out additional reinforcement in their environment. While BA has been shown to be effective as a stand-alone treatment, both basic and applied behavior analytic research indicate that a more efficient method of changing behavior would involve the immediacy and control that FAP techniques provide. Future research is needed to substantiate this claim and the applicability of this integrated treatment to relevant problems, including depressed clients with Axis II disorders and depressed clients with marital discord.

References

Beck, A. T., Ward, C. H., Mock, J., & Erbaugh, J. (1961). An inventory for measuring depression. *Archives of General Psychiatry, 4*, 561–571.

Billings, A., & Moos, R. (1984). Treatment experiences of adults with unipolar depression: The influence of patient and life context factors. *Journal of Consulting and Clinical Psychology, 52*, 119–131.

Blalock, J., & Joiner, T. (2000). Interaction of cognitive avoidance coping and stress in predicting depression/anxiety. *Cognitive Therapy and Research, 24*, 47–65.

Catania, A. (1998). *The taxonomy of verbal behavior*. New York: Plenum Press.

Coffman, S., Martell, C. R., Dimidjian, S., Gallop, R., & Hollon, S. D. (2007). Extreme nonresponse in cognitive therapy: Can behavioral activation succeed where cognitive therapy fails?. *Journal of Consulting and Clinical Psychology, 75*, 531–541.

Critchfield, K. L., & Benjamin, L. S. (2006). Principles for psychosocial treatment of personality disorder: Summary of the APA Division 12 Task Force/NASPR review. *Journal of Clinical Psychology, 62*, 661–674.

Cuijpers, P., van Straten, A., & Warmerdam, L. (2007). Behavioral activation treatments of depression: A meta-analysis. *Clinical Psychology Review, 27*, 318–326.

Dimidjian, S., Hollon, S. D., Dobson, K. S., Schmaling, K. B., Kohlenberg, R. J., Addis, M. E., et al. (2006). Randomized trial of behavioral activation, cognitive therapy, and antidepressant medication in the acute treatment of adults with major depression. *Journal of Consulting and Clinical Psychology, 74*, 658–670.

Ferster, C. B. (1967). Arbitrary and natural reinforcement. *The Psychological Record, 17*, 341–347.

Ferster, C. B. (1973). A functional analysis of depression. *American Psychologist, 28*, 857–870.

Gortner, E., Gollan, J. K., Dobson, K. S., & Jacobson, N. S. (1998). Cognitive-behavioral treatment for depression: Relapse prevention. *Journal of Consulting and Clinical Psychology, 66*, 377–384.

Hammen, C., & Brennan, P. A. (2002). Interpersonal dysfunction in depressed women: Impairments independent of depressive symptoms. *Journal of Affective Disorders, 72*, 145–156.

Holahan, C. J., & Moos, R. H. (1986). Personality, coping, and family resources in stress resistance: A longitudinal analysis. *Journal of Personality and Social Psychology, 51*, 389–395.

Hopko, D. R., Lejuez, C. W., LePage, J. P., Hopko, S. D., & McNeil, D. W. (2003). A brief behavioral activation treatment for depression. *Behavior Modification, 27*, 458–469.

Jacobson, N. S., Dobson, K. S., Truax, P. A., Addis, M. E., Koerner, K., Gollan, J. K., et al. (1996). A component analysis of cognitive behavioral treatment for depression. *Journal of Consulting and Clinical Psychology, 64*, 295–304.

Kanter, J. W., Busch, A. M., & Rusch, L. C. (2009). *Behavioral activation: Distinctive features*. London: Routledge Press.

Kanter, J. W., Callaghan, G. M., Landes, S. J., Busch, A. M., & Brown, K. R. (2004). Behavior analytic conceptualization and treatment of depression: Traditional models and recent advances. *The Behavior Analyst Today, 5*, 255–274.

Kanter, J. W., Manos, R. C., Busch, A. M., & Rusch, L. C. (2008). Making behavioral activation more behavioral. *Behavior Modification, 32*, 780–803.

Kanter, J. W., & Mulick, P. (2007, November). *Basic science foundations and new applications of behavioral activation*. Symposium accepted for the annual meeting of the Association of Behavioral and Cognitive Therapies, Philadelphia.

Kessler, R. C. (1997). The effects of stressful life events on depression. *Annual Review of Psychology, 48*, 191–214.

Kohlenberg, R. J., & Tsai, M. (1991). *Functional analytic psychotherapy: Creating intense and curative therapeutic relationships*. New York: Plenum Press.

Kuyken, W., & Brewin, C. R. (1994). Stress and coping in depressed women. *Cognitive Therapy and Research, 18*, 403–412.

Lejuez, C. W., Hopko, D. R., & Hopko, S. D. (2002). *The brief Behavioral Activation Treatment for Depression (BATD): A comprehensive patient guide*. Boston: Pearson Custom Publishing.

Lejuez, C. W., Hopko, D. R., LePage, J. P., Hopko, S. D., & McNeil, D. W. (2001). A brief behavioral activation treatment for depression. *Cognitive and Behavioral Practice, 8*, 164–175.

Lewinsohn, P. M. (1974). A behavioral approach to depression. In R. J. Friedman & M. M. Katz (Eds.), *The psychology of depression: Contemporary theory and research* (pp. 157–178). Washington, DC: Winston-Wiley.

Londahl, E. A., Tverskoy, A., & D'Zurilla, T. J. (2005). The relations of internalizing symptoms to conflict and interpersonal problem solving in close relationships. *Cognitive Therapy and Research, 29*, 445–462.

Lyubomirsky, S., & Nolen-Hoeksema, S. (1993). Self-perpetuating properties of dysphoric rumination. *Journal of Personality and Social Psychology, 65*, 339–349.

Martell, C. R., Addis, M. E., & Jacobson, N. S. (2001). *Depression in context: Strategies for guided action*. New York: Norton.

Mazure, C. M. (1998). Life stressors as risk factors in depression. *Clinical Psychology: Science and Practice, 5*, 291–313.

Mirowsky, J., & Ross, C. E. (1989). *Social causes of psychological distress*. New York: Aldine de Gruyter.

Monroe, S. M., & Depue, R. A. (1991). Life stress and depression. In J. Becker & A. Kleinman (Eds.), *Psychosocial aspects of depression* (pp. 1101–1130). Hillsdale, NJ: Erlbaum.

Murray, C. J. L., & Lopez, A. D. (Eds.). (1996). *The global burden of disease: A comprehensive assessment of mortality and disability from diseases, injuries, and risk factors in 1990 and projected to 2020* (Vol. 1). Cambridge, MA: Harvard School of Public Health on behalf of World Health Organization and World Bank.

Nolen-Hoeksema, S., Parker, L. E., & Larson, J. (1994). Ruminative coping with depressed mood following loss. *Journal of Personality and Social Psychology, 67*, 92–104.

Ottenbreit, N. D., & Dobson, K. S. (2004). Avoidance and depression: The construction of the Cognitive-Behavioral Avoidance Scale. *Behaviour Research and Therapy, 42*, 293–313.

Paykel, E. S. (1982). Psychopharmacology of suicide. *Journal of Affective Disorders, 4*, 271–273.

Pearlin, L. I. (1989). The sociological study of stress. *Journal of Health and Social Behavior, 22*, 337–356.

Tsai, M., Kohlenberg, R. J., Kanter, J. W., Kohlenberg, B., Follette, W. C., & Callaghan, G. M. (2008). *A Guide to functional analytic psychotherapy: Awareness, courage, love and behaviorism*. New York: Springer.

Zeiss, A. M., Lewinsohn, P. M., & Muñoz, R. F. (1979). Nonspecfic improvement effects in depression using interpersonal skills training, pleasant activity schedules, or cognitive training. *Journal of Consulting and Clinical Psychology, 47*, 427–439.

Zlotnick, C., Kohn, R., Keitner, G., & Della Grotta, S. A. (2000). The relationship between quality of interpersonal relationship and major depressive disorder: Findings from the National Comorbidity Survey. *Journal of Affective Disorders, 59*, 205–215.

Chapter 6
FAP and Psychodynamic Therapies

Irwin S. Rosenfarb

> *The question of the analyst's self-disclosure and self-revelation*
> *inhabits every moment of every psychoanalytic treatment.*
>
> (Levine, 2007, p.81)

The purpose of this chapter is to present a brief overview of current psychodynamic therapies and to show how these therapies may be understood within a Functional Analytic Psychotherapy (FAP, Kohlenberg & Tsai, 1991; Tsai et al., 2008) framework. As readers of this chapter are no doubt aware, FAP is a bit of an anomaly within the current therapeutic landscape. On the one hand, FAP is derived from radical behavioral epistemology. On the other hand, FAP is more similar clinically to psychodynamic approaches than to traditional behavioral therapies. Thus, FAP occupies a unique therapeutic space in that it is able to bridge both behavioral and psychodynamic worlds (see Kohlenberg & Tsai, 1991, Chapter 7). A clearer understanding, therefore, of current psychodynamic therapies may help FAP therapists become more effective in their clinical work.

As Gabbard and Westen (2003) recently pointed out, "Contemporary psychoanalysis is marked by a pluralism unknown in any prior era" (p. 823). Moreover, there is a recognition that "the either/or polarization of insight through interpretation versus change through experiencing a new kind of relationship has given way to the recognition that these components of change operate synergistically in most cases, with greater emphasis on one component for some patients and the other component in others" (Gabbard & Westen, 2003, p. 824). Psychoanalysts spend less of their time "digging for buried relics from the patient's past. Rather, much of our focus is on the way the here-and-now interaction between analyst and patient provides insight into the influence of the patient's past on patterns of conflict and object relations in the present" (Gabbard & Westen, 2003, p. 824). Current psychoanalytic and psychodynamic therapies may be characterized, therefore, by both the use of

I.S. Rosenfarb (✉)
California School of Professional Psychology, Alliant International University, San Diego, CA, USA
e-mail: irosenfa@alliant.edu

J.W. Kanter et al. (eds.), *The Practice of Functional Analytic Psychotherapy*,
DOI 10.1007/978-1-4419-5830-3_6, © Springer Science+Business Media, LLC 2010

interpretation to help clients develop insight into their problems and the fostering of a positive therapeutic alliance (Leichsenring & Leibing, 2007).

Transference and the Therapeutic Alliance

The most basic similarity between FAP and psychodynamic approaches is the emphasis on the therapeutic alliance or the therapeutic relationship. The focus on this relationship is at the core of both approaches and both therapies use the alliance to effect behavioral change. Central to both approaches is the idea of the corrective emotional experience (Alexander & French, 1946), the belief that through a therapeutic relationship with a positive other person, clients can learn new ways of interacting in the world (Gabbard & Westen, 2003).

In both psychoanalysis and FAP, therapists attempt to make clients aware of patterns of behavior exhibited with the therapist that also may be shown with significant others in clients' lives outside of therapy. Within psychodynamic approaches, this is known, of course, as "transference," which may be defined as the idea that clients repeat many of the same behaviors with their therapists that they have shown with significant others throughout their lives (Mitchell & Black, 1995). Transference interpretations by analysts are attempts to show clients how they are repeating these patterns, and how these patterns have led to many of their interpersonal difficulties.

Fonagy (2004), a prominent psychoanalyst, provided a good example of transference in psychoanalysis. Fonagy presented an in-depth review of one session with a client named "Miss A." In the prior session, Miss A had disclosed a traumatic hospitalization at age 4 after she fell down a flight of stairs. In the current session, Miss A began by talking about a project at work. Fonagy stated

> ... it felt as if Miss A was being very repetitive and superior, and a bit boring. My mind wandered and I could feel that I was about to switch off. I then remembered that when she described her accident the previous session, she had described her father's visits to the hospital. Although he visited her every day, she was resentful that he would merely listen to her complaints about the treatment she was receiving and would do nothing. I wondered to myself if he, like me, had switched off, perhaps unable to bear his child's suffering, and how she must have felt about this when she was in pain and frightened and if there was now a part of her that was genuinely unable to have interest in or feel her pain. I wondered how to suggest, without seeming critical and eliciting a defensive response, my sense that she almost expected to bore me because she wanted to prove that I, like her father, could not bear her pain. (p. 810)

Fonagy responded to Miss A by stating

> You speak to me as if you have no hope of my being interested in what you are saying ... It occurs to me that you are experiencing me at the moment as you said you used to experience your father when he came to visit you in the hospital. I think you are hopelessly used to people not doing anything about what is happening to you. (p. 810)

Through his interpretation, Fonagy is pointing out that the client is repeating the earlier experience she had with her father (i.e., acting in a boring manner, in FAP terms a CRB1 or a clinically relevant behavior that is an in vivo problem). In addition, by using the word "hopelessly" in the last sentence, Fonagy is implicitly stating that Miss A expects others to react in the same way as her father. Thus, Fonagy is using FAP Rule 5 ("provide functional interpretations of client behavior") to help the client develop a CRB3 (explanation of the causes of her behavior) in which she sees the connection between her "repetitive, superior, and boring" behavior and others' lack of interest in what she says. From a FAP perspective, it also would be important to know whether Fonagy's interpretation encouraged the client's direct expression of pain and distress within the session, and whether Fonagy then acted in ways that reinforced those behaviors. Interestingly, in an accompanying commentary, Irwin Hoffman, another prominent analyst, notes that it may have been better for Fonagy also to have expressed some regret for being bored. Hoffman (2004) states that Fonagy might have said, for example

> I feel bad because this aspect of your work is so important to you and you would like me to be interested, but I find my mind is drifting . . . It occurs to me that that's a bit narrow of me and that maybe I'm being a bit like your dad in that respect. (p. 818)

This self-reflection, Hoffman notes, may have served to further differentiate the analyst from the client's father (a use of Rule 5 in FAP). In addition, by responding in this way, Fonagy would be telling Miss A that being bored was *his* problem and that Miss A had a right to expect Fonagy to be interested in her work. Thus, this self-disclosure also might serve as a discriminative stimulus (a use of Rule 2 in FAP) to evoke more client CRB2s (in-session improvements such as the direct expression of pain and distress).

Hoffman (2004) furthermore points out that such therapist genuineness also models openness and vulnerability to the client (also a use of Rule 2). At one point in the session Miss A tells Fonagy, "You are so full of yourself, and then I don't like you." The analyst does not respond to this comment, but Hoffman notes that Fonagy might have said the following: "Really, I wasn't aware of that. Could you tell me more about what you mean?" In this way, the therapist not only responds positively to the client's expression of anger (using FAP Rule 3 to *reinforce* a potential CRB2), but he also implicitly lets the client know that he will try to change his own behavior (a use of Rule 2). Hoffman (2004) notes that if Fonagy were genuine with Miss A and showed her his vulnerability, the interaction may have become more "emotionally meaningful" (p. 820). This, in turn, may have served to encourage more emotionally meaningful exchanges in the future.

Transference, the Repetition Compulsion and Projective Identification

Transference and Stimulus Generalization

Some behaviorists have dismissed the concept of transference by stating that the concept can be understood through the behavioral principle of stimulus generalization. Behaviorists have noted that because therapists are similar to others in clients' lives, it is not surprising that clients react to therapists as they have reacted to significant others. It is possible, for example, that therapists are part of a stimulus class that includes all "authority figures" or all "older men" or all "women."

Stimulus generalization, however, merely describes the mechanism by which clients react to therapists as they have reacted to significant others in their life. The interesting part of the transference phenomenon though is *not* that stimulus generalization occurs but that stimulus generalization continues to occur even after clients have had repeated exposure to the therapist. A rat or pigeon, for example, can discern the difference between a dark red light and a light red light as a discriminative stimulus within a few trials. Yet, even after years of therapy, some clients may continue to act toward their therapists as they acted toward their parents. In addition, they may continue to do so despite the fact that therapists may consistently act very differently toward them than their parents did. Clearly, clients "know" verbally that therapists are very different from their parents (if they were not different, clients probably would not continue in therapy), yet they may continue to repeat the same behavioral patterns and treat their therapist as if he or she were their parent. From a behavioral perspective, stimulus features supporting generalization continue to be more salient to the client than those that would support discrimination

Thus, therapist attention to how discrimination can be achieved may be useful. For example, it may be that clients have not had enough exposure to their therapist to learn that he or she is different from their parents. It takes several trials, for example, for a rat or pigeon to learn that a bright red light signals different reinforcers than does a dark red light. In the same way, after decades of repeated exposure to one's parents, it may take several years (since the client may see the therapist only 50 min a week) for a client to learn that his or her therapist is a functionally different stimulus than his or her parents. The therapist also may be inadvertently reinforcing problematic behaviors that are similar to the behaviors reinforced by the client's parents. From a FAP perspective, the critical point is to understand the contingencies surrounding the client's behavior within the session and to examine how they are similar to and different from the contingencies that have operated on the client in the past.

The Repetition Compulsion and Projective Identification

Some psychodynamic theorists would say that there is a *need* for clients to treat therapists as significant others in their lives (Moore & Fine, 1990). Behaviorally, we would say that the tendency to treat a therapist as a significant other is a high-strength behavior. Psychoanalysts call this high-strength behavior the "repetition compulsion" (Leowald, 1971). From a FAP perspective, the repetition compulsion describes a pattern of problematic behavior that is repeating across several environments (O1s or outside life problems and CRB1s or in-session problems), so to understand the contingencies surrounding the behavior, the therapist should look for reinforcers that occur across several environments as well.

There are at least two reasons why clients may treat therapists as their parents. First, clients may want experiences that are familiar to them and second, clients may seek to "undo" past relationships that cause them distress. Repeating similar patterns may be comforting because they are familiar. This may be especially true when change and ambiguity are frightening or perceived as dangerous. Avoidance of change is an important and sometimes neglected CRB1.

A psychoanalytic concept related to the repetition compulsion is projective identification. Projective identification occurs when clients "project" certain thoughts, ideas, or feelings onto the therapist and the therapist actually behaves toward the client congruent with the behaviors that have been projected onto him or her (Ogden, 1979). Therapists do this because clients act in a manner that "pulls" for those behaviors. A client, for example, may see the therapist as "bossy" and, therefore, acts passive. The therapist then actually acts bossy in response to a passive client. Through the process of projective identification, clients may recreate interactions that occurred with significant others in their lives.

A second reason clients may react to their therapist as they did to significant others in their lives is to "undo" past relationships that cause distress. Imagine a client who grew up with a depressed mother who, at times, was unresponsive to his needs. It also may be that this client saw himself as responsible for his mother's depression and continually attempted to make his mother happy by "being the perfect little angel" she wanted him to be. This can be translated into behavioral terms. As Janoff-Bulman (1979) noted, seeing ourselves as responsible for negative events in our life may be adaptive when the alternative is to realize how powerless and helpless we are in the world.

Thus, even though the attempt to be perfect did not reduce his mother's depression, this client's behavior of trying to be perfect may have been negatively reinforced through avoidance of feelings of powerlessness and helplessness. It may have been preferable to believe that he could control his mother's depression than to believe that his mother was unresponsive to his needs. Moreover, the client may have been intermittently reinforced for trying to reduce his mother's depression and this may have resulted in the client feeling powerful and in control.

In therapy, the client's attempt to make his therapist happy and pleased is a high-strength behavior, and the client may do his homework diligently, for example, in an effort to accomplish with his therapist what he was unable to do with his mother. In addition, by recreating this pattern with his therapist and in other relationships, the client avoids being aware of painful, guilty, and angry feelings. In these situations, it may be essential for the therapist to avoid reinforcing behaviors that are indicative of the client's attempt to be "a perfect little angel" (a CRB1) and instead to reinforce behaviors that conflict with the therapist's wishes. Oppositional behaviors that do not please the therapist may be CRB2s for clients when their parents' conditional love and acceptance has been their most potent reinforcer.

It should be noted that there is very little empirical support for these concepts within psychoanalysis because needs, wishes, and desires are so difficult to assess. Behaviorists, for example, have done a very good job of specifying when something is or is not a reinforcer, but have done a poor job of specifying why that stimulus is reinforcing or how we can identify the significant reinforcers in a person's life. Thus, one's life experiences become critical in determining clients' CRB1s and CRB2 As Goldfried and Davison (1976) pointed out over 30 years ago, the expert behavior therapist must be a *Menschenkenner*, someone who understands people and is a "connoisseur" of human behavior.

Problems with Transference, the Repetition Compulsion and Projective Identification

For many analysts, transference involves a distortion of reality. Freud, for example, considered the client's reaction an "illusion" and thus ignored the therapist's "personality, behaviors, and role" (Langs, 1976, p. 27). A less extreme view was offered by Alexander and French (1946) who suggested that before a client reaction is classified as transference, the analyst must rule it out as a "normal reaction to the therapist and therapeutic situation as reality" (pp. 72–73). Clinically, a therapist who accepts the distorted reality aspect of transference may be less inclined to genuinely consider the possibility that a client's perception is valid when it differs from the therapist's. This, in turn, could deprive the client of an opportunity to learn how to resolve interpersonal conflicts in which each member of the dyad has a justifiable, but different view of the world. Similarly, a submissive client could be punished for being assertive when his or her view of reality is different from the therapist's. In situations where validation of clients' perceptions may be essential to their improvement, such needed validation may be limited or hampered by the distorted reality notion of transference. It may also be that the distorted reality notion will inadvertently reinforce an authoritarian or rigid stance for therapists who are already inclined in those directions.

In sum, transference is operant behavior that occurs because of similarity between the client–therapist relationship and past relationships the client has experienced. Furthermore, because it is an operant, there is no guarantee that such behavior will occur during the session. This FAP view of transference has the advantage of suggesting its causes, its relationship to the client's daily life problems, and how it is affected by the therapeutic process.

There are also many problems with the traditional psychoanalytic concept of projective identification In the projective identification of dependency, for example, (1) nothing is projected into someone else; the client is acting dependent because he or she was reinforced for it in the past, and was probably punished as a child for exhibiting more independent behaviors; (2) no conversion of an inner struggle into outer one takes place; the inner struggle is a side effect of both dependent and independent responses having been punished at different times; and (3) being this dependent has lost much of its past adaptive value; dependence now constitutes an avoidance behavior that prevents the client from contacting more positive contingencies associated with building in new behaviors (e.g., being assertive, taking control, having the ability to give and take).

More importantly, in terms of clinical implications, the designation of specific behaviors (i.e., dependence, power, sexuality, ingratiation) as projective identifications may be problematic. There may be an a priori judgment that when a therapist responds to the client's behavior with feelings of caretaking, incompetence, sexual arousal, or gratefulness, he or she is reinforcing the client's pathological behavior and this is, therefore, undesirable. Behavior, however, cannot be judged as problematic without considering the larger context; that is, although these client behaviors may be problematic (CRB1s), it is also possible that they are improvements (CRB2s) when considering the client's current repertoire. For instance, if a female client generally avoided relationships because she was afraid of being too dependent, then an emergence of dependence behavior would actually be a CRB2 and should be reinforced in the earlier stages of the therapy. Or, if dependence had been agreed upon as a CRB1, then improvements need to be shaped and reinforced rather than punished. An improvement might be the client's calling the therapist only once or twice a week as opposed to four or five times a week, or shortening her lengthy phone conversations to less than 10 min. The analytic view of the behavior as pathological might lead to the punishment of dependency behaviors, when such behaviors are CRB2s. In sum, the FAP position is that transference, the repetition compulsion, and projective identification are mentalistic constructs and clinicians, therefore, need to understand the specific client behaviors indicative of each.

Therapist Neutrality

Another important hallmark of classical psychoanalytic theory is the idea that the analyst never self-discloses and always maintains a "neutral" attitude (see Meissner, 2002). Stone (1981), for example, stated that "In general, the analyst does not answer questions. He gives no affective response to the patient's material or evident state of mind, nor opinions, nor direction, not to speak of active interest, advice or other allied communications" (p. 99). An example may help clarify why maintaining a neutral attitude and not giving a response to clients may be most beneficial. Imagine that an attractive client comes to therapy and frequently makes comments such as "I'm ugly" or "I'm unattractive." It would be natural for the therapist to want to tell the client, "I think you are attractive" but saying so may not be in the client's best interest. First, and most obviously, telling a client she is attractive may give the client the impression that the therapist was attracted to her. Yet, there may be a second, and more important reason why it may not be in the client's best interest to be told that the therapist thinks she is attractive.

One can imagine that this client has been told by many people in her environment that she is attractive. One can also imagine that since she has been an adult, the client has probably rarely if ever been told that she is ugly or unattractive. Yet, despite this, the client continues to "believe" she is unattractive. If the client has discounted the opinions of virtually everyone in her environment, why would not the client similarly discount the therapist's opinion?

One must also ask, though, why would a client continually view herself as unattractive when objectively she is attractive? Behaviorally, what is maintaining the client's statement that she is unattractive? There are several reasons why an objectively attractive woman may see herself as unattractive. First, it is possible that by viewing herself as unattractive, the client avoids dating situations. The client may be terrified of dating (or more directly, a sexual relationship) and the statement, "I am ugly" is part of a larger response class that is maintained by the avoidance of dating. A second possible reason why this client may see herself as unattractive despite objective evidence to the contrary is that her parents may have given her the message (either overtly or covertly) that she was not attractive. Her parents also may have reinforced behavioral repertoires consistent with not "acting attractive" (such as being affectionate or "acting cute" with her father). Thus, by seeing herself as and acting attractive, she is contradicting her parent's view of her, which may arouse much anxiety and fear. Furthermore, by seeing herself as unattractive, this client may be maintaining her ties to her family and their view of her. The client may fear that by seeing herself differently from the way her family sees her, she is losing those family ties and may be left feeling alone and isolated.

One can develop a similar scenario for clients who see themselves as "stupid" or "dumb" when objectively they have accomplished much in their lives. One must ask what is maintaining these statements when clearly these clients must have received much feedback that contradicts such a view. The maintaining contingencies may be outside of the client's awareness, but often may be tied to the client's family's view of the client and the avoidance of behavior that contradicts those views. Viewing oneself in a negative way, for example, may be part of a larger response class that serves, in part, as a way for clients to maintain family ties when breaking those ties is too frightening or painful. Moreover, viewing oneself as successful or accomplished may also be anxiety-provoking when the idea contradicts one's previous learning history.

On the other hand, at times it may be desirable to tell clients you think they are "attractive" or "bright" as it may force clients to deal with the discrepancy between your view of them and their own view of themselves. A client, for example, may think you are lying if you tell her she is attractive, bringing up issues of trust (a CRB1) that may be addressed within the therapeutic alliance. Another client may tell you she is unattractive because she hopes that you will tell her she is attractive and thus reassure her. In this case, the client's reassurance seeking would be an important CRB1. There are no clear right or wrong ways to deal with clients' negative views of themselves. It is probably most critical, though, for clinicians to try to understand the contingencies maintaining such behavior in order for them to be in a position to naturally reinforce client improvements.

Current Empirical Research in Psychoanalytic Therapy

Because much of psychoanalytic therapy is compatible with FAP, it may be helpful for FAP clinicians to be aware of some current empirical research in psychoanalytic therapy. Psychoanalysis and psychodynamic therapies are currently experiencing a renaissance. A Psychodynamic Diagnostic Manual (PDM Task Force, 2006) recently has been published by the Alliance of Psychodynamic Organizations, a collaboration of the major psychoanalytic organizations, and empirically supported psychodynamically oriented therapies have been developed to treat borderline personality disorder (Bateman & Fonagy, 1999; Levy et al., 2006), panic disorder (Milrod et al., 2000), post-partum depression (Cooper, Murray, Wilson, & Romaniuk, 2003), and cocaine dependence (Crits-Cristoph et al., 2003), among other disorders. Recent meta-analytic reviews of short-term psychodynamic psychotherapy (STPP; Leichsenring, Rabung, & Leibing, 2004) and long-term psychodynamic psychotherapy (LTPP; Leichsenring & Rabung, 2008) have found large pre-treatment to post-treatment effect sizes for both forms of therapy. In addition, patients receiving LTPP showed significantly better outcomes than patients receiving shorter forms of psychotherapy on measures of target problems, psychiatric symptoms, and social functioning. Furthermore, the average patient receiving LTPP was better off than 96% of the average patients receiving short-term treatments (Leichsenring & Rabung, 2008).

Although the analysis of transference is considered central to psychoanalysis and psychodynamic psychotherapy, surprisingly, there has been only one empirical study that has experimentally manipulated the number of transference interpretations within a randomly controlled clinical trial[1] (see Hoglend, 2004, for a review of transference research). Hoglend et al. (2006) randomly assigned 100 patients to one of two forms of psychodynamic psychotherapy. Both forms of therapy were identical except that in one, therapists were instructed to focus specifically on the therapeutic relationship (the transference group) whereas in the other treatment, therapists were instructed specifically not to focus on the therapeutic relationship (the non-transference group).

In the transference group, therapists were encouraged to explore clients' thoughts and feelings about the therapeutic relationship, and patterns of behavior shown in outside relationships were specifically linked to patterns shown with the therapist. In the non-transference group, therapists were told not to focus on the relationship and to not link any patterns of behavior to patterns shown with the therapist. In the non-transference condition, for example, the therapist might say, "You feel that your colleague is exploiting you at work and you have difficulty telling her directly, so your headache builds up" whereas in the transference group, the therapist might say, "You feel that your colleague is exploiting you at work and you have difficulty telling her directly, so your headache builds up. Could this also be related to a feeling

---

[1] Rosser et al. (1983) conducted the only other empirical study to manipulate transference interpretations. In this study, 32 patients with chronic obstructive airway disease (COAD) were randomly assigned to one of two forms of psychodynamic psychotherapy. In one form, therapists were instructed to "make free use of transference interpretations" while in the other form, therapists were told to withhold transference interpretations. Results indicated that patients that did not receive transference interpretations showed significantly more changes in psychiatric symptoms than patients who received transference interpretations. In addition, female patients who received transference interpretations rated the therapy as significantly more unpleasant. None of the patients, however, were seeking psychotherapy.

that I do not do my share of the therapeutic work?" (Hoglend et al., 2006, p. 1740). In both therapies, patients were seen weekly for 1 year.

Results indicated that, contrary to the authors' hypotheses, low-functioning clients (those with personality disorders) did better when they received transference interpretations whereas high-functioning clients (those without personality disorders) did equally well in both forms of therapy. Moreover, these results maintained over a 3-year follow-up period (Hoglend et al., 2008).

The authors interpret these findings as suggesting that low-functioning clients (those with long-standing problematic interpersonal relationships) may need the therapist to focus on their relationship. Not focusing on their relationship may be too anxiety-provoking. The client may need the therapist to be explicit about how he or she feels about the client. This may not be necessary for high-functioning clients. For these clients, focusing on their interpersonal relationship difficulties outside of therapy may be sufficient and it may not be necessary for the therapist to focus on the "transference." Thus, a focus on problems occurring within the relationship may be important for low-functioning clients whereas for high-functioning clients, important CRB2s may involve developing CRB3s – verbal behaviors that describe the functional relationship between the client's behavior and reinforcers in the natural environment.

Hogland et al.'s results are consistent with the robust finding that cognitive behavior therapy (CBT) is generally effective for the treatment of major depressive disorder even though CBT therapists do not emphasize attending to the therapist–client relationship (most CBT studies typically involve high-functioning clients). On the other hand, many correlational studies suggest that outcome is improved when attention is given to the therapist–client alliance, even when clients are high-functioning (Connolly et al., 1999; Kanter, Schildcrout, & Kohlenberg, 2005; Kohlenberg, Kanter, Bolling, Parker, & Tsai, 2002; Leichsenring & Leibing, 2007; O'Connor, Edelstein, Berry, & Weiss, 1994; Ogrodniczuk, Piper, Joyce, & McCallum, 1999). Decisions regarding when to focus on the therapeutic relationship are complex and poorly understood, and an idiographic assessment of each client may be critical in determining the best way to proceed in each situation.

Conclusion

Gabbard and Westen (2003), in their attempt to explain the mechanisms of change in psychoanalysis, concluded by saying, "Any time we are tempted to propose a single formula for change, we should take this as a clue that we are trying to reduce our anxiety about uncertainty by reducing something very complex to something very simple" (p. 837). At its most basic level, the therapeutic relationship is like any other close human relationship: two people are trying to connect with each other so that they each become more open, honest, and experiential. Psychoanalysis, for approximately 100 years, has been developing a theory to explain how this relationship can be curative of psychological problems. This theory, like any good theory, has evolved and has been refined through the experiences of psychoanalysts. Although the theory incorporates a very different world view from that of FAP, and defines its terms in ways that may be seen as problematic and unscientific by proponents of FAP, it would be foolhardy – given the obvious similarities between psychoanalysis and FAP in terms of technique – to argue that there is little to be gained from an examination of the principles and practices of psychoanalysts. After all, the theory stems from the real experiences of psychoanalysts in the therapy room with real clients. Psychoanalysts are trained to be exquisitely sensitive to the nuances of the therapeutic relationship and how client problems may unfold during the therapy hour in relation to the therapist. At the core of phenomena labeled transference or projective identification by psychoanalysts are real experiences so labeled.

Hopefully, FAP, through its emphasis on radical behavioral epistemology, may be able to help explain these nebulous and amorphous concepts within a scientific framework. FAP explanations may offer some useful operationalizations of psychoanalytic phenomena and may highlight certain therapist responses as particularly useful, thus offering some structure and guidance to a psychoanalytic theory that often leaves much to the judgement of the clinician. By doing so, FAP explorations of psychoanalysis can help our clients lead happier and more fulfilling lives.

References

Alexander, F., & French, T. M. (1946). *Psychoanalytic therapy: Principles and application.* Lincoln: University of Nebraska Press.

Bateman, A. W., & Fonagy, P. (1999). The effectiveness of partial hospitalization in the treatment of borderline personality disorder – a randomised controlled trial. *American Journal of Psychiatry, 156,* 1563–1569.

Connolly, M. B., Crits-Christoph, P., Shappell, J., Barber, J. P., Luborsky, L., & Shaffer, C. (1999). Relation of transference interpretations to outcome in the early sessions of brief supportive-expressive psychotherapy. *Psychotherapy Research, 9,* 485–495.

Cooper, P. J., Murray, L., Wilson, A., & Romaniuk, H. (2003). Controlled trial of the short- and long-term effect of psychological treatment of post-partum depression. 1. Impact on maternal mood. *British Journal of Psychiatry, 182,* 412–419.

Crits-Christoph, P., Siqueland, L., Blaine, J., Frank, A., Luborsky, L., Olken, L. S., et al. (2003). Psychosocial treatments for cocaine dependence: National Institute on Drug Abuse Collaborative Cocaine Treatment Study. *Archives of General Psychiatry, 56,* 493–502.

Fonagy, P. (2004). Miss A. *International Journal of Psychoanalysis, 85,* 807–814.

Gabbard, G. O., & Westen, D. (2003). Rethinking therapeutic action. *International Journal of Psychoanalysis, 84,* 823–841.

Goldfried, M. R., & Davison, G. C. (1976). *Clinical behavior therapy.* New York: Holt, Rinehart, & Winston.

Hoffman, I. Z. (2004). "Miss A": Commentary 2. *International Journal of Psychoanalysis, 85,* 817–822.

Hoglend, P. (2004). Analysis of transference in psychodynamic psychotherapy: A review of empirical research. *Canadian Journal of Psychoanalysis, 12,* 280–300.

Hoglend, P., Amlo, S., Marble, A., Bogwald, K. P., Sorbye, O., Sjaastad, M. C., & Heyerdahl, O. (2006). Analysis of the patient-therapist relationship in dynamic psychotherapy: An experimental study of transference interpretations. *American Journal of Psychiatry, 163,* 1739–1746.

Hoglend, P., Bogwald, K. P., Amlo, S., Marble, A., Ulberg, R., Sjaastad, M. C., et al. (2008). Transference interpretations in dynamic psychotherapy: Do they really yield sustained effects. *American Journal of Psychiatry, 165*, 763–771.

Janoff-Bulman, R. (1979). Characterological versus behavioral self-blame: Inquiries into depression and rape. *Journal of Personality and Social Psychology, 37*, 1798–1809.

Kanter, J. W., Schildcrout, J. S., & Kohlenberg, R. J. (2005). In vivo processes in cognitive therapy for depression: Frequency and benefits. *Psychotherapy Research, 15*, 366–373.

Kohlenberg, R. J., Kanter, J. W., Bolling, M. Y., Parker, C., & Tsai, M. (2002). Enhancing cognitive therapy for depression with functional analytic psychotherapy: Treatment guidelines and empirical findings. *Cognitive and Behavioral Practice, 9*, 213–229.

Kohlenberg, R. J., & Tsai, M. (1991). *Functional analytic psychotherapy: Creating intense and curative therapeutic relationships*. New York: Plenum Press.

Langs, R. (1976). *The therapeutic interaction* (Vol. 2). New York: Jason Aronson.

Leichsenring, F., & Leibing, E. (2007). Psychodynamic psychotherapy: A systematic review of techniques, indications and empirical evidence. *Psychology and Psychotherapy: Theory, Research and Practice, 80*, 217–228.

Leichsenring, F., & Rabung, S. (2008). Effectiveness of long-term psychodynamic psychotherapy: A meta-analysis. *Journal of the American Medical Association, 300*, 1551–1565.

Leichsenring, F., Rabung, S., & Leibing, E. (2004). The Efficacy of Short-term Psychodynamic Psychotherapy in Specific Psychiatric Disorders: A Meta-analysis. *Archives of General Psychiatry, 61*, 1208–1216.

Leowald, H. W. (1971). Some considerations on repetition and repetition compulsion. *International Journal of Psychoanalysis, 52*, 59–66.

Levine, S. S. (2007). Nothing but the truth: Self-disclosure, self-revelation, and the persona of the analyst. *Journal of the American Psychoanalytic Association, 55*, 81–104.

Levy, K. N., Meehan, K. B., Kelly, K. M., Reynoso, J. S., Weber, M., Clarkin, J. F., et al. (2006). Change in attachment patterns and reflective function in a randomized control trial of transference-focused psychotherapy for borderline personality disorder. *Journal of Consulting and Clinical Psychology, 74*, 1027–1040.

Meissner, W. W. (2002). The problem of self-disclosure in psychoanalysis. *Journal of the American Psychoanalytic Association, 50*, 827–867.

Milrod, B., Busch, F., Leon, A., Shapiro, T., Aronson, A., Roiphe, J., et al. (2000). Open trial of psychodynamic psychotherapy for panic disorder: A pilot study. *American Journal of Psychiatry, 157*, 1878–1880.

Mitchell, S. A., & Black, M. J. (1995). *Freud and beyond: A history of modern psychoanalytic thought*. New York: Basic Books.

Moore, B. E., & Fine, B. E. (1990). *Psychoanalytic terms and concepts*. New York: American Psychoanalytic Association.

Ogden, T. H. (1979). On projective identification. *International Journal of Psychoanalysis, 60*, 357–373.

Ogrodniczuk, J. S., Piper, W. E., Joyce, A. S., & McCallum, M. (1999). Transference interpretations in short-term dynamic psychotherapy. *Journal of Nervous and Mental Disease, 187*, 572–579.

O'Connor, L. E., Edelstein, S., Berry, J. W., & Weiss, J. (1994). Changes in the patient's level of insight in brief psychotherapy: Two pilot studies. *Psychotherapy: Theory, Research, Practice, Training, 31*, 533–544.

Rosser, R., Denford, J., Heslop, A., Kinston, W., MacKlin, D., Minty, K., et al. (1983). Breathlessness and psychiatric morbidity in chronic bronchitis and emphysema: A study of psychotherapeutic management. *Psychological Medicine, 13*, 93–110.

Stone, L. (1981). Notes on the noninterpretive elements in the psychoanalytic situation and process. *Journal of the American Psychoanalytic Association, 29*, 89–118.

Task Force, P. D. M. (2006). *Psychodynamic diagnostic manual* (*PDM*). Silver Spring, MD: Alliance of Psychoanalytic Organizations.

Tsai, M., Kohlenberg, R. J., Kanter, J. W., Kohlenberg, B., Follette, W. C., & Callaghan, G. M. (2008). *A guide to functional analytic psychotherapy: Awareness, courage, love, and behaviorism*. New York: Springer.

Chapter 7
FAP and Feminist Therapies: Confronting Power and Privilege in Therapy

Christeine Terry, Madelon Y. Bolling, Maria R. Ruiz, and Keri Brown

> *My schooling gave me no training in seeing myself as an oppressor, as an unfairly advantaged person, or as a participant in a damaged culture. I was taught to see myself as an individual whose moral state depended on her individual moral will. My schooling followed the pattern my colleague Elizabeth Minnich has pointed out: whites are taught to think of their lives as morally neutral, normative, and average, and also ideal, so that when we work to benefit others, this is seen as work that will allow "them" to be more like "us."*
>
> (McIntosh, 1988, p. 1)

The quote by McIntosh (1988) reflects a theme that weaves together this chapter on Functional Analytic Psychotherapy (FAP) and feminist therapies. Briefly, psychotherapy is comprised of a series of social encounters fraught with sources of behavioral influence that are subtle, indirect, and generally undetectable by those involved. We will examine the characteristic sources of influence on social behavior (Biglan, 1995; Glenn, 1988; Glenn & Malagodi, 1991; Guerin, 1994; Parott, 1986; Zimmerman, 1963) and make the case that their role within the therapeutic process should be of interest to therapists. As therapists we inevitably bring with us distinctive characteristics that identify us as members of social groups including, but not limited to, our race, ethnicity, gender, and socio-economic class, and we work with clients of different races, ethnicities, genders, and socio-economic classes. The social group memberships of the therapist and the client are inseparable components of the emergent therapeutic context. In this chapter we will explore how social group memberships participate in the therapeutic context and the influences of these on the emergent therapeutic relationship. McIntosh's above quote highlights our theme by alerting us that markers of our memberships in social groups can work their way into the context of the therapeutic encounter silently and invisibly, potentially impacting our behavior and our clients' behaviors in ways we had not imagined.

C. Terry (✉)
Palo Alto VA Healthcare System, Palo Alto, CA, USA
e-mail: christeineterry@gmail.com

J.W. Kanter et al. (eds.), *The Practice of Functional Analytic Psychotherapy*, DOI 10.1007/978-1-4419-5830-3_7, © Springer Science+Business Media, LLC 2010

As McIntosh suggests, it is entirely possible to be unaware of how we contribute to a context that confers unearned advantage to some based on sex, race, immigration status, sexual orientation, or physical or mental health abilities. She also makes us aware that it is possible that our views of what constitutes "normality" and the ways we work with others to help alleviate suffering may lead us to act in ways that perpetuate and promote one privileged view of normality to the detriment of other people whose realities are different from our own. The other person's reality remains invisible because, as Caplan (1995) reminds us, "the people who have the greatest power to impose their views of reality on others are those who are most likely to uphold the majority view of reality and normality" (p. 50).

McIntosh's quote also touches upon the concepts of power and privilege, processes that perpetuate certain views of reality as "neutral, normative, and average" (McIntosh, 1988, p. 1). Many of us have received little, if any, formal training or practice in identifying instances where power and privilege are operating as sources of behavioral influence. If we have learned to become aware of the influences exerted by power and privilege on behavior, we likely have not been taught how we can challenge it. We argue that as therapists we should become aware of power and privilege in the therapeutic context because without intention or awareness we may be engaging in behaviors that promote inequality and injustice at the expense of our clients. Further, our unintentional promotion of oppressive practices may produce iatrogenic effects for clients, violating the ethical mandate of doing no harm.

Feminist theories and therapies grew from an acute awareness of the systemic nature and daily effects of social injustice in people's lives and a passion to change societal imbalances. Feminist theories can be successfully integrated with behavior analysis (cf., Ruiz, 1998) and we propose a similar integration of feminist therapies with FAP. In this chapter we will consider ways that the contextual and systemic awareness fostered in feminist therapies can contribute to and enhance the practice of FAP. We discuss the constructs of power and privilege from a behavior analytic perspective and present a functional analytic view of these processes that can clarify our understanding of how they function and suggest ways to counteract their influence. Finally, we propose an alteration to FAP case conceptualization that will increase the salience of sociopolitical factors in the therapeutic relationship and aid therapists in identifying and working with issues of power and privilege both within and outside the therapeutic relationship to advance the therapeutic process.

Feminism and Behavior Analysis: Complementary Systems

Ruiz (1995) has discussed at length the points of convergence between the feminist perspective, broadly defined, and behavior analytic science. While the feminist community is highly diverse (cf., Herrmann & Stewart, 1994; Kirk & Okazawa-Rey, 1998; Reinharz, 1992), the orienting assumptions that guide feminist work and the themes woven through feminist discourse converge with the philosophical and conceptual terrain of radical behaviorism as articulated by Skinner (1945, 1953, 1969,

1974, 1978). For example, behavior analysts and feminists adopt a contextualistic view of behavior and reject psychological approaches that fail to take into account the conditions of people's lives. The two communities agree that scientific knowing is a relational process and reject the notion of the scientist as a privileged knower that is separate from the participant. That is, the perspectives the scientist brings to her work are important considerations given the social nature of scientific knowledge. Therefore, unlike models of science that search for universal and transcendental truths, feminists and behavior analysts agree that scientific work is a practical matter that aims at establishing effective solutions for the problems within a given context. The reader familiar with FAP will recognize elements of the foregoing discussion as "the conceptual foundations of applied behavior analysis [that] form the theoretical underpinnings for FAP" (Kohlenberg & Tsai, 1991, p. 7).

For years feminists have expressed the need for a feminist epistemology (Aebischer, 1988; Banaji, 1993; Harding, 1986; Marecek & Hare-Mustin, 1991; Unger, 1986) grounded in the experiences of women and other marginalized groups. Keller (1985), for example, has exposed the invisible but pervasive impact of gender ideology in science reflecting its masculinist perspective. As a result others have called for "woman-specific" knowledge (Aebischer, 1988) or feminist standpoint epistemologies (Harding, 1986) that recognize women's experiences as distinctly crucial in the development of alternative perspectives in science. The essential features of feminist epistemology include placing women at the center of inquiry, reducing or eliminating the boundaries between the scientist (knower) and the participant (known), and employing knowledge to challenge the subordination of women and other social groups marginalized on the basis of race, class, ethnicity, or other distinctions (Fee, 1986). Above all, feminist epistemology encourages the scientist to, in Keller's (1985) words, "listen to the material rather than assuming the scientific data self-evidently speak for themselves" (p. 134) because, she reminds us, the "data never do speak for themselves ... [as] all data presuppose interpretation" (Keller, p. 130).

In calling for a merger of feminist psychology and behavior analysis, Ruiz (1998) has noted the nature of transformative research that could emerge from the fusion. One such area is the study of gender as an "epistemological system" (Kaschak, 1992, p. 35). The behavior analyst's conceptual and methodological tools could be useful in this quest. One tool is the behaviorist's understanding of self-knowledge as being of social origin. Skinner (1974) stated,

> It is only when a person's private world becomes important to others [in the verbal community] that it is made important to him ... A person who has been made "aware of himself" by the questions he has been asked is in a better position to predict and control his own behavior (p. 31).

This understanding of self-knowledge and the focus of the analysis on the contingencies in the verbal community in its development may yield insights on the functions of gender (or race, class, sexuality, and other categories) as social and verbal classes. Moreover, a behavioral analysis of invisible social contingencies of discriminatory cultural practices and interpretive repertoires (see Hineline, 1992; Ruiz,

1998) of dominant (controller/scientist/therapist) and non-dominant (controllee/ participant/client) participants in social encounters (work setting/scientific research/therapy) may reveal useful information on the functional dynamics of power and privilege.

Feminist Therapies: A Brief Introduction

Feminist therapy emerged partially as a result of the consciousness-raising groups that arose within the women's movement of the 1960s and 1970s. In addition, feminists' criticisms of traditional therapy methods inspired the development of a therapy that was thought to better address the needs of women. Contemporary feminist therapy encompasses a wide variety of approaches. Unlike traditional forms of therapy, it does not have a standard, agreed-upon definition. It is a set of values or attitudes rather than a standard set of techniques or procedures. In fact, Marecek and Kravetz (1998) concluded

> Uniform standards of feminist practice would be nearly impossible to achieve. Just as there is no single definition of feminism nor one kind of feminist, there is no single meaning of feminist therapy, but rather a multiplicity of ideas about principles, processes, and therapy goals. (p. 35)

Despite the variability in forms of feminism and feminist therapy, several themes have been identified, including the importance of addressing sociopolitical factors, a focus on maintaining an egalitarian therapeutic relationship,[1] and balancing instrumental and relational strengths (Campbell & Wasco, 2000; Enns, 2004).

The emphasis on sociopolitical rather than intrapsychic factors as causes of women's psychological distress is central to feminist therapy (Park, 2004). Feminist therapists have been critical of traditional psychology for constructing women's symptoms as pathological. They reject the idea of individual psychopathology and instead endorse environmental or sociopolitical factors as potential causes of clients' distress (Gondolf, 1998; Walker, 1994). Thus, feminist therapists see women's symptoms as directly connected to their social and political contexts and as mechanisms for surviving within oppressive environments rather than as an individual "illness."

This emphasis on sociopolitical factors is reflected in a common idea from the second wave of feminist theory and activism, namely, that the personal is political (Gilbert, 1980). In the therapy setting, this view is bidirectional. That is, the client and therapist come to recognize that acting from their own received values about gender, ethnicity, class, sexual orientation, and other groupings affects society around them – that is, the personal is political. Conversely, they recognize that

---

[1]Establishing and maintaining an egalitarian therapeutic relationship are not accepted by all feminist schools of therapy (cf., Veldhuis, 2001). Some feminist writers have questioned the necessity and ethics of creating an egalitarian relationship, suggesting that it may inhibit successful therapeutic outcomes (Veldhuis, 2001).

these socially constructed values affect their personal lives – thus, the political is personal. In addition, the personal can become a direct part of the political realm when a person decides to take action toward societal change. This idea, which originated in the consciousness-raising groups of the 1960s and 1970s, represents quite a departure from traditional goals of therapy. Some feminist therapies promote social activism as a part of the therapeutic process for clients and consider activism integral to being a more effective feminist therapist (Enns, 2004). The connection between personal and political issues is core to feminist therapy, based on the fundamental belief that there is no real or lasting individual change without some type of social change (Sturdivant, 1980; Wyche & Rice, 1997). One criticism feminist therapists have of traditional psychotherapy is that therapists often encourage clients simply to adjust to their environment rather than challenge oppressive structures (Worell & Remer, 2003). Therefore, a major goal of feminist therapy is to help clients have an impact on their social and political environments, both for their own benefit and that of others.

Five techniques selected from feminist therapy procedures for highlighting sociopolitical factors include: (1) identifying and assessing the importance of clients' social locations (e.g., gender, ethnicity, social class, sexual orientation), (2) reframing clients' symptoms as strategies for coping with an unhealthy or oppressive environment (e.g., consciousness raising), (3) gender-role, cultural, and power analyses, (4) encouraging clients to initiate social change (at both macro and micro levels), and (5) therapist initiation of social change (Worell & Remer, 2003).

In addition, feminist therapists value an egalitarian relationship between the client and therapist (Brown, 1986; Enns, 2004; Gilbert, 1980; Marecek & Hare-Mustin, 1991; Park, 2004; Sturdivant, 1980; but see Veldhuis, 2001 for a dissenting view). Worell and Remer (1992) claim that power-sharing is a central concern for feminist therapy first because efforts to minimize the client–therapist power differential reduce the likelihood that therapy will serve as a further means of social control, and second, because the client–therapist relationship should not model the power differentials that women experience in their daily lives. Creating more egalitarian client–therapist relationships may also serve to keep clients in treatment, particularly those from "high-risk" groups who are reluctant to seek help from the mental health community due to prior experiences (and expectations of future experiences) of discrimination within psychotherapy (Worell & Remer, 2003).

Certain feminist therapy strategies are meant to reduce the power differential inherent in the therapy relationship and to increase client empowerment. Some of these strategies are (a) using appropriate self-disclosure, including making values explicit (so clients can choose to reject those values) and disclosing personal reactions and experiences when doing so is likely to be helpful to the client; (b) encouraging a consumer-oriented approach to therapy (i.e., demystifying the therapy process by informing clients of the process, rights, and responsibilities of therapy; encouraging clients to "shop around" for a therapist); (c) using caution in applying diagnostic labels, which may serve to position the client as "sick" and the therapist as "well"; (d) ensuring that goals are determined through a collaborative process; and (e) teaching clients skills that are consistent with the clients' stated goals (Brown & Brodsky, 1992; Brown & Walker, 1990; Sturdivant, 1980; Worell & Remer, 2003).

Feminist therapists also value the balancing of instrumental and relational strengths (Enns, 2004). Instrumental strengths are behaviors that have a primary function of completing tasks, whereas relational strengths are behaviors that have a primary function of maintaining relationships. Instrumental strengths are stereotypically associated with males and relational strengths (also known as expressivity) are stereotypically associated with females (Bem, 1981; Enns, 2004; Steiner-Adair, 1986). Feminist therapists encourage behavioral flexibility in all clients regardless of gender by challenging them to incorporate both instrumental and relational behaviors in their repertoires. In addition, they help clients understand how gender-role socialization has shaped their perceptions of agency (instrumentality) and communion (relational skills) in their own behavior as well as the behavior of others. Finally, feminist therapists help clients identify and value the relational aspect of their personalities, since in our society the relational realm has been considered less important than the instrumental realm.

Commonalities Between FAP and Feminist Therapies

Because functional analysis derives from a radical contextualist[2] worldview and feminist thinkers are deeply contextual by conviction, FAP and feminist therapies share aspects of an approach that differs fundamentally from mainstream psychology. The five feminist strategies to reduce power differentials listed above are also found in FAP (e.g., self-disclosure), though the rationale for pursuing them differs. The most theoretically salient of the commonalities is the endorsement of multiple causation for psychological difficulty, which in turn calls for a conceptual emphasis on function rather than topography. Both FAP and feminist therapies treat the person in context rather than treating symptom clusters or diagnoses.

As mentioned above, feminist therapists are critical of mainstream psychology's practice of assigning the causation of psychological difficulties to intrapsychic factors (e.g., personality factors such as aggressiveness and dependency) rather than to the sociopolitical contexts of which individuals are part. Radical contextualists also firmly reject intrapsychic models of causation for human behavior. Feminist therapists and behavior analysts recognize that intrapsychic models of causation may be useful ways of *describing* human behavior, but both deny that intrapsychic factors are causal mechanisms of behavior (Gondolf, 1998; Hayes & Brownstein, 1986; Park, 2004; Skinner, 1974; Walker, 1994). Instead, both feminists and radical

---

[2]In this chapter, the terms behavior analytic and radical contextualist will be used interchangeably. Both terms refer to the theory of behavior in which individual–environment relations, individual learning history, cultural history, and evolution are the proposed mechanisms of behavior change. This theory is often attributed to Skinner (1945, 1974), but has been expanded upon by Hayes, Barnes-Holmes, and Roche (2001), Sidman, Wynne, Maguire, and Barnes (1989), and many others.

contextualists propose models of behavior change that are based on multiple causation; that is, many factors and historical streams contribute to human behavior. As feminist writers Brown and Ballou (1992) state,

> Standard models of psychopathology have tended to look for a prime cause of the observed entity, rather than allowing for the possibility that similar phenomena may have multiple causations that interact with person and context in somewhat unique ways. (p. 113)

Behavior analysts propose that evolution (i.e., phylogenic selection), the environment, including an individual's learning history (i.e., ontogenic selection), and an individual's biology all contribute to determining behavior (Skinner, 1974), including the problematic behaviors that are typically seen in therapy.

In both FAP and feminist therapies this leads to an emphasis on function over topography. For example, Alice suffers from depression: a constant despairing mood, difficulty sleeping, loss of interest in food and favorite activities, withdrawal from social interaction, and difficulty thinking and concentrating. It came about in the context of her work environment, a welding company where she (the only female in the office) always finds herself in support-role tasks such as organizing company events, devising filing and tracking systems, and pacifying irate customers – in spite of the fact that she had been working there longer than the current management, had conceived and set up the business with her father, and often serves as management backup, where she performs admirably. A feminist might note one of the causal factors as the "glass-ceiling effect" – no matter how hard she works, Alice will not have access to higher positions in her company. Treatment then might focus on finding ways to address that form of workplace inequity. Note that this treatment does not address the topography of her presenting problem (e.g., sadness, sleeplessness) rather, the hypothesized function of her depression is withdrawal from an untenable situation rooted in long-standing societal patterns where Alice belongs to a subordinate group. In this case the hypothesis is that sexism is a systemic cause, and the glass-ceiling effect is the specific manifestation, so the problem is being addressed as a function of these phenomena.

A FAP therapist, on the other hand, may note that Alice treats him with considerable subservience during sessions, even though he is rather young and inexperienced. It is not that he thinks there is an intrapsychic cause (unassertiveness) for the depressive symptoms – rather, he may note that Alice is acting from a long history of being one of few women in a man's world, and has had no experience in changing what her experience tells her is "the way things are." Although this FAP therapist may shape assertive behaviors and direct communication in sessions with Alice (addressing what is apparently a problematic interpersonal pattern in her whole life), a FAP therapist with a deeper sense of the sociopolitical context might well combine such interactions with inquiry into steps Alice can take to remedy workplace inequities, while always noting her in-session reactions to him. For example, she may have difficulty articulating objections in the presence of a member of a dominant group.

Finally, both FAP and feminist therapies share the idea that the environment outside of therapy enters into the client–therapist interaction, as illustrated in the vignette above. Feminist writers have focused more on how the sociopolitical environment and learning based on one's cultural position influence client and therapist behaviors. FAP writers have focused more broadly on how the entirety of the environment and learning history impacts client and therapist behaviors.

A Rationale for Integration

By now, it is apparent that FAP and feminist therapies share a common foundation for a successful integration. Three additional reasons support this proposal. First, FAP therapists have recognized the need to identify and work with issues of power and privilege in the therapeutic situation (Rabin, Tsai, & Kohlenberg, 1996). In the first edition of the FAP book (1991), Kohlenberg and Tsai state,

> The therapist, however, as a member of the culture that supports subtle, and sometimes not so subtle, forms of prejudice and discrimination could have values consistent with the culture. Values refer to a person's reinforcers; this means that a sexist or racist therapist would continue to reinforce those client behaviors that have been shaped by a racist or sexist culture. We believe the most deleterious effect of oppression is that access to reinforcers is limited ... Consequently, a therapist who reinforces on the basis of sexism or racism would be interfering with repertoires that could increase long-term positive reinforcement and thereby compromise the goals of FAP. (p. 192)

However, FAP researchers and writers have been slow to take up the challenge presented by these suggestions; in the many years since the book was written, only one article on working with these issues has been published (Rabin, Tsai, & Kohlenberg, 1996) and only five presentations on the topic have been given nationally (Brown, 2009; Ruiz & Terry, 2006; Terry, 2005; Terry & Bolling, 2006; Terry & Bolling, 2007). Fortunately, feminist authors and therapists have written about issues of power and privilege since the 1960s and have proposed techniques for working with such issues in the therapeutic context. FAP could benefit greatly from the wisdom and methods feminist psychologists have developed in working with issues of power and privilege in the therapeutic encounter.

Second, the recommendations offered in the 1991 FAP text, although helpful, are neither exhaustive nor especially practical for therapists who lack time and resources to videotape and review sessions with "individuals sensitive to these issues" (p. 192). Finding such suitable consultants is actually more of a problem than anticipated, and is typically beyond the means of most therapists. Specifically, it is not sufficient simply to consult with a therapist who appears to belong to the same minority group as the patient one is treating. However well-intended, a request for this type of consultation based on the consultant's group membership is itself prejudicial (e.g., racist, sexist) and presumptuous. On the other hand, a colleague who specializes in sociopolitical issues would likely welcome a request for consultation. As noted below, many complex factors play into the sociopolitical position of every person. Incorporating the expertise of feminist therapists (conceptually and perhaps also in consultation) would be beneficial in dealing directly with these complexities.

Third, the 1991 recommendations presume that therapists are already aware of power, privilege and cultural contingencies in the groups to which the therapist and client belong. However, before a person can work with the "invisible knapsack" (McIntosh, 1988) of one's own assumptions about "the way things are," one must first become aware of those assumptions, and then realize that these issues will arise, however subtly, in the therapeutic relationship. FAP offers methods to specify which client and therapist behaviors that occur in daily life may enter into the therapeutic relationship and how those behaviors can be changed. Feminist therapies can enrich FAP by emphasizing the fact that the sociopolitical context is itself a source of clinically relevant behaviors, and as such will also inevitably enter into the therapeutic relationship. They offer techniques for becoming aware of and working with these issues as clinically relevant behaviors (see five of these techniques listed in the above section, Feminist Therapies: A Brief Introduction). As stated at the beginning of the chapter, everyone belongs to multiple socially constructed groups (in addition to our roles as client and therapist), and these groups' histories enter the therapy room as well. Thus, it is critically important that we become aware of the meanings inherent in belonging to socially constructed groups because those meanings will inevitably appear in the therapeutic context.

Power and Privilege: A Behavior Analytic Reconceptualization

Because FAP is based on a radical contextualist theory it is crucial that we understand power and privilege, central constructs in feminist therapies, in a manner that is consistent with the theory on which FAP is based. We believe that a behavior analytic view of power and privilege has certain advantages for psychological work in that it traces the origins of behavior patterns into the environment, including the historical environment that includes societal and cultural histories. This view of power and privilege eliminates reified constructs and makes interventions more direct. A behavior analytic view does not refer to internal entities or other mentalistic concepts for good reason: If one had to change *capacity to influence* or *unearned advantage*, for instance, how might one proceed? The second advantage of a behavior analytic view is that measurement is more direct and concise: it is based on behavior and consequences that can be tracked and measured directly and tailored to the individual, as might be done with the FAP case conceptualization form which we will describe in a later section.

Power and Privilege: Feminist Definitions

As stated earlier, feminist writers have focused on power and privilege as core issues in theory and practice. For example, feminists have addressed the impact of power and privilege in the lives of individuals, and how to change cultural and therapeutic practices to mitigate their unexamined effects. When feminist writers[3] speak of power they typically include Eagly's (1983) definition that power is "the capacity to influence the other person in a relationship" (p. 971). This influence can extend through many different systems and contexts and can include power in dyadic relationships, in a group(s), or in a society or culture. Feminist writers generally have focused on the functions of power within and across social groups and the position of groups within a certain society or culture (e.g., United States) (cf., Brown & Ballou, 1992; Campbell & Wasco, 2000; Enns, 2004). We will retain Eagly's definition of power as *capacity to influence* as we develop a behavior analytic perspective on social power and its functions in human relations.

Privilege is discussed in the feminist literatures as "unearned advantage . . . [and] . . . conferred dominance" (McIntosh, 1988, p. 1). A consequence of power is that members of the dominant group accrue privileges. One such privilege is easier access to higher-status social positions, neighborhoods, employment, and governance. Privilege therefore affords members of the dominant group with certain advantages. One example of privilege is facilitating or fast-tracking group members into positions from which they can exert their influence over others. Because the dominant group is in a position to set up normative practices within a social system (see Ballou & Brown, 2002; Brown, 1992; Brown, 1994; Fine, 1992), the privileges accrued by its members blend into the normative practices of the larger social system. Thus, privilege typically operates invisibly, undetected as a source of influence particularly by those who benefit from it (see Ruiz, 1998, 2003). Privilege is often embedded within institutions such as government and schools and the cycle of maintaining power within certain groups is continued (see Fine, 1992 for a detailed discussion).

A Behavior Analytic View of Power

The treatment of power and privilege by feminist writers is likely to be of interest to radical contextualists working to understand subtle forms of behavioral control. As discussed previously, Ruiz (1995, 1998, 2003) has made the case that merging feminist perspectives with the radical behaviorist conceptual framework promises a productive line of inquiry into important sources of social control. We believe that a feminist radical contextualist perspective has much to offer behavior analytic practices in its various domains of clinical work, including FAP. For example, one important line of questioning encouraged by a feminist radical contextualist perspective would be as follows. Consider a FAP therapist who is a Caucasian female, working with an African-American male client. This therapist may want to ask how

---

[3] Just as with feminist therapies, there is no one form of feminist theory, but there are common elements among the many feminist theories. One such shared element is the focus on socio-cultural contexts and how these contexts influence the behavior of women (cf., Campbell & Wasco, 2000; Enns, 2004).

her participation in one of the dominant groups (Caucasian) can potentially impact the social dynamics in psychotherapy with a client who participates in a social group (African-American) that has been marginalized in American culture. Additionally, the FAP therapist may want to ask how her participation in a non-dominant group (female) may impact the relational dynamics in therapy with the same client who is also a member of a dominant group (male). The FAP therapist operating from a feminist radical contextualist perspective could ask herself (and possibly her client) the following questions:

- What are the historical and current relationships between my ethnicity and my client's ethnicity? How might these relationships influence our therapeutic relationship? How might these relationships impact our ability to trust each other and to communicate with each other?
- What are the historical and current relationships between my gender and my client's gender? How might these relationships impact our therapeutic relationship? How might these relationships impact our ability to trust each other and to communicate with each other?
- How does the intersection of my ethnicity and my gender influence how I conceptualize my client's presenting problems, clinically relevant behaviors, and goals? How does this intersection influence my ability to form therapeutic relationships, maintain therapeutic relationships, and communicate with my clients?
- How does the intersection of my client's ethnicity and gender influence how he conceptualizes his problems and goals for therapy? How does this intersection influence his ability to form and maintain therapeutic relationships, engage in therapeutic activities, and communicate with the therapist?
- How do the intersections of my ethnicity and gender and of my client's ethnicity and gender impact the therapeutic relationship? How do these intersections influence therapeutic processes and tasks?

The above questions are just a small sample of the type of queries a FAP therapist informed by a feminist radical contexualist perspective might ask herself (and potentially her client) throughout the therapeutic encounter. Similar questions can be generated about other social group memberships (e.g., sexual identity) and about the impact of social memberships on other therapeutic processes and outcomes.

Behavior analytic definition of power. The behavior analytic theorist William Baum provided a concise interpretation of power as "the control that each party in a relationship exerts over the other's behavior" (2005, p. 235). The person with greater control over another individual's behavior is said to be the one "with power" and can be termed the "controller" (Baum; see also Skinner, 1974). The other person in the relationship, the one with less control over the controller's behavior, is termed the "controllee." Power is not an individual attribute, characteristic, or personality trait. Consistent with radical behavioral theory, power is found in the relationship between behavior and consequence, that is, the reinforcement relation. More specifically, Baum states that power is "the power of reinforcement relations by which that party controls the other's behavior" (p. 235). Consistent with Baum's interpretation, Guerin (1994, p. 284) states the following: "For behavior analysis, power is where the control lies, in either who arranges the consequences, who arranges the stimulus conditions which select behaviors, or who determines which behaviors can be shaped." Similarly, Biglan (1995) tells us that "the power to influence a practice can be conceptualized in terms of control of the consequences for the practice ... [and a] person or group with power can control people's access to both unconditioned and conditioned reinforcers" (p. 119).

The power of a reinforcement relation is determined by two factors: the importance of the reinforcer to the individual and the precision of control over the reinforcer (Baum, 2005). The importance of the reinforcer "depends not on its absolute value but on its value relative to other reinforcers in the controllee's life" (Baum, p. 231). For example, if an individual's most significant source of reinforcement is from her family members, then the reinforcement relations in the context of her family life will have more power than reinforcement relations from her employer (including salary) or from her neighbors. In this example, the individual may call in sick to work to take care of her child, may leave work early to attend a family event, and so forth. This illustration reminds us that the value of the reinforcers (in this specific example, the amount of money earned), is relative rather than absolute, and determined by the context of the individual's environment and learning history.

People who are called "powerful" are those who control the more important reinforcers in a relationship between parties. This is exemplified in employment situations in which the employer (controller) is considered the "one with power" because the employer is in control of the more important reinforcers in the employee–employer relationship, such as access to employment, health benefits, and wealth for the employee. The employee (controllee) does have control over reinforcers for the employer, but these reinforcers are typically not the more important reinforcers for the employer (e.g., prestige, money, and advancement in career are not in the purview of the employee). Moreover, the employer likely has easy access to other potential employees (controllees) that could serve equivalent reinforcing functions, including completing work with accuracy, meeting deadlines, and satisfying customers. What Baum highlights in his definition of power is that in the relationship the person who "has power" is the one who has control over the more important (i.e., difficult to access) reinforcers, while the person with "less power" has control over less important (i.e., easy to access) reinforcers. It is the disparity between those who have vs. those who do not have control over the important reinforcers that are difficult to access that constitutes the term we call "power."

Power is not just defined by control over the more important reinforcer relation, but also by the precision of control over the reinforcer (Baum, 2005). If the reinforcer relation is delayed or is inconsistent, then the relation is less powerful even if the reinforcer is more important. In therapy, this principle applies to the therapist's consequating of a client's behavior. For example, if a therapist tells a client to wait until the next session to talk about an improvement that occurred yesterday the therapist has less control over the client's behavior than if the therapist timed the discussion closer to the event.

Although Baum's discussion of power is about a relationship between two individuals, power can also be examined in the context of relationships between organizations, individuals and organizations, and for the purposes of this chapter, the relationships between socially constructed groups such as races, sexes, ethnic groups, and cultures. To understand power in the context of groups and organizations, we treat the group or organization as an individual. Although a group or organization is often comprised of multiple individuals, the "organizational functionaries are replaceable" (Baum, 2005, p. 216). The latter phrase refers to the fact that organizational functionaries (e.g., CEO's, judges, presidents) are not specific to any one individual, but are positions that can be filled with other individuals. Second, groups can also be thought of as individuals because the group remains stable even if the people who comprise the group do not (i.e., individuals can enter and leave the group, but the group continues to exist and has the same functions). What remains stable more specifically is the group's "mode of operation," that is, the reinforcement and punishment relations of the group (Baum). As with the relationship between two people, the individual can affect the behavior of the group and the group can affect the behavior of the individual.

As with power in the relationship between two individuals, power between an individual and a group or between two groups is determined by whichever party has control over the more important, or difficult to access, reinforcers, as well as the precision with which these are delivered. Historically, certain social groups have controlled the more important reinforcers for other groups. For example, traditionally, women's roles in society have been limited in comparison to men's more variable social roles which make available, for men, a wider range of alternative contingencies or social roles of power (Biglan, 1995). Thus historically, domination of women by men has meant "being restricted to a limited behavioral repertoire through historical power over arranging contingencies" (p. 284).

Another example is that of Western Europeans and descendants of Western Europeans in the United States. In the United States, Western Europeans and those of Western European descent have historically controlled land, money, and freedom (through their positions as employers and in government) – important reinforcers to most individuals. Control over the more important reinforcers by Western Europeans (i.e., generally considered today as Caucasians) in relation to other groups of non-Western Europeans and their descendants (i.e., people of color) can be considered a relationship of power. That is, Caucasians generally have easier access to important reinforcers than individuals of color and their accrued privilege nets Caucasians greater leverage over the more important reinforcers. Furthermore, historically Caucasians, through their positions of power as employers and through governmental positions, have managed reinforcement delivery with sufficient precision as to create effective controlling practices. An illustration of an effective management practice in the workplace is the employer who pays employees commissions for sales they generate. The government similarly selects timely cooperation of its citizens through taxation practices and its tax returns programs. The main power-differentiated groups in mainstream US culture (controller or advantaged group/non-dominant group) are male/female, white/non-white, adult/child, heterosexual/non-heterosexual, upper class/middle class/working class/unemployed-homeless, able-bodied/differently abled, English-speaking/non-English-speaking, Christian/non-Christian (Hays, 2001).

We have defined power as control over the more important reinforcers in a relationship between individuals, groups, or individuals and groups. Another aspect of power is the behavior of the individual termed the controller. Recall that the controller has control over and easier access to the more important reinforcers; additionally, the controller is reinforced for engaging in behaviors that influence or exert control over the other individual, the controllee. These may include behaviors such as silencing verbal expressions of beliefs that are not in agreement with the controller's, and asserting one's interests or needs at the expense of the interests or needs of others. The controller who has a history of being reinforced for exerting influence over individuals belonging to particular groups will be more likely to do so again in the future. Because our society tends to value members of certain groups (e.g., men, whites, heterosexuals) more than others, individuals belonging to these groups are more likely to be reinforced for exerting influence over others. These individuals have control over the more important reinforcers and have a history of reinforcement for behaviors that exert influence over others, therefore, these individuals are understood to "have power." In sum, power is the control over more important reinforcers and a history of reinforcement for behaviors that exert influence over others.

A final point to discuss that bears upon a behavioral understanding of power is the nature of social behavior and the social properties of contingencies that set the context for power relations. Behavior is considered social if "another person is involved as a stimulus context, a determinant of consequences or as part of the (group) behavior itself" (Biglan, 1995, p. 79). Social behavior is largely maintained by generalized social consequences and mediated by verbal contexts. Verbal behavior is a type of social behavior with powerful indirect effects deriving from extensive generalized social contingencies that emerge from our verbal communities. Social contexts are microcosms of the larger societal and cultural contexts, and as such they cannot be completely separated from them.

Therapy is a specific type of social context in which two individuals relate to each other and verbal contingencies are used to alter and maintain behavior. Therapy is a unique social context in that the relating behaviors of both parties are explicitly defined by each individual's role in the interaction (i.e., therapist or client) in addition to the goals of the interaction (i.e., to help the client get well or to behave in more adaptive ways). It is also a unique context in that it is viewed as one in which clients can reveal their innermost secrets and desires without the consequences that would be applied in most human interactions (e.g., rejection). The therapeutic encounter consists of social behavior and its context is vulnerable to the same cultural and societal practices that empower and privilege members of certain social groups while disempowering others. Therefore, therapy, as a social context, will inevitably evoke or elicit behaviors that are steeped in the societal and cultural context in which the therapy takes place.

Behavior analytic definition of privilege. Privilege is intimately related to power and as discussed earlier, is the result of certain groups "having power." Earlier we defined privilege as "unearned advantage ... [and] ... conferred dominance " (McIntosh, 1988, p. 1). Privilege from a behavior analytic perspective can be understood as differential access to more important reinforcers. The greater the access, the higher the probability that one will come into contact with reinforcers. Members of certain social groups have greater access to more important reinforcers, such as money, safety (e.g., living in a neighborhood that has less crime), and leisure (e.g., taking vacations, working 40 hours a week instead of 50 or 60 hours). For members of certain social groups, the probability of contacting these reinforcers is greater than for members of other groups, and these individuals therefore can be understood to "have privilege." In the United States, men typically earn more wealth for the same job as women even if both have similar educational and professional credentials (Marini & Fan, 1997; O'Neill, 2003; United States General Accounting Office, 2003). Thus, men in the United States are understood to "have privilege." Additionally, and perhaps more importantly, these reinforcers are not always contingent on the "privileged" individual's behavior. Thus, the reinforcers are "unearned" and based on membership in a certain social group.

Dealing with Sociopolitical Aspects of the Therapist–Client Relationship

As discussed earlier in the chapter, we believe that FAP therapists need to become more sensitive to how power and privilege can enter into the therapeutic context. To help FAP therapists become more aware of these phenomena, we propose that integrating FAP with feminist therapies will aid in increasing FAP therapists' awareness of their own participation as well as their clients' participation in systems of oppression and offer techniques for working with power and privilege in a therapeutic context. We now turn our attention to how FAP can be used specifically to help therapists identify and work with power and privilege in the therapeutic relationship.

   In most writings about FAP the focus is on the client's behaviors, but in FAP trainings and in supervision sessions there is extended discussion, examination, and analysis of the therapist's behaviors in the therapeutic relationship (Callaghan, 2006a, 2006b; Tsai, Callaghan, Kohlenberg, Follette, & Darrow, 2008). These authors have suggested a nomenclature and model for tracking therapist problematic behaviors (T1s) and therapist improved behaviors (T2s). The categories T1 and T2 are parallel to CRB1 and CRB2 for classifying client behaviors: CRB1s are problematic client behaviors that occur in the therapeutic context, T1s are problematic therapist behaviors that occur in the therapeutic context. Similarly, CRB2s and T2s are improvements in client and therapist behaviors, respectively, that occur in the therapeutic context. FAP therapists are trained to become aware of their own problematic behaviors and improvements that occur in the context of the therapeutic relationship, although they are not a target of treatment in the therapeutic context itself. Thus, the FAP therapist is not an objective, all-knowing expert, but an individual engaging with clients to help them move toward their goals in therapy. Any engagement with a client using FAP can be deeply personal, and all client interactions in FAP can evoke T1s and T2s.

An example of T1s and T2s may help to illustrate this more clearly. The first author (CMT) was working with a client who was very talkative and tended to dominate the therapy session by talking over her, interrupting her, or simply speaking for long periods of time. These behaviors constituted a CRB1 for the client and functioned to distance him from relationships and to avoid feelings of vulnerability. CMT had great difficulty interrupting the client, which was increasingly interfering with her ability to work effectively with him (e.g., interventions were not implemented or only partially implemented). CMT's hesitancy and avoidance of interrupting the client was a T1, a problematic therapist behavior that was occurring in the therapeutic relationship. After recognizing this behavior as a T1, CMT was able to notice her avoidance, and in time was able to change her behavior and interrupt the client when the discussion became tangential, a T2 (therapist improvement in the therapy relationship). This enabled CMT to begin implementing therapeutic interventions that were targeted to the client's treatment goals.

Just as with CRB1s and CRB2s, T1s and T2s can include a variety of behavior classes. We believe certain classes of behaviors, however, deserve particular attention and a unique designation to help make therapists more aware of these specific behaviors as they are emitted in the therapeutic context. The classes of behaviors focused on in this chapter are based on power and privilege exercised in the presence of individuals belonging to groups that are systematically oppressed and/or underprivileged. As discussed earlier, we believe that therapists are unwilling participants in promoting systemic and institutionalized practices based on racist and sexist (as well as other forms of discrimination and oppression) values inherent in the dominant culture. Because this type of power and privilege is embedded in the very contexts of which we are part, it can be extremely difficult for us to recognize our participation in prejudicial practices.

We believe that FAP, with its emphasis on examining therapist behaviors in the therapeutic context, can provide a method of identifying and examining how therapists and their clients may be unknowing participants in discrimination and oppression. However, we believe that it is not enough just to hope that FAP therapists will include these practices in their examination of their T1s and T2s and of their client's CRB1s and CRB2s. Rather a specific classification and method for doing so must be articulated. We propose the addition of a class of T1s/CRB1s and T2s/CRB2s called Sociopolitical 1s (SP1s) and Sociopolitical 2s (SP2s) that are based on therapist and client behaviors rooted in power and privilege associated with membership in specific socially constructed groups (e.g., race, ethnicity, gender). We will discuss SP1s, SP2s, and preliminary methods of identifying them in the section below.

SP1s and SP2s

SP1s are therapist or client in-session problematic behaviors (i.e., T1s or CRB1s) that reinforce or maintain power and privilege based on an individual's membership in a specific socially constructed group. As discussed earlier in the chapter, power is defined as the reinforcement relation that includes the more important reinforcers, and privilege is defined as access to the more important reinforcers. SP1s are behaviors that maintain certain reinforcement relations, namely those determined by a sociopolitical context in which members of specific socially constructed groups have increased access to the more important reinforcers. For example, the first author (CMT) was a treating a middle age female who was struggling with her desire to have a family and her desire to be successful in her career (a more detailed examination of this case with respect to SP1s and SP2s is presented below). CMT subtly encouraged the client to focus on her career by spending more time in therapy sessions on the client's vocational struggles and by redirecting the conversations toward the client's career issues instead of her concerns about family. These behaviors constituted a SP1 on the part of CMT because they functioned to maintain power for a specific socially constructed group (higher-educated individuals) and to decrease the client's access to a certain class of important reinforcers (reinforcers that are available by relating with intimate others). In this very brief example, the client tacted two competing sources of reinforcers: reinforcers related to her career and reinforcers related to intimate relating. CMT unknowingly reinforced talk about her own values (career) and subsequently punished talk about family (a value of her client's). It is not known which of the two sets of reinforcers was more important to the client, but what is clear from this illustration is that CMT, without awareness, promoted her own value system and the dominant culture's value system and in turn, silenced her client and punished talk about relational values (i.e., wanting to start a family) and possibly limited her access to a class of reinforcers that she tacted as important.

Therapist SP1s can result in culturally insensitive behaviors toward the client. Research in the area of multicultural counseling and therapy has shown that culturally insensitive practices can lead to treatment drop-outs (Brach & Fraserirector, 2000) and may be associated with lower therapeutic alliance or decreased client trust of the therapist (Brach & Fraserirector, 2000; Sue & Sue, 2002). Yet, as argued above, therapists are often unaware of their culturally biased behaviors. Thus, identifying the therapist's potential culturally biased behaviors as they may occur in therapy sessions is a critical first step in reducing their occurrence. Identifying SP1s may serve as an intervention in and of itself in that it helps therapists tact their culturally biased in-session behaviors, which may lead some individuals to change their behavior. However, mere awareness of SP1s may not be enough to change an entrenched repertoire. Research on implicit racial bias, for instance, shows that even when individuals can tact their bias against certain racial groups, this does not necessarily change their behaviors toward that group (Lane, Banaji, Nosek, & Greenwald, 2007).

Sociopolitical 2s (SP2s) may be therapist improvements (T2s) or client improvements (CRB2s) that reduce behaviors maintaining power and privilege. SP2s are behaviors that attempt to broaden access to the more important reinforcers to members of non-dominant groups. Because therapists are embedded within a social (and perhaps an institutional) context that grants power and privilege to particular groups of individuals and limits the power and privileges of other groups of individuals, shaping therapist SP2s is paramount. Although awareness of SP1s may not lead to behavior change, it may be a first approximation toward identifying and engaging in SP2s.

What can we as therapists do to remedy the situation, to avoid perpetuating the psychopathology of oppression? One element of a solution is to maintain a relentless emphasis on the functions of behavior in its context. If we can understand that a client's unhappiness or depression is, in part, an appropriate response to a larger social situation over which we and the client have little direct control, we may avoid blaming the victim for his/her suffering. Our interventions will acknowledge the self-maintaining nature of oppression and seek to focus the client's efforts (as well as our own) on areas and techniques for *effective* action in the given context.

Another critical element is to increase awareness of the sociopolitical antecedents of one's own behavior and the effect of those antecedents on others. Psychotherapy is a mainstream cultural phenomenon and as such participates in maintaining the invisible assumptions that *white color, male gender, educated, middle-to-upper-class, heterosexual values in general and Judeo-Christian views specifically* are normal and universally desirable. To the extent that these assumptions remain unexamined and unacknowledged as partial determiners of our behavior in session, we will remain blind maintainers of an oppressive system.

The ADDRESSING Model for Developing Therapist Self-Awareness

One useful tool for identifying potential SP1s and shaping SP2s is Patricia Hays' ADDRESSING model, described in her book, *Addressing Cultural Complexities in Practice* (2001). This model promotes an awareness of the complexities of social relationships: an individual may be dominant in some contexts and subordinate in others. Thus, it is more true to the actualities of the therapeutic situation than a more simplistic one-up, one-down model of power relations.

This model covers major areas of socially constructed group difference and is most useful for helping us become aware of the complex and contextual nature of power and privilege in an idiographic way. The acronym ADDRESSING is a mnemonic for: Age (effects of generation), Disability (born and acquired), Developmental, Religion, Ethnicity, SES (socioeconomic status, including occupation, education, income, rural or urban, family name), Sexual orientation, Indigenous heritage, National origin (immigrant, refugee, international student), and Gender. Effects of membership and status within these groups are *systemic processes* that manifest *between and among* groups. One may be privileged in one context and not in another. Awareness of these complexities will help us to negotiate the complexities of the therapeutic encounter as well as to help the client deal skillfully with daily life situations.

A Revised FAP Case Conceptualization Form

To further help with the identification of SP1s and SP2s, we have added columns to the FAP case conceptualization form for the therapist to note specific instances of each behavior class (see Fig. 7.1). The revised FAP case conceptualization form is intended to be a flexible working document that can be changed as evidence is gathered and hypotheses are tested, rejected, or kept. The two additions to the FAP case conceptualization form are the SP1 and SP2 columns, and the page containing Hays' ADDRESSING model as a means to identify SP1s and SP2s. Although our focus has primarily been on therapist behaviors as potential SP1s and SP2s, client behaviors can also be potential SP1s and SP2s, and therapists should note these along with their own SP1s and SP2s on the revised case conceptualization form.

A Clinical Case Example

A clinical case example may help clarify how these additions to the FAP case conceptualization play out in therapy. A[4] was a 35-year-old woman seeking treatment for anxiety and depression with the first author (CMT). She had recently graduated from a Ph.D. program and was currently looking for a job in her new career field when she entered treatment. A was the middle daughter of Eastern European immigrants who she said were "old fashioned." Although currently married, A described struggles with intimate relationships because of difficulty trusting others, as well as anxiety about her new career. CMT conducted cognitive behavioral therapy for depression and anxiety, and the client reported significant reductions in most of her depressive symptoms and some of her anxiety symptoms. As therapy progressed CMT worked with the client to begin tackling her core beliefs about trusting others as well as her competence/worth (for a discussion of FAP's perspective of working with core beliefs please see the chapter on FAP-Enhanced Cognitive Therapy by Kohlenberg, Kanter, Tsai, & Weeks, this volume).

The therapy at this time became much more focused on the therapeutic relationship with CMT as a means of identifying, processing, and countering her maladaptive core beliefs about interpersonal relationships and her competence/worth. One of A's problematic clinically relevant behaviors (CRB1s) was not expressing doubts or any negative comments about the therapy or the therapist because she was fearful that CMT would judge her negatively and think of her as a "bad client." A also had difficulties expressing her needs, particularly if she believed that they would lead CMT to construing her as a "bad or uncooperative client." Another of A's CRB1s was her difficulty in disclosing her emotions to CMT, in particular strong negative emotions of grief and anger, even when CMT actively encouraged her to do so. CRB2s (clinically relevant behaviors that move the client toward their therapeutic

---

[4]The demographics of the client and certain facts about the case have been altered to protect the client's identity.

For the Client

Relevant history (including sociopolitical factors that may affect the therapeutic relationship)	Daily life problems	In vivo problems/CRB1s	Daily life goals	In vivo improvements/ CRB2s
		SP1s		SP2s

For the Therapist

Relevant history (including sociopolitical factors that may affect the therapeutic relationship)	Daily life problems	In vivo problems/T1s	Daily life goals	In vivo improvements/ T2s
		SP1s		SP2s

Fig. 7.1 Revised FAP case conceptualization forms to include sociopolitical 1s (SP1s) and sociopolitical 2s (SP 2s). Adapted from the FAP case conceptualization form described in Kohlenberg, Kanter, Bolling, Parker, and Tsai (2002)

The ADDRESSING Framework can be used to help assess how sociopolitical histories may

impact client's and therapist's behaviors (SP1s & SP2s).

A = Age and age-related factors

D = Disability

D = Development (psychological, social developmental factors)

R = Religion

E = Ethnicity

S = Socioeconomic Status

S = Sexual Orientation

I = Indigenous heritage

N = Nationality

G = Gender

Fig. 7.2   The ADDRESSING framework (Hays, 2001, pp. 6–7)

goals) for A were being more open or more willing to contact strong emotions and to discuss her desire for avoidance of emotions. During this phase of therapy, A began to discuss an increasingly common conflict she experienced with her parents. The conflict was about her desire to have a career before having children, which was opposed to her parents' desires and beliefs that she should begin to have children in the near future and that she should stay at home to raise them. A described her desire to have both a family and a career, and expressed sadness about the effects of the conflict on her relationship with her parents, as well as the anxiety she experienced whenever she thought about the conflict.

CMT helped A examine the emotions of the conflict and promptly began working on ways to counteract any negative effects of the conflict on A's beliefs about her self-worth, working with A to help her come up with effective strategies to cope with the conflict. Soon after, A stopped discussing the issue and reported that although the conflict was still a source of anxiety, she did not wish to focus her time in therapy discussing it further. Although CMT wished to continue discussing the conflict and its effects on A, she refrained because she wanted to reinforce A for her CRB2 of expressing wants and needs. As CMT was preparing to give a presentation on SP1s and SP2s at a local conference, she returned to this case and began to realize that she may inadvertently have silenced the client. Upon further reflection on the interactions between A and herself, she realized that she focused more on the client's desire to have a career and did not investigate how the client's unique cultural standing and acculturation status may be influencing her understanding and reactions to the conflict. As discussed earlier, CMT's behaviors maintained power within a dominant group (higher-educated individuals) and may have denied the client access to important reinforcers (relating to others).

In addition to using the revised FAP case conceptualization form and the Hays' ADDRESSING model, therapists are encouraged to seek out information about multicultural counseling practices and research on diversity in clinical practices, and to talk openly with providers of similar and of different ethnicities, gender, and so forth to examine how their therapeutic behaviors are culturally biased. FAP practitioners often ask themselves "What is the function of the client's (or my) behavior?" and "Is that behavior a CRB1 (T1) or a CRB2 (T2)?" We propose that FAP practitioners also ask themselves the following questions: "Am I engaging in a behavior that is culturally biased toward my client?" "Am I making untested assumptions about my client based on my own sociopolitical background?" and "In what ways am I inadvertently silencing my client?" We believe the above actions will help therapists become more aware of power and privilege in the therapeutic context and help reduce the likelihood of engaging in behaviors that maintain oppression of specific socially constructed groups.

Additional Ways to Work with the Sociopolitical Aspects of the Therapist–Client Relationship

A mere intellectual acknowledgement of our biases may do nothing to remedy the situation. Awareness of privilege and power needs to be constantly renewed. This is a *practice* of countering oppression. We also propose that FAP therapists use feminist therapy techniques to help work with power and privilege in the therapeutic context, as discussed earlier. For example, therapists may choose to ask their clients about their experiences with oppression, discrimination, and prejudice. Therapists may also choose to examine with their clients how oppression, discrimination, and prejudice currently operate in their lives; how these phenomena influence their difficulties, their participation in therapy and the therapeutic relationship, and their work toward goals and values. If deemed therapeutic (as based on the case conceptualization and discussions with the client), therapists may work with clients to help them become involved in community activism or activities that work toward reducing oppression and discrimination.

Using the framework of the five FAP rules, the integration of FAP and feminist therapies may appear in the following manner:

- Rule 1: Watch for CRBs. Increased awareness of the sociopolitical aspects of the therapist–client relationship, the sociopolitical history of the therapist, and the sociopolitical history of the client will help the therapist begin to notice CRB1s, CRB2s, T1s, and T2s based on sociopolitical contexts and histories. Methods of increasing awareness were described above and include use of the revised case conceptualization form (SP1s and SP2s), Hays' ADDRESSING model, and discussion with colleagues about our biases.

- Rule 2: Evoke CRBs. We believe that therapists will not need to evoke SPs intentionally because the therapist–client relationship and the context of therapy are microcosms of the sociopolitical contexts operating outside of therapy, so the behaviors will occur naturally. Nevertheless, if therapists choose to evoke SPs intentionally they may do so by asking some of the questions posed above (e.g., asking clients how they believe oppression, discrimination, and prejudice affect their participation in therapy).
- Rule 3: Consequate CRBs. Therapists naturally consequate all client behaviors, but with an increased awareness of the sociopolitical context of therapy, they may choose to reinforce client behaviors that work toward increasing equality and reducing oppression (e.g., reinforcing a client's discussion about her cultural experiences).
- Rule 4: Notice your effect on the client. With increased awareness of the sociopolitical context of therapy, therapists can be more aware of how their behaviors may reflect bias and effect a subtle oppression of their clients, and they can begin to discern the impact of interventions to decrease oppression and increase equality in the therapeutic relationship.
- Rule 5: Provide rules to promote generalization. Therapists can provide rules about oppression and power and their effects on clients that may help them generalize their awareness of these factors outside of therapy. These rules may help encourage client behaviors that reduce oppression, increase equality, and/or promote social change.

Conclusion

Put simply, being human, therapists often unknowingly engage in behaviors that are culturally biased. This should come as no surprise to behavior analysts, as our behaviors are the products of long histories of reinforcement, our physiology, as well as ontogenic and phylogenic contingencies in the environment – contingencies that do not need to be tacted in order to affect our behavior. If we look more closely, we will see that it is not just our immediate environment that impacts our behaviors, but that larger social, political, and cultural environments – all with deep historical roots – impact our behaviors as well. We believe that FAP – in conjunction with feminist thinking – can offer practitioners interested in reducing culturally biased therapeutic practices a coherent and concise system with which to identify and modify problematic therapist behaviors that maintain the status quo in existing systems of oppression. We offer the beginning of an integration of FAP with feminist therapies and recognize that more can be done to further their integration. We agree with the feminist principle that the personal is political and the political is personal. It is time for FAP therapists to notice and act to decrease oppressive practices in the therapeutic context. It is time to work actively toward equal access to important reinforcers for all individuals.

References

Aebischer, V. (1988). Knowledge as a result of conflicting intergroup relations. In M. M. Gergen (Ed.), *Feminist thought and the structure of knowledge* (pp. 142–151). New York: University Press.

Ballou, M., & Brown, L. S. (2002). *Rethinking mental and health disorder: Feminist perspectives.* New York: Guilford Press.

Banaji, M. R. (1993). The psychology of gender: A perspective on perspectives. In A. E. Beall & R. J. Sternberg (Eds.), *The Psychology of gender* (pp. 251–273). New York: Guilford Press.

Baum, W. (2005). Relationships, management, and government. In *Understanding behaviorism: Behavior, culture, and evolution* (2nd ed., pp. 213–236). Malden, MA: Blackwell Publishing.

Bem, S. L. (1981). Gender schema theory: A cognitive account of sex-typing. *Psychological Review, 88*, 354–364.

Biglan, A. (1995). *Changing cultural practices: A contextualist framework for intervention research.* Reno, NV: Context Press.

Brach, C., & Fraserirector, I. (2000). Can cultural competency reduce racial and ethnic health disparities? A review and conceptual model. *Medical Care Research and Review, 57*, 181–217.

Brown, L. S. (1986). From alienation to connection: Feminist therapy with Post-Traumatic Stress Disorder. *Women and Therapy, 5*, 13–26.

Brown, L. S. (1992). Feminists perspectives on psychopathology: Introduction. In L. S. Brown & M. Ballou (Eds.), *Personality and psychopathology: Feminist reappraisals.* New York: Guilford.

Brown, L. S. (1994). *Subversive dialogues: Theory in feminist therapy.* New York: Basic Books.

Brown, K. (2009). *Development of a behavior analytic treatment for depressed women: Integrating principles of feminist therapy.* Unpublished doctoral dissertation, University of Wisconsin, Milwaukee, WI.

Brown, L. S., & Ballou, M. (Eds.). (1992). *Personality and psychopathology: Feminist reappraisals.* New York: Guilford Press.

Brown, L. S., & Brodsky, A. M. (1992). The future of feminist therapy. *Psychotherapy: Theory, Research, Practice, Training, 29*, 51–57.

Brown, L. S., & Walker, L. E. A. (1990). Feminist therapy perspectives on self-disclosure. In G. Stricker & M. Fisher (Eds.), *Self-disclosure in the therapeutic relationship* (pp. 135–154). New York: Plenum Press.

Callaghan, G. M. (2006a). Functional analytic psychotherapy and supervision. *International Journal of Behavioral and Consultation Therapy, 2*, 416–431.

Callaghan, G. M. (2006b). Functional assessment of skills for interpersonal therapists: The FASIT system: For the assessment of therapist behavior for interpersonally-based interventions including Functional Analytic Psychotherapy (FAP) or FAP-enhanced treatments. *The Behavior Analyst Today, 7*, 399–433.

Campbell, R., & Wasco, S. M. (2000). Feminist approaches to social science: Epistemological and methodological tenets. *American Journal of Community Psychology, 28*, 773–791.

Caplan, P. J. (1995). *They say you're crazy: How the world's most powerful psychiatrists decide who's normal.* New York: Addison-Wesley.

Eagly, A. H. (1983). Gender and social influence. *American Psychologist, 38*(9), pp. 971–981.

Enns, C. Z. (2004). *Feminist theories and feminist psychotherapies: Origins, themes, and diversity* (2nd ed.). New York: Haworth Press.

Fee, E. (1986). Critiques of modern science: The relationship of feminism to other radical epistemologies. In R. Bleier (Ed.), *Feminist approaches to science* (pp. 42–56). New York: Pergamon.

Fine, M. (1992). *Disruptive voices: The possibilities of feminist research.* Michigan: University of Michigan Press.

Gilbert, L. A. (1980). Feminist therapy. In A. M. Brodsky & R. T. Hare-Mustin (Eds.), *Women and psychotherapy* (pp. 245–266). New York: Guilford Press.

Glenn, S. S. (1988). Contingencies and metacontingencies: Towards a synthesis of behavior analysis and cultural materialism. *The Behavior Analyst, 11*, 161–180.

Glenn, S. S., & Malagodi, E. F. (1991). Process and content in behavioral and cultural phenomena. *Behavior and Social Issues, 1*, 1–14.

Gondolf, E. W. (1998). *Assessing woman battering in mental health services*. Thousand Oaks, CA: Sage.

Guerin, B. (1994). *Analyzing social behavior: Behavior analysis and the social sciences*. Reno, NV: Context Press.

Harding, S. (1986). *The science question in feminism*. Ithaca: Cornell University Press.

Hayes, S. C., Barnes-Holmes, D., & Roche, B. (2001). *Relational frame theory: A post-Skinnerian account of human language and cognition*. New York: Kluwer Academic/Plenum Publishers.

Hayes, S. C., & Brownstein, A. J. (1986). Mentalism, behavior-behavior relations, and a behavior analytic view of the purposes of science. *Behavior Analyst, 9*, 175–190.

Hays, P. (2001). *Addressing cultural complexities in practice: A framework for clinicians and counselors*. Washington, DC: American Psychological Association.

Herrmann, A. C., & Stewart, A. J. (1994). *Theorizing feminism: Parallel trends in the humanities and social sciences*. Boulder, CO: Westview.

Hineline, P. (1992). A self-interpretive behavior analysis. *American Psychologist, 47*, 1274–1286.

Kaschak, E. (1992). *Engendered lives: A new psychology of women's experience*. New York: Harper Collins.

Keller, E. F. (1985). *Reflections on gender and science*. New Haven, CT: Yale University Press.

Kirk, G., & Okazawa-Rey, M. (1998). *Women's lives: Multicultural perspectives*. Mountain View, CA: Mayfield.

Kohlenberg, R. J., Kanter, J. W., Bolling, M. Y., Parker, C., & Tsai, M. (2002). Enhancing cognitive therapy for depression with Functional Analytic Psychotherapy: Treatment guidelines and empirical findings. *Cognitive and Behavioral Practice, 9*(3), 213–229.

Kohlenberg, R. J., & Tsai, M. (1991). *Functional analytic psychotherapy: Creating intense and curative therapeutic relationships*. New York: Plenum Press.

Lane, K. A., Banaji, M. R., Nosek, B. A., & Greenwald, A. G. (2007). Understanding and using the Implicit Association Test: IV. What we know (so far). In B. Wittenbrink & N. S. Schwarz (Eds.), *Implicit measures of attitudes: Procedures and controversies*. New York: Guilford Press.

Marecek, J., & Hare-Mustin, R. T. (1991). A short history of the future: Feminism and clinical psychology. *Psychology of Women Quarterly, 15*, 521–536.

Marecek, J., & Kravetz, D. (1998). Putting politics into practice: Feminist therapy as feminist praxis. *Women and Therapy, 21*, 17–36.

Marini, M. M., & Fan, P. L. (1997). The gender gap in earnings at career entry. *American Sociological Review, 62*(4), 588–604.

McIntosh, P. (1988). White Privilege and Male Privilege: A personal account of coming to see correspondences through work in women's studies. *White Privilege: Unpacking the Invisible Knapsack*. Retrieved July 1, 2005, from http://www.case.edu/president/aaction/UnpackingTheKnapsack.pdf

O'Neill, J. (2003). The gender gap in wages, circa 2000. *The American Economic Review, 93*(2), 309–314.

Park, S. M. (2004). Feminism and therapy. In C. Negy (Ed.), *Cross-cultural psychotherapy: Toward a critical understanding of diverse clients* (pp. 281–300). Reno, NV: Bent Tree Press.

Parott, L. J. (1986). On the differences between verbal and social behavior. In P. N. Chase & L. J. Parrott (Eds.), *Psychological aspects of language* (pp. 91–117). Springfield, IL: Charles C. Thomas.

Rabin, C., Tsai, M., & Kohlenberg, R. J. (1996). Targeting sex-role and power issues with a functional analytic approach: Gender patterns in behavioral marital therapy. *Journal of Feminist Family Therapy, 8*, 1–24.

Reinharz, S. (1992). *Feminist methods in social research*. New York: Oxford.

Ruiz, M. R. (1995). B. F. Skinner's radical behaviorism: Historical misconstructions and grounds for feminist reconstructions. *Behavior and Social Issues*, 5(2), 29–44.

Ruiz, M. R. (1998). Personal agency in feminist theory: Evicting the illusive dweller. *Behavior Analyst*, 21(2), 179–192.

Ruiz, M. R. (2003). Inconspicuous sources of behavioral control: The case of gendered practices. *The Behavior Analyst Today, 4*, 12–16.

Ruiz, M., & Terry, C. M. (2006). *Enhancing behavior analytic principles with feminist principles*. Paper presented at the meeting of the Association for Behavior Analysis (ABA), Atlanta, GA.

Sidman, M., Wynne, C. K., Maguire, R. W., & Barnes, T. (1989). Functional classes and equivalence relations. *Journal of the Experimental Analysis of Behavior, 52*, 261–274.

Skinner, B. F. (1945). The operational analysis of psychological terms. *Psychological Review, 52*, 270–277.

Skinner, B. F. (1953). *Science and human behavior*. New York: Macmillan.

Skinner, B. F. (1969). *Contingencies of reinforcement–A theoretical analysis*. New York: Appleton-Century-Crofts.

Skinner, B. F. (1974). *About behaviorism*. New York: Alfred A. Knopf.

Skinner, B. F. (1978). *Reflections on behaviorism and society*. Englewood Cliffs, NJ: Prentice Hall.

Steiner-Adair, C. (1986). The body politic: Normal female adolescent development and the development of eating disorders. *Journal of the American Academy of Psychoanalysis, 14*, 95–114.

Sturdivant, S. (1980). *Therapy with women: A feminist philosophy of treatment*. New York: Springer.

Sue, D. W., & Sue, D. (2002). *Counseling the culturally diverse: Theory and practice*. New York: Wiley.

Terry, C. M. (2005, August). *FAP and the sociopolitical: Power and oppression in therapy*. Paper Presented at the 1st annual FAP Summit, Seattle, WA.

Terry, C. M., & Bolling, M. Y. (2006, August). *Sociopolitical issues and FAP: Unconscious assumptions, silenced voices*. Paper presented at the 2nd annual FAP Summit, Seattle, WA.

Terry, C. M., & Bolling, M. Y. (2007, May). Functional Analytic Psychotherapy (FAP): A context to analyze and work with issues of power and privilege. In C. M. Terry (Chair), *Power and privilege: Synthesizing behavior analytic theories and feminist theories*. Symposium conducted at the meeting of the Association for Behavior Analysis (ABA), San Diego, CA.

Tsai, M., Callaghan, G. M., Kohlenberg, R. J., Follette, W. C., & Darrow, S. M. (2008). Supervision and therapist self-development. In M. Tsai, R. J. Kohlenberg, J. W. Kanter, B. Kohlenberg, W. C. Follette, & G. M. Callaghan (Eds.), *A guide to Functional Analytic Psychotherapy: Awareness, courage, love and behaviorism* (pp. 167–198). New York: Springer.

Unger, R. K. (1986). Looking toward the future by looking at the past: Social activism and social history. *Journal of Social Issues, 42*, 215–227.

United States General Accounting Office. (2003). *Women's earnings: Work patterns partially explain difference in men's and women's earnings*. Retrieved February 22, 2008, from http://www.gao.gov/news.items/d0435.pdf

Veldhuis, C. B. (2001). The trouble with power. *Women and Therapy, 23*(2), pp. 37–56.

Walker, L. E. A. (1994). *The abused woman and survivor therapy: A practical guide for the psychotherapist*. Washington, DC: American Psychological Association.

Worell, J., & Remer, P. (1992). *Feminist perspectives in therapy – An empowerment model for women*. Chichester: Wiley.

Worell, J., & Remer, P. (2003). *Feminist perspectives in therapy: Empowering diverse women* (2nd ed.). New York: Wiley.

Wyche, K. F., & Rice, J. K. (1997). Feminist therapy: From dialogue to tenets. In J. Worell & N. G. Johnson (Eds.), *Shaping the future of feminist psychology: Education, research, and practice* (pp. 57–72). Washington, DC: American Psychological Association.

Zimmerman, J. (1963). Technique for sustaining behavior with conditioned reinforcement. *Science, 142*, 682–684.

Part II
FAP Across Settings and Populations

Chapter 8
FAP-Enhanced Couple Therapy: Perspectives and Possibilities

Alan S. Gurman, Thomas J. Waltz, and William C. Follette

A Functional Analytic Psychotherapy (Kohlenberg & Tsai, 1991) approach to couple therapy or a FAP-enhanced approach to other variants of behavioral couple therapies (Integrative Behavioral Couple Therapy, Cognitive Behavioral Couple Therapy, Traditional Behavioral Couple Therapy) may seem to have been inevitable in the context of the rapidly evolving "third wave" of behavior therapy (Functional Analytic Psychotherapy, Acceptance and Commitment Therapy, Dialectical Behavior Therapy). And yet, in the broader world of couple and family therapy, it seems ironic that a FAP-enhanced style of therapy rarely has been addressed (cf. Lopez, 2003; Rabin, Tsai, & Kohlenberg, 1996).

All the two dozen or more major approaches to couple and family therapy that have emerged and evolved since the 1950s explicitly have emphasized context (e.g., the context of symptoms, the context of meaning). Ironically, probably none of these approaches have ever explicitly identified that what may be operating in their methods is nearly identical to the most fundamental principle and goal of FAP, whether in individual therapy or couple therapy: the changing of behavior in its natural environment in order to improve the generalization of therapy-induced change to life beyond the consultation room.

It may be that while FAP-relevant (e.g., operant or behavior analytic) principles readily can be demonstrated to be at work in the therapy of such varied methods as structural family therapy, emotionally focused couple therapy, and object relations couple therapy (Gurman, 2008a), therapists of such persuasions do not identify the operations of behavior analytic principles in their work because few of them have had training in, or often even any substantial exposure to, behavioral therapies of any sort.

Earlier behavioral couple therapies (Traditional Behavioral Couple Therapy, Jacobson & Margolin, 1979; Baucom, Epstein, LaTaillade, & Kirby, 2008) generally do not harness the potential power of a FAP case conceptualization

A.S. Gurman (✉)
University of Wisconsin School of Medicine and Public Health, Madison, WI, USA
e-mail: asgurman@wisc.edu

J.W. Kanter et al. (eds.), *The Practice of Functional Analytic Psychotherapy*,
DOI 10.1007/978-1-4419-5830-3_8, © Springer Science+Business Media, LLC 2010

or specifically use contingent responding to within-session clinically relevant behaviors (CRBs), which we discuss below. Early behavioral couple therapies (e.g., Jacobson & Margolin, 1979) decidedly were focused on helping couples more closely approximate idealized standards for "healthy" couple behavior. Those approaches rested on the so-called matching-to-sample philosophy: through research, identify what reliably and validly differentiates "healthy" or "happy" from "unhealthy" or "unhappy" married couples and then develop and apply clinical treatment methods to help "unhappy" couples look (behave) more like "happy" couples. That is, the overwhelming emphasis in those earlier behavioral couple therapy methods was on shifting, shaping, and modifying the *form* of couples' interactions. These approaches were heavily prescriptive of both the couple's target behaviors and the therapist's facilitative behavior.

More recently, Integrative Behavioral Couple Therapy (IBCT) (e.g., Christensen, Jacobson, & Babcock, 1995; Dimidjian, Martell, & Christensen, 2008) has renewed an emphasis on more FAP-consistent behavioral principles for therapy with couples by (a) tailoring treatment goals to the couple and (b) calling upon greater use of natural (versus arbitrary) reinforcement and contingency-shaped (versus rule-governed) interventions (Berns & Jacobson, 2000).

Still, a FAP-enhanced couple therapy requires a therapist to work quite differently than the pioneers of behavioral couple therapy, including IBCT, have proposed. In this chapter, we suggest some of the major differences from the practice of common behavioral couple therapies and highlight changes that would be required by a FAP-enhanced approach to working with clinical couples.

Brief Overview

FAP-enhanced couple therapy brings an interpersonally focused behavior analytic approach to the assessment, conceptualization, and treatment of relationship distress. This chapter starts with a discussion of the assessment and case conceptualization process in FAP-enhanced couple therapy. This process is similar to that of FAP in individual therapy with the very significant added benefit of an important element of each partner's environment being present in each session (i.e., the other partner). We then discuss the structure of FAP-enhanced couple therapy. As a process-oriented approach, this discussion of structure is provided to help distinguish the approach from others that are more prescriptive of what particular actions the therapist is expected to take and the types of outcomes sought. This is followed by a discussion of FAP-enhanced couple therapy as a process. In this process-focused section, the establishment of rapport is discussed, followed by several guiding principles that are specific to this approach. Some techniques are discussed that, while not unique to FAP, illustrate how existing therapeutic approaches can take on a new life within a FAP-consistent case conceptualization. The final section helps therapists conceptualize their therapeutic interactions in terms of the underlying philosophy that guides FAP.

Assessment and Case Conceptualization in FAP-Enhanced Couple Therapy

The assessment process of FAP-enhanced couple therapy is very flexible and varies widely depending on the presenting relationship and the skills and stimulus properties that the therapist brings to the relationship. Like all FAP therapists, FAP-enhanced couple therapists need to be able to conceptualize interpersonal interactions in terms of behavioral principles (i.e., functional analysis). The following points aim to help orient newcomers to this approach in applying FAP to couple therapy; however, these points will not absolve newcomers of the need to increase their abstract and practical knowledge of behavior analysis.

1. *In assessing with a couple the nature of their major concerns and what maintains those concerns, no particular domains of behavior are privileged over others.* A functional analytic perspective on therapy with couples is not grounded in any particular set of standards for relational health. Still, couple therapists do not practice in a knowledge vacuum, and inevitably are informed by their awareness of the types of dimensions of couple relationships that may contain the central clinical problem. Thus, for example, communication and problem solving, sexuality, role expectations, attachment security, and capacity for other- and self-regulation of affect are reasonable (descriptive, not functional) domains to wonder and inquire about early in therapy as a source of hypotheses about what may be maintaining the couple's difficulties (cf. Hayes & Toarmino, 1995). The point is that the therapist must be sensitive to what is and is not working for the couple, instead of what "ought" to be working for them.
2. *In FAP-enhanced couple therapy, couple difficulties are not assumed to reflect fundamental skill deficits,* as is true of much traditional behavioral couple therapy. Therapists and partners often assume that relationship-enhancing repertoires are missing from the couple's relationship (i.e., constitute problems of acquisition). FAP-enhanced couple therapists, on the other hand, see these putative deficits as being more likely to reflect performance problems, i.e., situationally specific low-probability repertoires that are under unfortunate stimulus control. This is often made evident, for example, when one partner is described by the other as "lacking feeling," or "unempathic," as if those were broad personality traits, yet there is ample evidence that this partner shows such interpersonal effectiveness skills in other relationships. Several studies (e.g., Birchler, Weiss, & Vincent, 1975) of couple interactions strongly support this more functional perspective. A number of behavioral marital therapy researchers, including the late Neil Jacobson (Holtzworth-Munroe & Jacobson, 1991; Lawrence, Eldridge, Christensen, & Jacobson, 1999) have acknowledged the relevance of this acquisition–performance distinction with couples.
3. *In FAP-enhanced couple therapy, it is essential to think of couple problems in terms of functional classes,* i.e., that behaviors of similar form can have different functions in different contexts, and especially that different behaviors can have the same function. Identifying and understanding idiographically

relevant functional classes for a couple is mostly the responsibility of the therapist, although couples in effective therapy probably become better at such functional identification over time. These functional classes are identical to what IBCT refers to as "themes." Compared to IBCT, however, FAP-influenced couple therapy is much more likely to attend to the appearance of "events" within a response class during the therapy session itself, whereas IBCT is more likely to include more discussion of the varied ways (forms) in which a functional class is manifested outside the consulting room.

4. *The identification of functional classes requires the observation of patterns of behavior over time.* Although an explicitly experimental approach to conducting a functional analysis rarely occurs in the course of therapy, the therapist does have the opportunity to observe and experience the impact each partner has on each other and on the therapist over time. A descriptive functional analysis of these interactions provides a provisional working hypothesis that is continuously updated and/or revised as the therapist has the opportunity to observe and participate in larger samples of behavior as therapy progresses. It is important for the therapist to continuously review her hypotheses in light of ongoing interactions. This can keep previous interactions from excessively biasing hypotheses since the function of behavior may shift over the course of therapy.

5. *The FIAT (Functional Idiographic Assessment Template;* Callaghan, 2006*) categories can be used to facilitate identification of functional classes of behavior.* The FIAT looks at five categories of behavior that have high base rates of involvement in suboptimal interpersonal functioning.

   a. *Problems with identification and assertion of needs* can be a significant source of relationship distress. Such problems may exist either because such relationship-enhancing behavior is not historically in the repertoires of the partner(s), such behavior is punished within the current relationship, or such behavior is excessive and aversive to the partner.
   b. *Problems of impact and feedback* frequently contribute to relationship distress, for example, when a partner is excessively sensitive to the feedback from her partner or when a partner is insufficiently sensitive to his impact on his partner, commonly seen in coercive cycles of the pursuer–distancer relationship.
   c. *Problems of emotional experience and expression* also can take many forms, for example, individual difficulty in describing one's such experience can be relationally distancing (e.g., "stonewalling"), or excessive emotional disclosure can be experienced as aversive or become mutually dysregulating.
   d. *Problems of interpersonal closeness/intimacy* are very common sources of couple distress, for example, discrepant needs for and comfort with intimate relating, or differing expectations of what constitutes intimate relating.
   e. *Problems of interpersonal conflict*, such as verbally aggressive (e.g., criticism, contempt) or physically abusive behavior, are very common in couple therapy, and must be addressed or blocked to ensure each partner's willingness to continue in therapy.

The FIAT was developed for use in individual therapy, and is but one approach to identifying functionally relevant classes of problem behavior with couples. Any clinical approach that facilitates the identification of controlling relational themes can be used (e.g., Dimidjian et al., 2008).

Conceptualizing Clinically Relevant Behavior (CRB)

As with individual FAP, FAP-enhanced couple therapy focuses on three broad classes of behavior.

> *CRB1s*: These are behavior patterns that contribute to suboptimal relationship functioning. CRB1s can be characterized in three broad ways:
>
> a. *Behavioral excesses*: Some behavior patterns may work well in a relationship only in moderation (e.g., talking about work), while others may be considered excessive if they occur at all (e.g., any form of abuse). CRB1 behavioral excesses are those whose moderation or elimination would result in improved relationship functioning and satisfaction for the couple.
> b. *Behavioral deficits*: Some partners lack the skills to behave effectively. Occasionally, this involves an outright skills deficit in which an individual has no practical experience of a skill being supported by his social community (e.g., emotional disclosure). More often, an individual may have insufficient response variability/flexibility. It is often necessary to be able to communicate the same idea in several different ways to impact effectively the other partner. Limitations in the range of effective responding also can be conceptualized as a behavioral deficit.
> c. *Problems of stimulus control*: Perhaps it is most often the case that individuals have the skills they need to be interpersonally effective but fail to use them at appropriate times. Failure to use a skill in an appropriate situation can be conceptualized as a CRB1. Moreover, responses that work in other situations may not with the partner. This often happens when one partner's disclosure results in the other engaging in problem-solving behavior instead of providing emotional support (or vice versa depending on the relationship). This also happens when one partner solicits emotional disclosure from the other when the latter is seeking quiet time alone. In both of these situations, each partner's behavior is under the influence of what each would want in the situation independent from the other partner's needs.

> *CRB2s* are behavior patterns that are effective in themselves or as alternatives to CRB1s. This may involve developing a new skill or using an existing skill in a difficult situation. It may also involve the tempering of a behavioral excess – the first step of which simply may involve not emitting a CRB1 when presented with an opportunity. The therapist–partner relationships play

an exceptionally strong role in the identification of CRB2s. The therapist is better able to notice and appreciate small improvements in behavior. In contrast to an individual's partner, part of the therapist's role is to appreciate small improvements in behavior even though they may not be of sufficient magnitude to improve the couple's relationship. The special importance of therapist–partner interactions is explored later in this chapter.

CRB3s are client descriptions of situation–behavior–outcome relationships related to CRB1s and CRB2s. When clients can make these types of functional analyses they are in a better position to predict and influence their own behavior. These statements about the relationship include an adequate description of the types of situations or contexts that precede the behavior (e.g., "the therapist said something that I experienced as critical"), the behavior itself (e.g., "I crossed my arms, averted my gaze, and appeared disinterested"), and the outcome (e.g., "the therapist shifted the conversation to my partner instead of continuing to engage with me"). Early in therapy, this type of functional analysis may take a few minutes, that is, the partner notices what had just transpired after the moment is over. As the skill of noticing these functional relationships improves, clients can increasingly use them in real time.

A major caveat about CRB3s is that they can become a way of talking about therapy rather than engaging in the therapy. They also can be used as tools to blame the other partner for problems (e.g., "every time we visit my mother, I do 'X' (reasonably) and you in turn do 'Y' and you know that makes me angry"). CRB3 talk about out-of-session behavior should be monitored closely to ensure that it does not develop counter-therapeutic functions. CRB3 talk about in-session behavior affords the therapist access to the situational variables accompanying the statement where conventionality can be assessed.

The identification and exploration of CRBs serve several purposes. The purpose of identifying and exploring CRB1s is to determine interaction patterns (brief and broad) that negatively impact the relationship or that are likely to maintain dissatisfaction, distance and/or resentment. The purpose of identifying and exploring CRB2s is to determine interactional patterns that are likely to improve the relationship or maintain improvements. Training clients to engage in CRB3-related functional analyses should allow such talk to work as a tool to increase the likelihood of generalizing the personal work on CRB1s and CRB2s outside of the therapy session.

Presentation of the Case Conceptualization

After one or two sessions, the therapist presents an initial case conceptualization to the couple. It is important for the therapist to collaboratively present the formulation. It is not necessary to discuss CRBs as such although it is important to discuss what behavior patterns have not been working well (i.e., CRB1s) for each individual. The therapist should use what she noticed about the patterns of behavior that did not seem to work well to guide each partner to discuss what each notices that he or she does that is not working well. It is far better to have each partner identify these on his or her own than for the therapist to present a laundry list of ineffective responses. If the therapist has noticed a problematic behavior pattern that an individual does not identify, the therapist should describe the behavior and ask the individual how that pattern seems to be working for her. The therapist should allow the client's experience of his behavior patterns to guide the CRB identification process; it sometimes takes clients time to notice that a particular pattern is a CRB1. Thus, the first step involves finding where there is agreement between the therapist and the client over which behavior patterns are not working. Such agreement is important for the treatment contract because working on CRB1s in light of a mutually agreed upon case conceptualization frames the work as a form of therapist caring. Thus, skillfully done, the presentation of a case conceptualization frames future therapist in vivo CRB1 feedback as a type of caring intended to help the client move toward doing what is more likely to work in her relationship. Skillful discussion of CRB1s can enhance the intimacy of the therapeutic relationship and set a true collaborative tone for the course of therapy. Discussion of CRB1s should have the effect of communicating empathy, understanding, and compassion.

It is also important to consider discussing what types of responding may be considered improvements (i.e., CRB2s). This does not have to be an exhaustive discussion, but partners often can note that they are able to engage in some forms of more effective behavior in other relationships. This discussion also provides an opportunity to discuss what small improvements actually may look like since they are at high risk for not being noticed by either partner within their interactions.

It is important to place nearly equal emphasis on each partner's CRB1s. A generous and skillful discussion of CRB1s should strengthen the therapeutic relationship and the therapist should aim to have a strong and collaborative relationship with each partner. Neither partner should become the "project" or "broken one." The relationship is a system and partners typically respond to each other's CRB1s in kind. If one partner seems to have more egregious examples of CRB1s than the other, the therapist may present them in terms of broader functional categories (e.g., dismissing feedback, failing to reciprocate affection) rather than a litany of individual behaviors. The individual behaviors should be used as examples of the functional classes rather than in place of them. As therapy progresses, it will be useful for partners to be able to conceptualize novel examples of these classes as they occur.

Finally, if a partner disagrees with a therapist's initial conceptualization of a CRB1, the therapist should not dismiss the disagreement as resistance. A great deal can be learned about the partner's experience of the relationship by asking her to describe the workability of the suspected problematic behavior pattern. Therapist hypotheses are not always correct and collaborating over a disagreement can enrich the therapeutic relationship. If the therapist maintains a generous as opposed to authoritative stance through the disagreement process, most clients will agree that it will be perfectly acceptable for the therapist to bring the issue up again if the behavior occurs in session and its effectiveness is in question. It is important to note that the discussion of CRBs involves provisional hypotheses about how particular patterns of behavior are likely to function in the relationship. As with all forms of FAP, the case conceptualization should be revisited and revised throughout the course of therapy. It is inevitable that some hypothesized functional relationships are not confirmed or will need to be modified and that new classes of problems will reveal themselves when older patterns of behavior are altered.

The Structure of FAP-Enhanced Couple Therapy

The most obvious and compelling notion that significantly would influence what a FAP-enhanced couple therapy would look like is this: in couple therapy, everything a couple does in the therapy room, whether dyadically or individually, is potentially a CRB! Although couples generally do not behave toward each other in therapy as they do when not being observed by others, they do provide a much larger sample of their actual problem-maintaining behavior in their relationship than can be gleaned from self-reports about behavior outside therapy sessions. FAP-oriented couple therapists, unlike FAP-enhanced individual therapists, usually do not have to wonder how their responses to patients' behavior will map onto the community of likely responses in their clients' natural (out-of-therapy) environment. In couple therapy, the natural environment is in the office, or, at least much more of it than in any individual therapy. Certainly, the couple does not live in a bubble. They interact with their children, families of origin, friends, and people in places such as schools, work, and churches. However, there is no therapy that provides more of the natural environment in which identified problems occur than couple (and family) therapy.

This obvious observation carries significant implications for the structure of FAP-enhanced couple therapy. Some important comparisons and contrasts to other behavioral couple therapies can be identified as the following:

1. *In FAP-enhanced couple therapy, the couple likely is to be encouraged to set the initial agenda for each session* (after the evaluation and joint setting of treatment goals). Whatever the couple selects to focus on in a given session either will be about CRBs (i.e., presumably CRB1s early in therapy) or will provide opportunities for CRBs to occur. The agenda setting itself may even be a CRB depending on the process the couple uses to arrive at the agenda or whether it is set with the purpose of minimizing contacting a difficult issue. Therapist-driven agendas, including therapy manual-driven agendas, risk redirecting the session away from the higher base-rate CRBs that could be targeted in session.
2. *FAP-enhanced couple therapy is much more process-oriented than traditional behavioral couple therapies.* While the couple and the FAP-enhanced therapist certainly will talk "about" important things (e.g., recounting last night's argument at home), more attention will be paid to the live, real-time, observable interaction in the therapy room. While FAP-enhanced couple therapy certainly

can and should include, as appropriate, maintaining a clear and consistent focus on treatment goals, using homework and other tasks to promote CRB2s and evoke avoided CRB1s, much of the power of a FAP perspective is diminished if the therapist aims at influencing the content of the session more than the process.

3. *FAP-enhanced couple therapy rarely includes sessions held with either spouse alone.* In addition to the potential strategic and alliance-damaging potential of such individual meetings (Gurman, 2002, 2008a), they inherently reduce the amount of the natural couple environment available for working toward change.

4. *While the focus of FAP-enhanced couple therapy sessions will usually be on the couple's interaction, the relationship itself need not be the sole focus of treatment.* Intrapersonal or individual issues, problems, and concerns, while not necessarily about the relationship, often carry enormous implications and consequences for the couple. Thus, addressing aspects of a partner's individual "disorder," (e.g., depression or anxiety, extramarital stressors such as workplace conflicts, family-of-origin concerns or tensions, medical health challenges, child's disruptive behavior), is not outside the purview of FAP-enhanced couple therapy. They fall within its purview largely to the extent to which such presumptively individual or non-couple matters are involved functionally in the maintenance of the couple's central difficulties that constitute the focus of treatment, as initially set forth in, or later revised for, the case conceptualization.

5. *In FAP-enhanced couple therapy, the therapist takes a more active and personal role in all in-session interactions.* The matter in couple therapy of who speaks to whom elicits a wide range of views within the couple therapy field (Gurman, 2008a). There are decided advantages to supporting therapist–partner talk, for example, modeling new behavior, clarifying matters in a behavioral analytic chain analysis, and fostering a partner's successive approximations to addressing painful feelings. Therapist–partner talk often will occur more frequently at the beginning of therapy, while partner–partner talk should become relatively predominant as more effective repertoires develop.

The Process of FAP-Enhanced Couple Therapy, with Special Emphasis on the Role of the Therapist

In individual FAP, the therapist takes on a decidedly different role than in traditional behavior therapy. In traditional behavior therapy, the therapist, besides being an expert on psychopathology and psychological difficulties, serves as a "social reinforcement machine" (Krasner, 1962) not of in-session clinically relevant behavior, that is, CRB1s and CRB2s, but of important changes that occur outside the consultation room. In addition, in traditional behavioral therapy, the therapist often arranges for experiences in the office that simulate the real-life conditions under which the patient's problem occurs, such as the use of behavior rehearsal or assertiveness training with socially anxious patients.

In FAP, by contrast, the therapist's main role is to stand in for the community in which the client lives, thus fostering the generalization of positive treatment effects achieved in the therapy itself. In this way, the relationship itself between the therapist and the client provides the mechanism of beneficial therapeutic change (Follette, Naugle, & Callaghan, 1996). Therein lies the power of couple therapy, in having the potentially naturally healing environment in the room. And therein also lies the major reason why FAP-enhanced couple therapy will look rather different from, and perhaps be more complex than, FAP with individuals. The healing relationship in individual FAP is between client and therapist. In all couple therapies (Gurman, 2001, 2008b), the ultimate central healing relationship is that between the relationship partners. And yet, the therapist–client relationship (Therapist–Partner A, Therapist–Partner B) initially will have an equally central role in the practice of FAP-enhanced couple therapy, as we now explain.

Conceptualizing Therapeutic Interactions

There are three therapeutic relationships in couple therapy: Therapist–Partner A, Therapist–Partner B, and Partner A–Partner B. Effective Partner A–Partner B interactions have the highest therapeutic value for distressed couples, but these types of interactions are least likely to occur between the partners early in therapy. As therapy progresses, the likelihood of Partner A–Partner B interactions leading to positive therapeutic outcomes increases.

Given our perspective that the central healing mechanism in couple therapy centers on the partner–partner relationship, not, as in individual FAP, on the client–therapist relationship, it may seem odd to some to place a strong emphasis on the therapist–partner relationships. However, especially at the beginning of therapy it is more important for the partners to be participating directly in a therapeutically beneficial relationship than the target relationship. A genuine and engaged therapist–partner therapeutic relationship will have several qualities similar to the partner–partner relationship (i.e., evoke similar CRBs) with the added benefit that the therapist should be more likely than the other partner to respond to CRBs therapeutically and in line with the case conceptualization. These Therapist–Partner A interactions serve several functions such as the following:

1. Being "outside" the couple's relationship, the therapist should be able to notice and appreciate small magnitude CRB2s at a higher rate than either partner. For example, the therapist is more likely to try to "flip" a CRB1 into a CRB2 by highlighting small improvements that Partner B has not noticed. This may hasten the use of these skills in the relationship with Partner B.
2. The therapist is likely to occasion a different and more adaptive interactional repertoire than Partner B, providing Partner A the opportunity to use these more adaptive skills in the presence of Partner B. This plants the seeds for

generalization and establishes a more relationship-proximal social standard for
using these skills within the partner–partner relationship.

3. The therapist can facilitate CRB3 talk about what differs between the Therapist–
   Partner A relationship and the Partner A–Partner B interactions.

4. Partner B is provided the opportunity to observe Partner A's CRBs without
   immediately responding. This helps extinguish impulsive reactions to Partner
   A's CRBs. This type of inhibition of dysfunctional responding is a prerequisite
   to engaging in more farsighted types of interaction with Partner A.

5. When the therapist supports CRB2s, this serves a modeling function for Partner
   B. We comment further on this modeling function below.

One role of the FAP-enhanced couple therapist is to intervene on dysfunctional
partner–partner interactions and redirect them to partner–therapist interactions. As
discussed earlier, early partner–partner interactions are less likely to be therapeutic
than therapist–partner interactions. How the partners interact with one another does
have an impact on the therapist. A distinguishing feature of FAP-enhanced couple
therapy is that the therapist will use her relationship with the partner to process
the impact partner–partner interactions have on her. These redirections allow the
therapist to better pace the dynamics of the session, block partners from engaging
in an escalating reciprocal series of CRB1s, and allow CRBs to be directly engaged
within the therapist–partner relationship in line with the case conceptualization.

It is important to consider how the role of the therapist in individual FAP com-
pares to the role of the therapist in FAP-style couple therapy. To facilitate this
important comparison, we will examine the place of the basic five rules of FAP
(Kohlenberg & Tsai, 1991) in a FAP-style couple therapy. We also address some
variations of basic FAP rules that we have added to manage the unique complexities
of therapy with couples.

The Early Therapeutic Alliances

Although couple therapy is usually brief, so that active change induction needs to
be addressed rather early, a working alliance with the couple must be established
to create a safe environment in which change can begin (Gurman, 1981). Thus,
early therapist interventions must be aimed at both establishing such an alliance
and increasing optimism about problem-relevant change. Beginning with the first
conjoint meeting, each partner must feel that something of personal value has been
gained. The pathway by which such felt satisfaction occurs varies from individual
to individual. And on this score, a FAP-oriented couple therapist has an important
initial advantage over many other therapists in that he will necessarily be idiographically "tuned into" individual differences between the partners. For example, a FAP
couple therapist particularly should be able to recognize when a partner feels allied
with the therapist as the result of (a) her offering of empathy and warmth; (b) her giving more structuring or feedback (e.g., the therapist identifies a problematic couple

pattern of which they had been unaware); or (c) her providing direction for behavior change that is consistent with their goals for therapy.

The therapist's need to respond differentially to individuals in establishing the early therapeutic alliance is hardly a novel proposition. What makes this self-evident principle more complex in couple therapy is that Partners A and B of the same couple may (functionally speaking) require different experiences to feel that a positive client–therapist relationship is developing, especially early in therapy.

The FAP couple therapist works to establish himself early on as a caring provider of general noncontingent reinforcement. But since couple therapy is typically quite brief (Gurman, 2001) and there is often a significant discrepancy between the partners' levels of readiness to change, he usually must incorporate some change-oriented interventions early in therapy. Doing so will help to strengthen the therapeutic alliance.

Using the Five Rules of FAP with Couples

Rule 1. Watch for CRBs. Often in couple therapy CRBs are easily observed, especially CRB1s early in therapy. But because couple therapy is a three-person situation, many CRB1s occur in more subtle and disguised ways than in individual therapy dyads, making them harder to detect, mostly because there are multiple contingencies controlling the behavior. For example, an emotionally distant husband who shows great difficulty with affective expression to his wife (who complains about this), tries to follow the rule of "being more open" in therapy by engaging in relatively more self-disclosing chitchat with the therapist, perhaps about something they have in common, e.g., sports. This could be a CRB2, speaking more about his feelings and thoughts (which the therapist may want to support/reinforce), but its competing, and maybe stronger, function may be to "kill time" in the session as a temporary avoidance (CRB1) of direct conversation with his partner. It also may function to induce the therapist to feel more warmly toward him (e.g., two men talking about sports) in the hope that the therapist will "feel" for him more subsequently and protect him (therapist-reinforced CRB1) when he is feeling more affectively dysregulated, and perhaps the therapist may even punish his wife when she challenges her husband to talk to her more openly. Since maintaining balanced therapeutic alliances with both partners is a common strategic challenge throughout therapy for couple therapists of any theoretical orientation, being mindful of trying to draw in the less-motivated partner may ironically reinforce that partner's CRB1 (e.g., avoidance of experiencing and expressing emotion). In fact, in the emotionally intense atmosphere that often occurs in couple therapy, trying to engage the less-motivated partner may even interfere with the therapist's likelihood of observing/noticing the avoidance-reinforcing function of the partner's behavior. Moreover, in the example above, the husband's football banter may actually constitute a CRB1 rather than a CRB2 by virtue of its power to engage with the therapist more, but in a predictably safe way.

Rule 1A. Remember that each partner's private (internal) experience (e.g., negative attributions about the partner, increases in arousal or discomfort) is as relevant to functional analysis as is their public (overt) behavior. The therapist only can indirectly observe private CRBs, whether CRB1s or CRB2s, by observing some collateral behavior (e.g., shifting in chair, averting a gaze, rolling of eyes, smiling) or recognizing a likely context for a private response (Skinner, 1945). However, since they regularly are part of the couple's mutually regulating and dysregulating feedback loops, the FAP couple therapist will need to *inquire about* the partners' internal experiences (responses to the other partner's behavior and to the therapist's behavior). For example, Partner B's inadvertent reinforcement of Partner A's CRB1 (laughing when Partner A avoids emotional contact by clever joking) is itself influenced by internal experience (e.g., feeling hurt by the joking, but fearing to express her hurt feeling, arising from a history with Partner A of being ignored and/or punished in her family of origin for expressing "soft" feelings). More specifically, the therapist may *wonder aloud* about Partner B's internal experiences, based on what Partner A's behavior has stimulated *in the therapist*. Thus, in FAP couple therapy, Rule 1, "Watch for CRBs," must be expanded to the private domain of the partners' experience (behavior) in order to more adequately capture relevant variables in the couple's problem-maintaining cycles. As Follette and Hayes (2000) have emphasized, in "constantly conducting a functional analysis of the client's behavior. . . the therapist is required to postulate response classes, (and) hypothesize about controlling variables. . . ." (p. 401).

Rule 1B. To Watch for CRBs, Watch The Partner. Since the natural environment of the couple is in the therapy room, a rich source of possibilities for identifying CRBs is to be found by the therapist's watching Partner B's response to (whatever) Partner A (is doing). This multiperson clinical context provides a unique opportunity for the therapist to see clinically relevant contingencies and sequences "live" in addition to those about which she speculates. Since the partners have a long history of mutual influence and regulation and dysregulation, it is common for subtle cues (discriminative stimuli) and subtly delivered consequences to escape the observation of the therapist. Thus, when struggling to identify *CRB sequences,* therapists would be wise to remember that the first time, it's an observation; the second time, it's a possibility; the third time, it's a pattern.

Rule 2. Evoke CRBs. Beyond the many inherent aspects of therapy that can evoke CRBs (e.g., session scheduling, fee-setting) there are numerous ways in which the use of standard behavioral or other therapeutic interventions may evoke CRBs, e.g., directing a partner to summarize the central thrust of what her partner has just said before expressing her own thoughts on the subject (communication training), or encouraging the receiving partner to "hear" the fear behind the sending partner's ill-temperedness toward her in order to help her experience him in a different light (acceptance training).

First, and most obviously, most of the kinds of *questions* the individual FAP therapist might present to the client *about the therapy, the therapist, or the therapeutic relationship* will need to be re-oriented to address (evoke descriptions of) the same types of behavior (thoughts, feelings) toward the relationship partner. For example, the question, "What do you think I'm thinking about you/what you did/what you just said?" becomes, "What do you think (your partner) thinks. . .?" Or, instead of, "What's your reaction to what I just said?" the therapist asks, "What's your reaction to what your partner just said?" (Landes, Busch, & Kanter, 2006, p. 36). Or, more subtly, the therapist might inquire, "What do you think your wife is feeling now, as she hears you express to me that you are feeling sad?"

Second, when the therapist calls upon common couple therapy interventions, it is important to watch for *how the partners respond to each other* as well as how they respond to the therapist when the therapist proposes that they do something different, for example, try to sustain a conversation about a "hot topic" in a way that calls upon their own resources, or try to match the therapist's specification of the "something different" (e.g., "Let's try that again, but this time, Bob, I'd like you to ask Sue a couple of clarifying questions about her views on this before you tell her your own").

Thus, even when the therapist attempts to evoke CRB2s by specifying the form of rule-governed behavior she is trying to increase between the partners (in the hope that its appearance will be well received and reinforced by the partner), she must balance her noticing of possible CRBs of each partner toward both her *and* possible CRBs of each partner toward the other partner.

Rule 3. Actively respond to CRBs. The matter of how to respond effectively to CRBs probably poses the most complex and challenging aspect of doing a FAP-enhanced couple therapy. As Kohlenberg and Tsai (1991) note, "It is difficult to put Rule 3 into practice" because "the only natural reinforcers available in the adult therapy situation are the interpersonal actions and reactions between the client and therapist" (p. 29). Obviously, there is no such limitation in conjoint couple therapy. Rather, the difficulty of putting Rule 3 into practice, and dealing with other aspects of consequating CRBs, has different sources and requires different principles for the therapist to follow in working with couples.

Responding to CRB1s. We propose these guiding principles to enhance the therapist's effective responding to CRB1s in couple therapy:

1. The therapist must remain alert to how she is responding to dyadic patterns and sequences of couple behavior in addition to specific actions of the individual partners.
2. The therapist must be alert to (aware of, notice) the response of each partner to the CRB1s of the other partner. At times, the therapist will merely note (Rule 1) these responses, especially early in therapy or when a topic of concern that has never been discussed before in the therapy is brought to a session. At other times, the therapist will respond overtly to them. Such therapist noticing is especially important when the couple has entered therapy because of both couple difficulties and the psychiatric symptoms of one partner, e.g., depression, and particularly when it is known or assumed that there is a recursive interplay between the couple conflict and the individual's symptoms.
3. The therapist may, and usually should, use his "self" to shift the couple's problematic (clinically relevant) interaction. Herein lies the biggest difference

between this approach and the practice of other behavioral approaches to couple therapy, including IBCT. What is called for from the FAP-enhanced couple therapist is to use his experiencing-of-the-interaction to promote change by sharing with Partner A the impact a CRB1 has just had on him. Therapist–partner relationships are influenced by how each partner interacts with the other and it is the therapist's role to share this impact when it is in the best interest of the relationship and fits within the collaboratively developed case conceptualization. In this light, the impact of the CRB1 on the therapist can then be compared or contrasted with what Partner B was experiencing. This stance is consistent with the therapist's overriding aim in FAP-enhanced couple therapy to change behavior in its natural context. The therapist–partner relationships are natural relationships that can be compared and contrasted with the couple's relationship.

4. The therapist may respond to Partner B's response to Partner A's CRB1 by modeling new or prompting alternative (especially non-punishing) behavior. The therapist needs to monitor the impact such modeling and prompting have on the couple's relationship to ensure it has the intended effect.

Although modeling may serve a secondary function of the therapist's consequating CRBs, there is a risk in couple therapy of overemphasizing this function. To the extent that the therapist may be better at noticing and responding to CRB2 approximations in Partner A than Partner B is, such consequating/modeling may be experienced by Partner B as taking the side of A, or by Partner B as having been inadequate in not noticing the positive change in A. Of course, therapist modeling of positive consequation of CRB2s should be balanced toward both partners over time, but still does have the potential for creating immediate alliance ruptures.

Responding to CRB2s. Early in therapy, obvious CRB2s may be hard to come by. A skill the therapist needs to develop is "flipping" a CRB1 into a CRB2 by noticing any (no matter how small) varied dimension of a CRB1 that could be considered an improvement. This involves a type of generosity that is often lacking in the couple's relationship and the therapist needs to genuinely appreciate such variation. Therapist responses to CRB2s are often slightly exaggerated early in therapy when trying to shape CRB2s. As therapy progresses and CRB2s increase in frequency, the more natural consequences of effective interpersonal commerce will take over.

Rule 3a. In addition to consequating CRB1s and CRB2s in the form of individual partners' behaviors, also consequate dyadic partner–partner sequences that are central to the case conceptualization.

Rule 3b. In deciding at a given moment whether to consequate the behavior of Partner A, Partner B, or the sequence of behavior between Partners A and B (Rule 3a), be accepting of one's own errors, confusion, and uncertainty. This may involve being "therapeutically loving" (Tsai et al., 2008, p. 83) to ourselves as well as to our clients.

Couple therapy is many times more complex than individual therapy, and, though tempting, it is very difficult to set forth "decision rules" for the therapist's consequation of CRBs. This is especially so because so often, in a given couple sequence, even a brief one, (a) there are numerous CRB1s provided by both partners; (b) there is often, in a given couple sequence, even a brief one, a mixture of both CRB1s and CRB2s; and (c) as therapy progresses, there are increasingly more sequences with CRB2s from both partners. We may be able to rationalize or explain/justify after the fact our moment-to-moment decision making regarding which elements in the three-way couple therapy we consequate. Still, the reality of couple therapy is that so much that is clinically relevant is happening at virtually the same time between, among, and within the participants, that, in the end, the therapist must ultimately rely on her broadly usable, though often implicit, skill repertoires for sorting out (discriminating among) what is most important at a given moment, and having, as Landes et al. (2006) put it, "a considerable degree of interpersonal sensitivity and empathy" (p. 16). These therapist repertoires, they understatedly note, are "difficult to operationalize behaviorally" (p. 16).

Rule 3c. Be aware that different emphases on therapist–partner interactions versus partner–partner interactions are called for at different phases of therapy and with different types of couples.

In other types of behavioral couple therapy, the lion's share of the therapist's attention is on the partner–partner relationship. FAP-enhanced couple therapy balances this emphasis with an emphasis on intentionally using the therapist–partner relationships as a significant force for change. As suggested earlier, a greater emphasis on therapist–partner interaction than partner–partner interaction may appropriately characterize the opening phase of much FAP-style couple therapy. But there are also common situations in which an early therapist–partner emphasis may be either unnecessary or contraindicated, for example, when both partners are very responsive to the therapist's early efforts to shift partner–partner interaction; the couple's primary difficulty involves a highly focal concern or limited aspect of their relationship; or whatever the presenting problem or the couple's interaction around it, their individual and joint behavior evokes little in the way of personal reactions in the therapist.

It is essential to always keep in mind that the ultimate purpose of focusing on the therapist–Partner A/B interaction is to ultimately influence future partner–partner interactions, which are the healing centerpiece in couple therapy.

Consider the following clinical scenario to illustrate the relevance of "Rule 3a" (consequating sequences as well as individual behaviors) and "Rule 3b" (being mindful and accepting of one's own confusion as a couple therapist) and the inherent complexity of couple therapy and its seeming arbitrariness sometimes.

Bob and Sue, married 11 years, have seen three previous couple therapists to little avail. Sue is now at the brink of possibly leaving Bob, having discovered that he has been "meeting real women online," going to "gentlemen's clubs," and watching pornography on the internet, having promised to stop such behavior several years earlier. Bob, highly skilled in his line of work, has suffered from major depressions his entire adulthood, and has now been unemployed for almost 3 years. He also has intense social anxiety and avoids all forms of interpersonal conflict. Sue, an energetic "doer," works full time while also studying to finish her master's degree at a local college. The eldest and most parentified of the several children in her family of origin, she regularly takes on the major role of arbitrating family conflicts and "mentoring" her most poorly functioning siblings. Bob is almost totally cut off from his family of origin and longs for the closeness of Sue's family for himself. At the same time, he is easily hurt with feelings of abandonment and neglect, with which he had "become pretty familiar," he says understatedly, in his family of origin. He fears asking Sue for what he needs emotionally, both because "she's almost never available" and because "it's just hard for me to ask [anyone for anything]."

In the therapy, Sue pursues, and Bob distances (avoids). The therapist has been working to support all of Bob's small changes (even some brief kind words toward Sue) toward closeness, blocking Sue's well-learned pattern of "taking over" relationships, and often having difficulty coping with the ensuing frustration, disappointment with others, and rapid affective dysregulation (which, in turn, further turns Bob away from her).

In session four, the topic of the couple's spending little time together is once again brought up. Sue just recently has been "deluged" by family-of-origin problems over the Christmas period, and Bob, in still one more failed effort to connect with his viciously critical father over the holidays, has just been "castigated for being alive."

They both want more couple contact. Sue turns to Bob, and in a gentle voice says simply, "Bob, we really need to find a way to spend more time together." Bob, who, with his considerable intelligence and wit, has managed interpersonal tensions for nearly 4 decades by using humor, often tinged with sarcasm, half-smilingly responds, "I'll have to check with your secretary to see if there's any time on your calendar." The words are sarcastic, and yet his voice is also soft, his facial expression is inviting, and there is good eye contact between the partners.

Sue responds to Bob, "God damn you! Can't you even drop your fuckin' 'humor' and sarcasm with me for a minute?" Bob turns away from Sue, slides down on his end of the sofa on which they are both sitting, and averts his gaze. The sequence perfectly illustrates the couple's central dilemma and its major components, appearing as they do in couple therapy, in varied forms: Sue's relationship-initiation, Bob's rejection sensitivity, Sue's affective volatility, and Bob's retreating.

All of this has taken about 15 seconds. Given the rapid shift of tone from a soft one to a very angry/withdrawn one, the therapist may decide to redirect the couple, as discussed earlier. But in what way? He justifiably could focus on specific observable elements in the brief couple exchange, identify the feelings arising in himself upon witnessing the couple's exchange, or comment on the entire exchange. Or, he could do nothing and simply wait to see what happens next. His choices included (but were not limited to) the following:

1. Reinforce Sue (Partner A) for reaching out to Bob (CRB2).
2. Reinforce Bob (Partner B) for his half-hearted acceptance of Sue's invitation ("I'll check with your secretary. . .").
3. Ignore Bob's "humor" (consequence Partner B's CRB1) and encourage him to respond directly rather than sarcastically to Sue's invitation (prompt CRB2).
4. Ignore or punish Sue's (understandable, but not helpful or adaptive) angry outburst at Bob (consequence Partner A's CRB1).

5. Encourage Bob to move out of the hiding/attacked position and stay in emotional contact with Sue (block CRB1, prompt CRB2), her anger notwithstanding.
6. Ignore both Bob's sarcastic response and Sue's angry counter-response (consequate both CRB1s), and invite Bob to express what he felt toward Sue initially upon hearing her invitation (prompt CRB2).

OR,

The therapist could focus on the 15-seconds *sequence*. She could

1. Comment on or inquire about Sue's reaction to Bob's reaction to the initial invitation.
2. Comment on or inquire about Bob's reaction to Sue's reaction to Bob's reaction to the initial invitation.

Where the therapist would punctuate this clinically relevant sequence is quite arbitrary, and would be largely a result of both his case conceptualization-based and intuitive sense of which partner is more likely, *in that brief moment*, to be influence-able by the therapist; in what direction the conversation is seen as likely to go if left uncommented upon by him (e.g., "Do I predict that either Sue or Bob will make any un-therapist-prompted attempt to repair their immediate rupture?"), and whether he decides to focus on coaching the couple's obviously needed communication and affect-regulation skills, and if so, whose?

While it might be tempting to consequate any of several elements in the 15-seconds exchange (e.g., Sue's invitation for closeness, Bob's sarcastic but gentle acceptance of that invitation, Sue's rageful reaction to that half-acceptance), it would be probably be an error to do so. Consequating interactional sequences provides more options to facilitate out-of-session generalization than "de-contextually" focusing on single elements in a recurrent interactional chain. Of course, consequating the longer sequence inherently would include consequating multiple elements in that sequence, and not risk alliance-damaging therapist side-taking. Thus, the therapist might say, "I really got a hopeful feeling seeing the two of you moving in the same direction, trying to get closer, but then I felt sad when I saw how the vulnerability in each of you to doing that got in the way and created such tension between you so quickly." Perhaps followed by, "How could you do that exchange over (prompts CRB2s) so that just the safe, connecting part shows up?"

The therapist might also consequate the sequence by inquiring about internal factors likely to have affected this brief exchange, influenced by his awareness of aspects of the couple's relationship that were *not* being shown or verbally expressed at the moment. Reasonable candidates for such a commentary or "wondering aloud" could include the following:

1. Ask Bob if it was difficult for him to simply accept Sue's invitation, since he clearly was missing their contact, for fear (avoidance of) that she would "back out of our plans at the last minute," as she so often had to respond to the needs of a sibling.

2. Ask Sue if she is, in disguised form, beseeching Bob to rescue her from her family-of-origin involvements (a therapist inference based on previous sessions) by "giving her a good reason to say 'no' to her siblings" because she has a (justifiable) reason to do so, i.e., have a date with Bob.

There are many such organismic variables and establishing operations rooted in the couple's history together and in their individual family learning histories that the therapist may speculate as to their functional role at the moment in this 15-s exchange. Doing so would constitute a variation of Rule 5, "provide statements (here, tentative) of functional relationships/give interpretations of variables that affect (both) client(s') behavior." Wondering aloud about "hidden meanings" (Tsai, Kohlenberg, Kanter, & Waltz, 2008, p. 66) in partners' verbal behavior is an important therapist role in couple therapy and constitutes a valuable way of consequating patient behavior that is intended not to evoke CRB1s or to reinforce CRB2s, but to prompt and call forth awareness of the links between private and public behavior.

It is important to remember that in FAP-enhanced couple therapy, useful therapist consequation of client behavior need not involve personal disclosure, and that evoking, shaping, and reinforcing "interpersonally vulnerable behavior" (Kohlenberg, Kohlenberg, & Tsai, 2008, p. 135) in the couple's relationship usually should be given a higher priority than efforts to promote therapist-partner (client) intimacy, as in individual FAP. Such vulnerabilities have been described compellingly by Scheinkman and Fishbane (2004).

If the therapist follows the Rule 5 option, does he address his words to Bob, to Sue, or to Bob and Sue? To be more inclusive, as suggested above, he should address both of them, but what if he senses that one of them at that moment seems likely to be more responsive than the other partner to the therapist's input? What if he sees no cues that would suggest which partner may be more responsive right now, but, instead plays the odds that Sue will more easily connect because typically that has been the case in earlier sessions?

Commenting on the longer sequence with Bob and Sue would be appropriate, but what if the therapist senses that Bob may not engage with this commentary since he is feeling put down (punished) by Sue for his semi-warm, semi-sarcastic response to her invitation. Keep in mind that the therapist already knows, from the initial evaluation by a staff psychiatrist and by first session couple history-taking, that when Bob feels "really dissed" or "attacked" by Sue, he intermittently retreats to his bed, at times for several days, does not eat, and occasionally threatens suicide.

How does the FAP couple therapist decide, in a matter of seconds (and with composure in the face of Sue's red-faced rage), to which of these functionally, clinically relevant pieces of the couple's interaction he might most usefully respond, and in what manner (e.g., reinforce CRB2s, punish CRB1s, block CRB1s and prompt CRB2s, invoke Rule 5)? Unlike the football quarterback who can call a time out to plan the next "intervention," the couple therapist is more like the soccer player who, having no timeouts available, must "consequate" (the opposing team's) behavior on the basis of disciplined intuition and implicit understanding of the immediate situation. Aspects (controlling variables) of the immediate situation that might usefully influence the therapist's course of action would include her sense of which partner seems to be more immediately accessible and likely to be responsive to her actions, and her awareness of the overall depth of her working alliance with each partner while being careful not to place undue responsibility on one partner.

In addition, reviewing the "game plan"/case conceptualization before each session with the couple may function as a kind of establishing operation for the therapist to discriminate and respond more reliably to the "correct" class of behavior. Of course, different case conceptualizations may lead the therapist to respond differently to the same couple behavior.

Rule 4. Notice Your Effect on each Partner. As in individual FAP, the couple therapist must watch to see whether his behavior toward each partner is actually having its desired effect, the opposite effect, or no discernible effect. But since couple therapy is about the dyadic system, not just individuals, the FAP couple therapist should also note Rule 4a: notice the effects of your behavioral efforts in relation to Partner A on Partner B, and vice versa.

Rule 5. Interpret Variables that Affect Client Behavior and Implement Generalization Strategies. Applying FAP Rule 5 with couples is identical, in both its intent and effect, to what one of us (Gurman, 2008a, p. 407) calls "the teaching of systemic awareness" via "functional analytic awareness training." The enhancement of partners' functional relational-systemic awareness may be the most salient way in which the FAP-enhanced couple therapist provides a model that facilitates generalization of in-session changes to everyday life. Following the core FAP principle of the therapist's responding naturally, such interpretive awareness training (providing the couple statements of functional relationships about their interaction) is rarely imported into FAP-enhanced therapy sessions as a module or predetermined and planned therapist activity. Rather, when it fits the emerging therapeutic conversation, sometimes at a compelling moment for enhancing partners' skill at understanding what maintains their difficulties, sometimes near the end of a session to cement an important teaching moment about what has happened in session, the therapist may call upon Rule 5. In fact, probably the major use of Rule 5 occurs at a given moment of couple exchange, with the therapist seeking to amplify (by clearly describing and summarizing, usually interactional sequences) the partners' awareness of the variables the therapist notes to be central to both the maintenance of their shared difficulty and its amelioration.

In a FAP-influenced couple therapy, the therapist invoking Rule 5 will include her identifying, in effect, in the form of a (non-technically stated) behavioral chain analysis both the external, observable elements in the particular sequence *and* the internal, private experience that also constitute links in the chain, similar to what Gurman (2008a, p. 407) calls "linking individual experience and relational experience."

Of course, the collaborative construction of "homework assignments" is commonplace among couple therapies (Gurman, 2008b), and is called upon in FAP-enhanced couple therapy to facilitate generalization of in-session CRB2s.

Therapeutic Techniques in FAP-Enhanced Couple Therapy

Kohlenberg and Tsai (1991) have noted that, in the pursuit of applying Rule 1, "Any method or concept that can help in CRB detection... has a place in FAP..." (p. 47). In this pragmatic and functional spirit, as is true of the practice of individual FAP (e.g., Kohlenberg, Kanter, Bolling, Parker, & Tsai, 2002), in principle any method (or technique) that may have some likely utility to promote desired couple change is potentially relevant to the practice of a FAP-enhanced couple therapy. Of course, commonly used social learning theory-based techniques from Integrative Behavioral Couple Therapy (e.g., acceptance training), Cognitive Behavioral Couple Therapy (e.g., reattribution training) and Traditional Behavioral Couple Therapy (e.g., behavioral exchange) readily fit with the practice of FAP-style couple therapy. But perhaps less obviously, such varied interventions as "softening" and "empathic conjecture," from Emotionally Focused Couple Therapy (Johnson, 2008), and interpretation of partner motivation and meaning in Object Relations Couple Therapy (Scharff & Scharff, 2008), also are likely to be pragmatically compatible with the emphases of FAP-style couple therapy on modifying in-session partner behavior and experience. Likewise, enactment, the "centerpiece of the change process" in Structural Couple Therapy (Simon, 2008), has much in common with the FAP-enhanced couple therapy emphasis on observing, eliciting, and consequating CRBs. The structural couple therapist helps to transform problematic interaction patterns through "personal participation" in "the reality of their (the family's and the therapist's) mutual experience" (Aponte, 1992, p. 271).

These conceptually disparate methods illustrate the proposition that form follows function. FAP's functional (i.e., behavior analytic) orientation allows it to provide a compelling conceptual base for a genuinely integrative approach to couple therapy (Gurman, 2002, 2008b). This integration, to be meaningful, needs to be driven by a behavior analytic conceptualization of the functional aspects of the integrated approaches. Many therapies make use of similar techniques. It is the coherent understanding of when and why to use a particular technique that is important. Technical eclecticism should not be confused with theoretical eclecticism.

Therapist Caveats

FAP-enhanced couple therapy is difficult as one can readily see in the Bob and Sue example. As mentioned earlier, many behavioral couple therapies have designed interventions by trying to teach what appear to be useful behavioral topographies and then presume that will function for most people. Anyone who has done much couple therapy comes to appreciate that couples can be happy together even if the therapist cannot imagine himself or herself in such a relationship. Ultimately, those relationship behaviors that function well for a particular couple are what is important even if the topography is very different for what would work in the therapist's own relationship. It is hard to conceive of the way the farmer's daughter from Grant

Wood's portrait "American Gothic" would prefer to function in a relationship compared to Cher's character Loretta in the 1987 movie "Moonstruck." Presumably both fictional characters could be happy in relationships, but what therapist could predict the relevant functional classes to which to attend in therapy. It takes an open mind and keen observational skills to recognize and idiographically shape functional repertoires for people with such disparate histories.

A second caveat to consider is that ultimately it is the partner–partner dyad that matters. Each therapist–partner dyad can be very powerful in establishing conditions for new behavior to emerge that will work in the partner–partner dyad. It is not the therapist's task to directly transfer therapist–partner behaviors to the partner–partner relationship. What needs to get transferred is the sensitivity to how one's behavior affects the other person. When Partner A acts with caring attention to the impact he or she has on Partner B, and Partner B can accurately assess that impact and report back to Partner A, then the power of the in vivo nature of couple therapy can work with incredible positive mutual influence. It is the task of the therapist to bring about this type of interaction rather than prescribe or proscribe specific behavioral topographies.

References

Aponte, H. J. (1992). Training the person of the therapist in structural family therapy. *Journal of Marital and Family Therapy, 18*, 269–281.

Baucom, D. H., Epstein, N. B., LaTaillade, J. J., & Kirby, J. S. (2008). Cognitive behavioral couple therapy. In A. Gurman (Ed.), *Clinical handbook of couple therapy* (4th ed.). New York: Guilford Press.

Berns, S., & Jacobson, N. S. (2000). Marital problems. In M. J. Dougher (Ed.), *Clinical behavior analysis* (pp. 181–206). Reno, NV: Context Press.

Birchler, G., Weiss, R. L., & Vincent, J. P. (1975). A multidimensional analysis of social reinforcement exchange between martially distressed and nondistressed spouse and stranger dyads. *Journal of Personality and Social Psychology, 31*, 349–360.

Callaghan, G. M. (2006). The Functional Idiographic Assessment Template (FIAT) system. *The Behavior Analyst Today, 7*, 357–398.

Christensen, A., Jacobson, N. S., & Babcock, J. C. (1995). Integrative behavioral couple therapy. In N. S. Jacobson & A. S. Gurman (Eds.), *Clinical handbook of couple therapy* (2nd ed., pp. 31–64). New York: Guilford Press.

Dimidjian, S., Martell, C. R., & Christensen, A. (2008). Integrative behavioral couple therapy. In A. S. Gurman (Ed.), *Clinical handbook of couple therapy* (4th ed.). New York: Guilford Press.

Follette, W. C., & Hayes, S. C. (2000). Contemporary behavior therapy. In C. R. Snyder & R. E. Ingram (Eds.), *Handbook of psychological change: Psychotherapy processes & practices for the 21 st century* (pp. 381–408). New York: Wiley.

Follette, W. C., Naugle, A. E., & Callaghan, G. M. (1996). A radical behavioral understanding of the therapeutic relationship in effecting change. *Behavior Therapy, 27*, 623–641.

Gurman, A. S. (1981). Integrative couple therapy: Toward the development of an interpersonal approach. In S. H. Budman (Ed.), *Forms of brief therapy* (pp. 415–462). New York: Guilford Press.

Gurman, A. S. (2001). Brief therapy and couple/family therapy: An essential redundancy. *Clinical Psychology: Science and Practice, 8*, 51–65.

Gurman, A. S. (2002). Brief integrative marital therapy: A depth-behavioral approach. In A. S. Gurman & N. S. Jacobson (Eds.), *Clinical handbook of couple therapy* (3rd ed., pp. 180–220). New York: Guilford Press.

Gurman, A. S. (2008a). Integrative couple therapy: A depth-behavioral approach. In A. S. Gurman (Ed.), *Clinical handbook of couple therapy* (4th ed.). New York: Guilford Press.

Gurman, A. S. (2008b). A framework for the comparative study of couple therapy: History, models and applications. In A. S. Gurman (Ed.), *Clinical handbook of couple therapy* (4th ed.). New York: Guilford Press.

Hayes, S. C., & Toarmino, D. (1995, February). If behavioral principles are generally applicable, why is it necessary to understand cultural diversity? *The Behavior Therapist, 18,* 21–23.

Holtzworth-Munroe, A., & Jacobson, N. S. (1991). Behavioral marital therapy. In A. S. Gurman & D. P. Kniskern (Eds.), *Handbook of family therapy* (2nd ed., pp. 96–133). New York: Brunner/Mazel.

Jacobson, N. S., & Margolin, G. (1979). *Marital therapy: Strategies based on social learning and behavior exchange principles.* New York: Brunner/Mazel.

Johnson, S. (2008). Emotionally focused couple therapy. In A. S. Gurman (Ed.), *Clinical handbook of couple therapy* (4th ed.). New York: Guilford Press.

Kohlenberg, R. J., Kanter, J. W., Bolling, M. Y., Parker, C. R., & Tsai, M. (2002). Enhancing cognitive therapy for depression with functional analytic psychotherapy: Treatment guidelines and empirical findings. *Cognitive and Behavioral Practice, 9,* 213–229.

Kohlenberg, R. J., Kohlenberg, B., & Tsai, M. (2008). Intimacy. In M. Tsai, R. J. Kohlenberg, J. W. Kanter, B. Kohlenberg, W. C. Follette, & G. M. Callaghan (Eds.), *A guide to functional analytic psychotherapy: Awareness, courage, love and behaviorism.* New York: Springer.

Kohlenberg, R. J., & Tsai, M. (1991). *Functional analytic psychotherapy: Creating intense and curative therapeutic relationships.* New York: Plenum.

Krasner, L. (1962). The therapist as a social reinforcement machine. In H. H. Strupp & L. Luborsky (Eds.), *Research in psychotherapy* (Vol. 2, pp. 61–94). Washington, DC: American Psychological Association.

Landes, S. J., Busch, A. M., & Kanter, J. W. (2006, August). *Translating theoretical into practical: A functional analytic psychotherapy treatment manual.* Unpublished manuscript, University of Wisconsin-Milwaukee, Milwaukee, WI.

Lawrence, E., Eldridge, K., Christensen, A., & Jacobson, N. S. (1999). Integrative couple therapy: The dyadic relationship of acceptance and change. In J. Donovan (Ed.), *Short-term couples therapy* (pp. 226–261). New York: Guilford Press.

Lopez, F. J. C. (2003). Jealousy: A case of application of functional analytic psychotherapy. *Psychology in Spain, 7,* 86–98.

Rabin, C., Tsai, M., & Kohlenberg, R. J. (1996). Targeting sex-role and power issues with a functional analytic approach: Gender patterns in behavioral marital therapy. *Journal of Feminist Family Therapy, 8,* 1–24.

Scharff, J. S., & Scharff, D. E. (2008). Object relations couple therapy. In A. S. Gurman (Ed.), *Clinical handbook of couple therapy* (4th ed.). New York: Guilford Press.

Scheinkman, M., & Fishbane, M. D. (2004). The vulnerability cycle: Working with impasses in couple therapy. *Family Process, 43,* 279–299.

Simon, G. (2008). Structural couple therapy. In A. S. Gurman (Ed.), *Clinical handbook of couple therapy* (4th ed.). New York: Guilford Press.

Skinner, B. F. (1945). The operational analysis of psychological terms. *Psychological Review, 52,* 270–277.

Tsai, M., Kohlenberg, R. J., Kanter, J. W., Kohlenberg, B., Follette, W. C., & Callaghan, G. M. (2008). *A guide to functional analytic psychotherapy: Awareness, courage, love and behaviorism.* New York: Springer.

Tsai, M., Kohlenberg, R. J., Kanter, J. W., & Waltz, J. (2008). Therapeutic technique: The five rules. In M. Tsai, R. J. Kohlenberg, J. W. Kanter, B. Kohlenberg, W. C. Follette, & G. M. Callaghan (Eds.), *A guide to functional analytic psychotherapy: Awareness, courage, love and behaviorism.* New York: Springer.

Chapter 9
FAP with Sexual Minorities

Mary D. Plummer

The landscape of psychotherapy with lesbian, gay, and bisexual (LGB) clients has evolved so dramatically in recent history it would seem unrecognizable to those who defined the field only five decades ago. The first edition of the Diagnostic and Statistical Manual of Mental Disorders (DSM, American Psychiatric Association, 1952) described "homosexuality" as a sociopathic personality disturbance requiring long-term treatment. Almost three decades later, catalyzed partly by the gay liberation movement as well as research on the prevalence and psychological correlates of same-sex attraction and sexual behavior (Hooker, 1957; Kinsey, Pomeroy, & Martin, 1948; Kinsey, Pomeroy, Martin, & Gebhard, 1953), the DSM-III shifted direction, re-categorizing "homosexuality" as a "sexual orientation disturbance" (American Psychiatric Association, 1980). It was not until 1987 that the profession removed all remnants of its earlier characterizations of "the homosexual" as disturbed, pathological, arrested, regressed, or from the DSM (DSM-III-R, American Psychiatric Association, 1987).

Since the psychological debate concerning sexual minorities climaxed and receded, mainstream interest in treatment for LBG clients has dwindled and research on the topic has been ghettoized. Over the past 2 decades, LGB mental health research has been conducted largely by researchers who themselves identify as LGB and has been disseminated in niche-specific publications, special editions, and books devoted to the topic. This has resulted in a significant gap between policy and practice (American Psychological Association, 2000) such that graduate students report inadequate if not blatantly heterosexist training experiences in psychology programs, with even less preparation for working with bisexual clients (Phillips & Fischer, 1998). Practicing clinicians also report feeling professionally incompetent in working with lesbian and gay clients (Bieschke, McClanahan, Tozer, Grzegorek, & Park, 2000), admit to a general lack of familiarity with common difficulties faced by sexual minorities, and manifest a heterosexist bias in a variety of therapy contexts including problems in understanding, assessment, and intervention

M.D. Plummer (✉)
University of Washington, Seattle, WA, USA
e-mail: maryplummer@gmail.com

J.W. Kanter et al. (eds.), *The Practice of Functional Analytic Psychotherapy*,
DOI 10.1007/978-1-4419-5830-3_9, © Springer Science+Business Media, LLC 2010

(Garnets, Hancock, Cochran, Goodchilds, & Peplau, 1991). These findings suggest that while therapist anti-gay bias seems to have decreased, it continues to impact treatment of sexual minority clients in substantive ways.

There are a number of reasons why this should concern the professional community. First and foremost, ethical standards outlined by the American Psychological Association mandate that psychologists "are aware of and respect cultural, individual, and role differences, including those based on ... sexual orientation ... [and] try to eliminate the effect on their work of biases based on those factors" (American Psychological Association, 2002). Furthermore, the *APA Guidelines for Psychotherapy with Gay, Lesbian, and Bisexual Clients* (APA, 2000) encourage psychologists to increase their awareness of challenges faced by sexual minorities across the lifespan and across cultures, recognize and mitigate personal biases, and respectfully understand the variety of norms, values, and family structures represented in this diverse population.

Beyond the ethical standards and values of the profession, service utilization statistics provide another reason for special attention to therapy with sexual minority clients. Sexual minorities, particularly lesbians, appear to be more likely than their heterosexual counterparts to seek therapy at some point in their lives (e.g., Cochran, Sullivan, & Mays, 2003; Jones & Gabriel, 1999). A variety of hypotheses exist to explain this finding. Many suggest that sexual minorities experience higher levels of stress deriving from daily exposure to micro-aggressions, subtle and overt discrimination, rejection or alienation from family and religious institutions, unique legal and financial burdens, internalized homophobia, identity concealment, stigma consciousness, and hate crimes. Stress and coping theorists link these types of chronic stressors with psychopathology insofar as external conditions tax individuals' psychological resources, rendering them more vulnerable to mental or somatic illness (Dohrenwend, 2000). At the same time, sexual minorities often have less access to the social support that might help mitigate the effects of chronic stress (Safren & Heimberg, 1999). From a behavioral perspective, the chronic stressors translate into increased likelihood for punishing contingencies for behaviors that are functional for non-LGB individuals such as the acceptance and expression of one's identity and the pursuit of one's personal values. Likewise, the relative deficit of social support translates into decreased access to interpersonal reinforcers for these same functional behaviors. It is not surprising, therefore, that a growing body of research points to higher incidence of psychopathology among sexual minorities including mood and anxiety disorders (Gilman et al., 2001), suicidality (Fergusson, Horwood, & Beautrais, 1999; Herrell et al., 1999), social anxiety (Safren & Pantalone, 2006), and body image disturbances (Siever, 1994), which may bring them to the therapy office more frequently.

Considering the overwhelming likelihood that therapists will count LGB clients within their caseloads (Garnets et al., 1991), and that their work with these populations ought to comply with the aforementioned ethical standards and guidelines, it is imperative that FAP treatment considerations with sexual minorities be included in this volume.

FAP with Special Populations: A Caveat

While the title of this chapter may imply differences between "standard" FAP and FAP with sexual minorities, the central message is that FAP is *not* to be practiced any differently with these populations. That is to say, (1) the five "rules" of FAP, (2) its focus on function rather than topography, (3) the application of a thorough case conceptualization, (4) the development of a therapeutic relationship that evokes clinically relevant behavior (CRB), and (5) the importance of therapist awareness, courage, therapeutic love, and genuineness all hold true regardless of the identity of the client. The idiographic philosophy underpinning FAP requires this sort of equality in its application across demographic categories. Furthermore, FAP's radical behavioral foundations eschew any preconceived definitions of psychological health with regard to sexual orientation or any other aspect of identity. Rather than attempting to reinforce a defined set of healthy behaviors, the FAP therapist defines treatment targets in collaboration with the client, and in general, aims to weaken repertoires under aversive control (e.g., repertoires defined by the goal of minimizing exposure to potential discrimination, rejection, or heterosexism) and strengthen repertoires that increase access to positive reinforcers.

What is the purpose of this chapter, then? Rather than leading the reader to practice FAP differently with sexual minorities, this chapter aims to assist the therapist in upholding the same dictums of practice in their work with these populations. In order to create the requisite therapeutic environment that fosters trust and openness, FAP therapists working with sexual minorities may need to bolster their awareness of this population's unique contexts (e.g., individual, group, political, historical, religious, ethnic, and generational contexts). Additionally, in order to minimize therapeutic mistakes when reacting to sensitive client issues, and to recognize and create therapeutic opportunities when a mistake occurs, FAP therapists may need to invest more energy into self-exploration and developing awareness of their own biases. These aims are pursued in this chapter by (1) reviewing environmental and historical factors common to many sexual minorities, (2) considering issues in the mutual determination of therapy targets (client life problems), (3) suggesting potential CRBs resulting from these common historical/environmental factors, and (4) highlighting therapist fears and biases which, if left unexamined, could inhibit treatment effectiveness of FAP or distort its fidelity.

Considering the Case Conceptualization

The effective practice of FAP rests substantially on the careful development of an idiographic case conceptualization specifying relevant history, client life problems, in vivo problems (CRB1s) and improvements (CRB2s), and outside life goals (Tsai et al., 2008). In keeping with this approach to treatment, the following sections review important considerations and common themes that arise in each of these categories when working with sexual minorities.

Relevant History

According to FAP, client problems are controlled by historical and current environmental factors. Thus, the specification of these contextual factors is paramount to structuring treatment in service of behavior change. While FAP therapists always focus their assessment of relevant history on each client's report of his or her individual experiences, greater awareness of the multiple environmental systems frequently encountered by certain groups of clients (nomothetic information) can highlight potentially important variables to assess and help establish a favorable psychotherapeutic environment.

Environmental Systems. The FAP contextualist worldview is reflected in Bronfenbrenner's (1979) Ecological Systems Theory, which posits that all individuals exist within a variety of environmental systems including the microsystem (the client's immediate environment, e.g., family, work, school), mesosystem (comprised of connections between immediate environments), exosystem (external environments which indirectly affect the client, e.g., parents' religious affiliation), and macrosystems (larger cultural systems, e.g., ethnic community, political culture). It is useful for FAP therapists to consider all of these environmental systems as they assess for relevant history and controlling variables (discriminative stimuli exercising behavioral control; see Chapter 4 of Kohlenberg & Tsai, 1991) experienced by LGB clients.

Identity Development. During this process of assessment, it is essential also to consider LBG clients' phase of identity development. Though there are important differences among the many LGB identity development models in the literature (e.g., Cass, 1979; Fassinger & Miller, 1996; Troiden, 1979), taken together they suggest a basic framework of "identity confusion, identity comparison, identity assumption, and identity commitment" (Dworkin, 2001, p. 672). Noteworthy critique of these models has pointed out that while they imply a linear progress through stages of identity recognition, coming out, and identity integration, it is more accurate to conceptualize the identity process as a non-linear and bi-directional movement through phases which can be re-entered as LGB individuals encounter various environmental systems throughout their lifetimes (e.g., Myers, 2000).

During each of these phases, LGB individuals will typically contact particular environmental systems and therein face common intra- and/or interpersonal challenges. In the earliest phases – before LGB individuals first begin to question their sexual orientation – they are likely to observe aversive contingencies (e.g., verbal harassment, social rejection, physical assault) operating in the environment upon sexual minorities and indeed anyone who is "different." Furthermore, they may begin to derive rules based on witnessing these homonegative contingencies within their micro-, meso-, exo-, and macrosystems. As they begin to recognize their own same-sex attraction and question their sexual orientation they may experience an internal struggle – a conflict between what is naturally reinforcing for them (i.e., sexual interaction with same-sex partners, whether real or imagined) and the fear of contacting the aversive contingencies they have observed in their environment if they do identify as LGB. This conflict may result in aversively controlled rule-governed behavior. That is, despite their attractions, they may choose to date members of the opposite sex based on rules specifying the contingencies they have witnessed, e.g., *If I act on my same-sex attractions, my family will reject me, whereas if I date someone of the opposite sex I will be accepted.* Similarly, they may reject their attractions internally (e.g., thinking, *I know what lesbians are like and there's no way I'm one of them*) or externally (e.g., rejecting others who identify as LGB to escape the consequences of being labeled as LGB themselves).

As the process of identity development continues, LGB individuals face other challenges, most likely being subjected to some of the punishing contingencies they previously witnessed, feared, and avoided at earlier stages of development. As individuals begin to accept their sexual orientation and incorporate related behaviors into their repertoires of affiliation, identity expression, and sexuality, they are likely to experience a host of punishing consequences within many, if not all, environmental systems. For example, friends may reject them, family members may ignore or minimize their new identity, school environments may subtly or overtly punish expression of their identity, and religious institutions may warn them of future "eternal" punishment. Furthermore, larger cultural systems may punish and negatively reinforce them in a multitude of ways including invalidation of their very identity and relationships and denial of certain benefits and rituals afforded heterosexual couples and families.

In addition to these damaging experiences, bisexual individuals often face unique challenges and punishing contingencies as they recognize their identity and come into contact with contradictory macrosystems: the homonegative environment of mainstream culture as well as the heteronegative environment of the LGB community. Subjected to the opposing contingencies of these two worlds, bisexual individuals going through the public coming out process may need to develop even greater private control in order to engage in self-determination. That is, just like their gay and lesbian peers going through the coming out process, they face invalidation and punishment for self-determination based on private stimuli (same-sex attractions) that are unacceptable to the greater homonegative environment in which they live. But unlike their gay and lesbian peers, when they publicly choose an identity that does not conform to the rules of a dichotomous society, they become targets of punishment from other sexual minorities who may invalidate their chosen identity, viewing them as uncertain, scared to come out as gay/lesbian, or even traitors.

Therapists who are aware of these common aspects of the personal and group history of sexual minorities, as well as the nuanced interplay between phases of identity development and relevant environmental conditions, are in a position to complete a more thorough and accurate case conceptualization. These informed therapists would assess for their LGB clients' levels of sexual identity development and their rules specifying environmental contingencies with respect to sexuality (e.g., *If I tell my lesbian friends I date men as well as women, they will reject me*). If their clients' sexuality appears at all relevant to their presenting problem(s), they would specifically inquire about any relationship between the two. Furthermore, they would recognize and possibly explain to their clients that while it is not uncommon for such a relationship to exist (e.g., stigmatized identity correlates with higher levels of stress and decreased social support which may increase the likelihood for developing psychological problems as described above), it is unlikely that sexual orientation forms the etiological root of their presenting problems. This issue is further discussed below in terms of the conceptualization of client life problems.

Client Life Problems

The majority of LGB clients present in therapy with concerns very similar to those of their heterosexual peers, such as mood disorders, somatic difficulties, eating disorders, chronic stress, and substance abuse (Caitlin & Futterman, 1997; Meyer, 2003). In addition to these common themes, other issues linked to sexuality may prompt an LGB client or couple to seek therapy including homophobia, problems with identity development, coming out, parenting issues, HIV/AIDS-related issues, sex and intimacy, or coping with major life events which may not be recognized or validated by the larger heterosexual community. When seeing LGB clients, therapists often make one of two mistakes in framing these presenting problems. Either impelled by explicit homonegative attitudes or influenced by unconscious bias, some therapists attribute any presenting problems exclusively to their clients' sexual orientations. For example, imagine a lesbian client who attributes her presenting symptoms of low mood, anhedonia, withdrawal, and feelings of worthlessness to the recent breakup of a long-term same-sex relationship. Her therapist might conceptualize this same array of symptoms as major depression due to arrested sexual development, reducing the client's psychological suffering to the inevitable consequences of an unsatisfying, superficial lesbian relationship. The therapy that proceeds from the therapist's incompatible perceptions of the presenting problem and its etiology is likely to punish the client's attempt to seek help and may not only alienate the client from that particular therapist, but may contribute to a generalized distrust of the psychotherapy process.

At the other end of the spectrum, well-intentioned therapists, perhaps motivated out of political correctness, can minimize the relevance of sexual orientation in their clients' presenting problems fearing they might be seen as homophobic if they assess for any relation between the two. Under such aversive control, compelled by their own fears, therapists may avoid asking if and how their clients' identity or the struggles they have experienced because of their identity contribute to their low mood, social withdrawal, social anxiety, or other difficulties. It is crucial for FAP therapists to explore their own fears and underlying biases in order to minimize any such avoidance within the assessment process, both because the assessment itself would otherwise be incomplete, and because avoidance or minimization of the topic so early in therapy may result in clients learning (whether consciously or not) that discussion of sexuality in therapy will be punished or ignored. Ideally, therapist self-exploration will result in therapists developing an understanding of the functional relationship between their fears and their avoidance in session. The therapist is then better positioned to explore the possible relevance of sexuality and associated environmental conditions on the client's presenting problems.

In some cases, the therapist's hypothesis may not be accepted by her/his client, and the client may suggest that the therapist's inquiry is evidence of her/his heterosexist or homonegative bias. When this occurs (as such mistakes are virtually inevitable at some point) the interaction can be utilized as a therapeutic opportunity in a variety of ways. Depending entirely on the case conceptualization of the client, this mistake could evoke CRBs to be reinforced, provide an occasion for deeper mutual understanding, initiate the therapist's use of self-disclosure, and/or lead to further exploration of how the client responds to perceived bias in his/her life.

In Vivo Occurrences of Client Problems (CRB1s) and Improvements (CRB2s)

A core aspect of FAP assessment is the ongoing appraisal of the client's life problems and improvements occurring within the context of therapy. When client problems involve their sexual identity, the FAP therapist will be watching for, evoking, and reinforcing related clinically relevant behaviors (CRBs) related to sexual orientation or same-sex relationship dynamics. CRBs are always defined in functional terms and therefore cannot be predicted on a group level. Nevertheless, it can still be helpful and stimulating to consider concrete instances of CRB related to the life problems LGB clients sometimes bring into therapy. To this end, Table 9.1 provides examples of client life problems related to LGB identity and potential

Table 9.1 Potential client life problems related to sexual orientation and associated CRBs

Client life problems related to sexual orientation or same-sex relationship dynamics	Potential CRB1s	Potential CRB2s
Client avoids discussing sexuality-related topics (e.g., mentioning her/his relationship status) with others for fear of judgment or rejection	Client avoids bringing up sexuality-related topics in session	Client initially engages in discussion of topics related to sexuality and eventually initiates these discussions in session
Client is highly stigma-conscious, likely to assume homo-/biphobia on the part of others who have not proven themselves trustworthy, and is more likely to assume the world is viewing her/him through the lens of sexual orientation	Client is highly stigma-conscious in session, likely to assume homo-/biphobia on the part of the therapist, particularly early in therapy, and is more likely to assume the therapist is negatively judging her/him through the lens of sexual orientation. Client may also repeatedly inquire about the therapist's opinion or esteem for her/him	Client develops a more flexible and accurate attributional style. When she/he does perceive stigma or bias on the part of the therapist, she/he directly investigates this perception with the therapist (e.g., via direct questioning)

Table 9.1 (continued)

Client life problems related to sexual orientation or same-sex relationship dynamics	Potential CRB1s	Potential CRB2s
Avoiding eye contact with others in daily life when discussing anything related to sexuality	Avoiding eye contact with the therapist in session when discussing anything related to sexuality	Client initially makes sporadic eye contact, and eventually sustains eye contact with the therapist while discussing sexuality-related topics
Rigidly heterosexual or gender-conforming self-presentation across all environments in daily life for fear of outing oneself or appearing effeminate or "butch"	Rigidly heteronormative or gender-conforming self-presentation in sessions (e.g., dress & grooming, gesticulation, expressions of emotion, assertive-ness/submissiveness, vocal characteristics)	Client develops useful discriminative functions with regard to self-presentation, resulting in his/her flexible expression of sexual orientation and gender in session
Difficulty following through with a plan to come out to parents due to fear of being judged or rejected, despite this being a core value of the client	Avoiding disclosure of sexual orientation to therapist for fear of therapist judgment or rejection	Client might initially broach the topic of relationships or attractions and only later come out to therapist. Eventually the client may become more and more able to discuss specific sexual activities with the therapist
Distancing from GLB individuals and culture due to internalized homophobia	Choosing to work with a heterosexual therapist or distancing from a therapist who is (or is perceived as) GLB	Becoming closer to or aligning with a therapist who is (or is perceived as) GLB
Difficulty developing or maintaining emotional intimacy within gay relationship as both partners have been socialized against intimacy-enhancing repertoires	Gay client avoids interactions with therapist that would build therapeutic intimacy, particularly if working with a male therapist	Gay client initially allows therapist to initiate intimacy-building interactions, and eventually initiates these interactions
Difficulty maintaining a sense of self or expressing individuality within long-term lesbian relationship	Always aligning with the therapist, difficulty expressing differences or disagreement, adopting characteristics of therapist, particularly if female/lesbian	Initially, simply questioning the therapist; eventually challenging the therapist and acknowledging differences and disagreement in session

CRB1s and CRB2s to watch for in session (which may or may not be relevant for an individual LGB client).

This table presents only a handful of examples of client life problems and associated CRB1s and CRB2s related to or stemming from sexual minority identity. As tempting as it may be to use these ideas as a template for working with LGB clients, it is crucial that FAP therapists see these ideas as a springboard for case conceptualization possibilities. In undertaking this task, FAP therapists must reference their LGB clients' own perceptions of their life problems and therapy goals, while respecting each client's unique cultural background and values. To illustrate this point, consider a client who comes to therapy wishing to deal with his growing awareness of bisexual attractions. This client reports that he is no longer in denial of his attraction to men in addition to women, but he is unsure how to integrate this aspect of himself in certain domains of his life, particularly in his family life. He worries that if he comes out he would be emotionally distanced by his family, if not outright disowned. It is for these reasons, he explains, that he is considering remaining "closeted" and attempting to pursue only his attractions to women.

Knowing nothing else about this client's therapy goals and cultural context, we might rely upon existing identity development models to conceptualize the client's life problems and ascertain appropriate treatment goals. Following that approach, this client's desire to remain closeted to his family might be taken as evidence that he has not fully accepted his sexual identity or orientation, or perhaps indicate some hindrance in his identity development process. With this conceptualization, the therapist might become an advocate for the client working toward disclosure of his sexual orientation to his family. But, if we add crucial contextual information about the client's family and cultural background, different conclusions emerge. What if the client were raised in a Hasidic Jewish or Muslim community? What if he reports that his membership in his religious subculture has reinforced the importance of strong familial bonds and social networks with other members of his religious community? This client's access to support from the wider bisexual or queer community may be limited because he lives in a rural Hasidic enclave or, as a recent immigrant, speaks only a minimal amount of English. When viewed through this lens, the impact of culture on the client's values becomes clear, highlighting how indiscriminant application of predetermined treatment goals for all sexual minorities is inappropriate and potentially can be harmful. The FAP therapist's responsibility is to work collaboratively with each LGB client to determine if and how their current behaviors (both in and out of session) and treatment goals represent adaptive responses to given environmental conditions. Likewise, together the therapist and client can determine if active attempts to change their environment (e.g., through activism or engagement with a more supportive community) would provide greater access to reinforcement in their lives.

Therapist Work: A Look in the Mirror

Having explored GLB considerations with various aspects of the FAP case conceptualization, I now turn to a discussion of a crucial variable in FAP, the therapist. Before focusing the discussion exclusively on therapist issues with GLB clients, I begin with a discussion of more general therapist issues that will later be applied to working with sexual minorities.

Therapist Issues in Evoking and Responding to CRBs with Clients of All Sexual Orientations

The central mechanism of change in FAP is the therapist's natural, contingent responding to client in-session behaviors. The effectiveness of FAP, then, rests largely on the variable of the therapist – not only insofar as it matters in any other type of therapy, but even more so in FAP because the therapist's own personhood, stream of learning history, T1s (therapist in-session problem behaviors) and T2s (therapist in-session target behaviors), values, and personal mission will together determine the fidelity of the instrument upon which the client's progress depends. This is why therapists utilizing FAP must engage in an ongoing process of self-exploration and growth, expanding their own behavioral repertoire to include the extensive network of behavioral classes their clients also work to develop.

FAP therapists are obligated to increase their awareness of and enhance their own repertoires for a number of reasons. Therapists with broader repertoires relevant to the therapy process are more likely to notice, evoke, and naturally reinforce client CRBs. To put this in more concrete terms, imagine a therapist whose own emotional and interpersonal behavioral repertoire is limited. In her outside life she may tend to avoid contact with intense emotions resulting from interpersonal closeness and vulnerability; in particular, relationships in which the other person becomes extremely important to her. Perhaps this therapist avoids contact with controlling variables (discriminative stimuli for interpersonal closeness and vulnerability) by intellectualizing her emotions, remaining in a "one-up" position in most relationships, focusing on others' needs and feelings, presenting herself as emotionally self-sufficient, and masking aversive emotions with a convincing smile. Imagine too that this therapist has not reflected on these personal tendencies and has not considered how they show up in her work as a therapist. Completely outside of her awareness her avoidance patterns may inhibit many of her clients' progress. When her clients begin to contact their own controlling variables (when CRBs are evoked), this therapist is likely to respond with behaviors that distance her from these stimuli, inadvertently punishing her clients' progress. For example, if a client were to engage in a CRB2 of expressing raw emotions, she might attempt to contain her own discomfort by translating them into intellectual terms. When a client risks sharing deep pain, which would move most people in her outside life, this therapist might appear unaffected in any personal way. When a client asks her what she personally thinks or feels about him, she may don her convincing smile while giving a "canned" textbook answer, rather than taking the risk of sharing with the client how much impact he truly has on her and how moved she really is to see him working so hard.

Contrast this example with another therapist who has the same T1s, but is consistently undertaking the task of recognizing and changing her own avoidance behaviors in life and in session. As her avoidance shrinks (requiring risk-taking, courage, vulnerability), and she increases contact with her controlling variables in the context of a supportive social environment (e.g., a consult group or an FAP supervisor), her T2s are reinforced and her repertoires expand. Over time she becomes more likely to gain an awareness of avoidance behaviors in her clients, more likely to reinforce their approach toward controlling variables, and more likely able to tolerate the intense emotions associated with presenting discriminative stimuli for clients (evoking).[1]

As mentioned at the outset of this chapter, ideal FAP with heterosexual clients is no different than ideal FAP with LGB clients in its overall process. So it is true with the responsibility of personal work on the part of the therapist. The remainder of the chapter is devoted to discussion of specific types of self-exploration, awareness building, and repertoire enhancement by therapists that can benefit work with sexual minority clients.

Therapist Issues When Treating Sexual Minority Clients

What should FAP therapists do to expand their relevant repertoires when working with sexual minorities? How can they contact the relevant controlling variables and develop new behavior that is more affirmative of their LGB clients? While there is no comprehensive formula for this process, I have provided a loose structure that can guide the reader to consider a variety of aspects of self including one's fears, attitudes, biases, sexual attractions, and experiences. Although all of these domains are clearly interrelated, they are explored in separate sections for organizational purposes.

Therapist Discomfort with and/or Avoidance of Content Related to Sexuality

Therapists whose behavior was shaped within a homonegative and generally sex-negative environment (i.e., the overwhelming majority of therapists, *including* LGB therapists) are likely to be somewhat uncomfortable with open and direct exploration of same-sex attractions and/or discussion of sexual behavior. Regardless of one's best intentions or consciously held values, reinforcing CRBs related to sexuality will require willingness to contact one's own controlling variables, and therein, will require courage.

Consider a male client who is in the earliest stages of recognition and acceptance of his same-sex attractions working with a male FAP therapist whose T1 is avoidance of sexual content in sessions. The client's CRBs will take a multitude of forms many of which would likely elicit/evoke aversive private experiences on the part of the therapist. Hopefully, when CRBs are fairly obvious, (e.g., *I'm beginning to realize that my whole life I have felt more drawn to men than women* – likely an obvious tact and CRB2; see Chapter 3 in Kohlenberg & Tsai, 1991 for a discussion of the relevance of verbal behavior concepts such as "tacts" and "mands" in FAP), most

---

[1]This is why FAP supervisors often tell trainees that before asking their clients to complete any assignment or engage in an experiential exercise, they themselves must undertake the task.

therapists would feel compelled to pursue the issue even in the face of their own discomfort (e.g., by saying *"Tell me more about that"*), thereby reinforcing the client's CRB2 of exploring his attractions. Much of the time, however, clients struggling at this stage of identity development exhibit subtler CRBs. For example, a male client who has not yet acknowledged his attraction to men might say to his therapist, *I hate that my sister is always checking up on my dating life and trying to set me up with her girlfriends!* This statement that appears to be an obvious tact could also be a disguised mand (i.e., an indirect request) that the therapist stop making heterosexual assumptions about him in their therapy. In this case, a therapist who is avoidant of sexual content could very easily miss the hidden meaning as he chooses to follow up on the more comfortable topic of the client's expression of anger toward his sister.

LGB clients who are no longer struggling to acknowledge their sexual orientation or identity may still be reluctant to discuss their sexual activities with their therapists, especially when working with cross-gender therapists and/or those perceived to be heterosexual. Depending on their case conceptualization, clients' sexual activity and/or in-session disclosure thereof may be very relevant to the therapy. Therapists who collude with their clients' circumnavigation of this territory, or punish/extinguish clients' attempts to enter it, run the risk of inhibiting their progress.

Consider a client who has consistently avoided discussing his sexual activities in therapy. While describing the events of his weekend he somewhat indirectly indicated the extent of his sexual activities for the first time in his therapy:

Client: *This weekend was just like all the others. I went out to the bars, cruising. You know what I mean, right?*

Rather than being guided by the client's case conceptualization, a therapist might give in to her discomfort in a variety of ways. She might lead the conversation in a less aversive direction:

Therapist 1:   *Mm-hmm. So what else happened this weekend?*

Fearful of appearing ignorant or getting into the details of "cruising," the therapist might subtly foreclose the client's entrée into this conversation about sexual behavior by disingenuously stating:

Therapist 2:   *Cruising? Oh, sure, I know what you mean.*

Or conversely, the therapist might problematize or pathologize the client's sexual behavior based on her own values and biases:

Therapist 3:   *Why do you think you end up doing that every weekend? You know you're not going to find happiness that way.*

Any of these responses are likely to decrease the client's likelihood to engage in further CRB2s to the extent that the client sees that his therapist is uncomfortable or disapproving of his behavior. Contrast this with the outcome of responding genuinely and openly:

Therapist 4:   *I'm really glad you're clarifying this, Glen. You told me about going to the bars, but no, it wasn't clear that you were out cruising. Tell me more about your experiences cruising – I don't want to make any assumptions here.*

While this natural reinforcer will likely deepen the discussion and reveal further potentially relevant information, it can be augmented by a follow-up discussion prompted by the therapist:

Therapist 4:   *Glen, you hadn't told me very much about your sex life before today. So what was it like to bring that up with me? How did you feel about my response?*

Here the therapist shifts the focus of discussion from daily life to the therapeutic relationship, creating an opportunity for in vivo shaping of CRB2s.

In summary, clients will contact their controlling variables (i.e., be provided with new learning opportunities) only insofar as their therapists are willing to do the same. If therapists are only comfortable speaking about sexuality in sterile, scientific terms, they are likely to shape their clients to do the same, or to avoid talking about sexuality entirely – inside and outside of session. If they avoid using direct and clear language about sex and sexuality, their clients' progress equally will be limited. If they hold negative attitudes about certain types or frequency of sexual behavior, they may inadvertently shape their clients to withhold information about their sexual interactions from their therapists. By putting in the effort to expand these repertoires, however, therapists can serve as models, block their clients' avoidance, and be more naturally reinforcing of client CRB2s. In FAP, both clients and therapists are asked to push the boundaries of their comfort zones, to take risks, to lay bare their vulnerabilities, and to reveal their humanity. In the real relationship that results, genuine, natural reinforcement of client CRBs becomes possible.

Therapist Explicit and Implicit Attitudes

Attitudes have been defined by behaviorists as the learning process by which people come to evaluate stimuli in the environment favorably or unfavorably (Fishbein & Ajzen, 1975). Each individual's pattern of evaluations or biases is thought to result from her/his respondent and operant learning history in the context of particular social environments. Research in the field of attitudes and behavior suggest that *explicit attitudes* (in behavioral terms: the affective responses, behavioral biases, or predispositions that are within awareness and can be described) are merely the tip of the iceberg (Dovidio, Kawakami, & Beach, 2001). *Implicit attitudes* (in behavioral terms: affective responses, behavioral biases, or predispositions outside an individual's awareness) result from operant and respondent conditioning processes that may or may not be directly taught or even noticed by the individual therapist (Olson & Fazio, 2001). Similar to explicit attitudes, they can reflect the myriad favorable and unfavorable representations of stigmatized groups available in his/her social, political, and cultural environment. Unlike explicit attitudes, however, these automatic biases typically go unnoticed by even the most earnest, well-intentioned individuals who attempt to "introspect" their prejudices. Implicit attitudes and explicit attitudes are discussed separately below as they can be measured and manipulated in differing ways.

Exploring Explicit Attitudes. In the domain of explicit prejudice against LGB individuals, a number of studies reveal that these types of personal bias predict overt behaviors both within and outside of the therapeutic context. Looking specifically within the therapeutic context, a study by Hayes and Gelso (1993) revealed that male therapist homophobia (as measured by a self-report attitude questionnaire) predicted a pattern of avoidant and punishing therapist responses (e.g., disapproval, silence, selective ignoring) that diverted attention away from issues related to sexuality or inhibited further exploration thereof. In a follow-up analogue study regarding therapist reactions to lesbian clients, the same relationship was found between male and female therapists' explicit homophobia and avoidance responses while counseling lesbian clients. Additionally, more cognitive errors were made by female therapists in recalling sexual content presented by these lesbian clients (Gelso, Fassinger, Gomez, & Latts, 1995).

Given such data on the effects of explicit attitudes on therapist behavior, readers are encouraged to reflect on the ideas and questions about sexuality posed in Table 9.2, for an informal assessment of explicit attitudes about LGB issues.

Table 9.2 Questions and probes to explore explicit attitudes

(1) Do I feel that same-sex relationships are somehow "less than" cross-gender relationships?
(2) Do I believe that sexual orientation is a social construction or a biologically determined and fixed aspect of an individual?
(3) When I meet someone who identifies as bisexual, do I often try to figure out if they're "really" gay or lesbian?
(4) Am I more curious about someone's sexual and/or abuse history if I know they are a sexual minority?
(5) Do I get distracted by someone's gender presentation if it is atypical?
(6) Despite the research findings, do I worry more about children raised in non-traditional relationships or family structures?
(7) Do I assume that a client who chooses to be in an open or polyamorous relationship must have intimacy problems or perhaps must really desire a monogamous relationship "deep down"?
(8) How does my body react to descriptions or images of same-sex sexual behavior? How is this different or similar to how I react to descriptions or images of cross-gender sexual behavior?
(9) How would I react to discovering that a close relative was bisexual, lesbian, or gay?
(10) How do my religious affiliations and spiritual beliefs inform my attitudes about sexual minorities?
(11) Do I believe that same-sex couples should have the right to marry? Why or why not?
(12) Do I tend to actually favor the sexual minorities among my friends, or attempt to gain their approval and acceptance?
(13) Do I believe that there are no differences between cross-gender and same-sex relationships?
(14) What experiences have I had with LGB individuals and how have these informed my group stereotypes?

We are all well intentioned and aware of social norms and rules; therefore when conducting this exercise you are encouraged to explore and allow for socially undesirable responses. Note that these questions are intentionally evocative and do not necessarily have a "right," consistent, or foolproof answer.

This list only scratches the surface of attitudes and beliefs meriting exploration. Nevertheless, these verbal stimuli may have precipitated some aversive private events in the reader such as increased heart rate, sweat gland activity, and changed breathing patterns consistent with reports of uncertainty, anxiety, and shame. This group prediction is based on the assumption that while the overwhelming majority of readers were conditioned in social environments which reinforced heterosexism and paired sexual minorities with negativity, these readers also identify with the "rules" (verbal discriminative stimuli) of their professional community such as the APA Ethics Code and "Guidelines for psychotherapy with lesbian, gay, and bisexual clients." Because the conditions for reinforcement differ substantially in these two different contexts, therapists may experience discomfort related to contradictions between their own contingently shaped behaviors and the rules they have developed to govern their behavior. If the task of balancing these competing and contradicting rules and discriminative stimuli is sufficiently aversive, it may lead to avoidance of stimuli related to sexual orientation in our professional and personal lives. It is here that FAP therapists are urged to move forward into any discomfort they experience to acknowledge and begin to challenge their biases. More detailed discussion of this process is offered later in the chapter.

Exploring Implicit Attitudes. Before moving on with that task, how can we include our implicit (not verbally tacted) behaviors in the process? Is it even necessary to do so? Research suggests that indeed it may be useful for therapists to consider their implicit bias when working with stigmatized or minority clients: the link (though not causal) between implicit prejudice and explicit behavior has been demonstrated in a growing body of research focusing primarily on racial bias (for a review, see Dasgupta, 2004). This literature reveals that implicit bias predicts subtle observable behaviors toward stigmatized racial groups (e.g., eye contact, body posture, speech errors) better than explicit attitudes (e.g., Fazio, Jackson, Dunton, & Williams, 1995). It is quite likely then, that the same would be true with regard to implicit homonegative bias.

Emerging from the debate surrounding the measurement of implicit biases are response latency measures such as the Implicit Association Test (IAT; Greenwald & Banaji, 1995), an experimental paradigm developed to explore automatic cognitive and affective behaviors outside awareness. The IAT asks the test-taker to rapidly pair binary sets of stimuli (e.g., pairing a heterosexual image with the word "good," or a gay/lesbian image with the word "good"). Based on the individual's history of reinforcement for pairing the two concepts together, he/she will be more or less likely to respond to them as a single unit. If pairing gay/lesbian stimuli with "bad" has been more strongly reinforced in the test-taker's history, it should be easier for the test-taker to respond faster when asked to pair the two versus pairing gay/lesbian stimuli with the word "good". The response latency in pairing each set of stimuli gives a measure of, in the test developer's terms, one's implicit attitude and, in behavioral terms, the strength of the historical relation between the two concepts. The more related, the more rapidly one is able to respond.

While the IAT has primarily been used to collect data on a group level, it can also be used as a tool to gain greater awareness about an individual's implicit biases and preferences. Interested readers are encouraged to investigate their own implicit biases regarding sexual orientation as measured by the IAT for Sexuality (available through the "Demonstration Test" portal at https://implicit.harvard.edu/implicit/demo/). Though the IAT cannot be said to be a perfectly accurate test of implicit bias (for example, you may find that your exact results vary across two trials) this 15-min test can be extraordinarily useful in terms of opening one's eyes to bias that may be outside awareness. As these biases enter awareness one is already in a better position to predict and control them.

It takes willingness and courage for anyone to acknowledge bias – whether explicit or implicit – and to commit to perpetually challenge this bias. The good news is that preliminary research suggests that while these biases cannot be directly "unlearned," our implicit and explicit behaviors are malleable, that is, they can be altered by repetitive exposure and reconditioning (e.g., Pettigrew & Tropp, 2006; Rudman, Ashmore, & Gary, 2001; for a review, see Blair, 2002). The task of challenging bias via exposure and reconditioning is expounded upon at the conclusion of the chapter.

Exploring Therapist Sexuality and Experiences

A logical next step in an FAP therapist's self-exploration is in the domain of one's own sexuality. For some fortunate therapists, graduate training included coursework that invited exploration of one's sexual attractions, fantasies, and identity. The majority of us, however, may never have questioned or examined these aspects of self, or perhaps were forced to examine these issues as part of our own coming out process. Rather than accepting any default assumption of sexuality, or conceptualizing one's sexuality as a fixed entity that can be fully known at any one time, therapists benefit from actively engaging in an open and ongoing self-exploration conducted in the spirit of curiosity and compassion. In this process, one may ask oneself to consider both lived experiences as well as chosen identity, considering any gaps or differences between the two. If heterosexually identified, one may ask oneself about our same-sex feelings and approach these non-judgmentally, opening toward any internal conflicts that arise. If bisexually identified, one may also ask oneself about any discrepancies between real and conceptualized feelings and non-defensively consider how and why one identifies as bisexual. If gay or lesbian identified, one contemplates both same-sex and other-sex attractions, non-defensively opening to the full spectrum of sexual feelings and gently acknowledging any discrepancies or conflicts therein. As part of this process, we open to memories of personal experiences – both sexual and social – with sexual minorities and heterosexually identified individuals that may have shaped how we identify ourselves, with whom we affiliate, and how we conceptualize "straight," bisexual, gay, lesbian, and "queer" individuals. All of these avenues of exploration can provide rich information about our biases, the conflicts that might obstruct empathic connection, and potential obstacles we need to overcome in order to be naturally reinforcing to our sexual minority clients.

Another aspect of therapist identity and self-awareness which merits attention in this discussion is the match between therapist and client sexual orientation. While heterosexually identified therapists must be on the lookout for the obvious distortions inherent to "outsider" status, therapists who themselves are sexual minorities face other obstacles in treating LGBs, which, if not countered, pose potential hazards in FAP therapy. Therapists who are "insiders" may view their LGB clients through a lens of assumed similarity, over-identification, or idealization, running the risk of under-assessing the client's idiographic presentation and/or ignoring dysfunction. LGB-identified therapists may consciously or unconsciously assume their sexual minority clients will (or should) proceed through the same course of identity development as they have themselves. They may subtly or directly encourage their clients to adopt their personal philosophy of sexuality – as a dichotomous, fixed, or fluid characteristic. Likewise, they may assume that what has worked best for them will work best for their LGB clients in terms of coming out, responding to homophobia, choosing to be monogamous or negotiating open relationships, and merging with or remaining emotionally independent in relationships. For these reasons it is imperative that LBG therapists be mindful of, and combat, the pitfalls of their "insider" status.

Overcoming Therapist Fear of Appearing Prejudiced

Most therapists aspire to hold some degree of conscious egalitarian beliefs with regard to LGB populations. When treating LGB clients, then, it is highly likely that therapists would desire their clients to recognize their open-mindedness and awareness. As much as this desire may reflect one's best intentions, the fear of appearing prejudiced, homophobic, or ignorant can easily become a barrier in treatment. These fears can lead therapists to miss important information because they choose not to acknowledge the limits of their familiarity with clients' LBG experiences and identity. When clients use culture-specific terminology or refer to experiences unfamiliar to some therapists, rather than asking for clarification these therapists may try to deduce their clients' meaning from context or may hope the clients will provide further clarification during the session. Another problem arises when therapists avoid conceptualizing anything related to sexuality as relevant or dysfunctional even if it appears so. If these therapists do consider sexuality or identity-related information in the functional analyses of LGB clients, they may be reluctant to bring up their functional hypotheses with their clients. Finally, wary therapists who do not share their clients' sexual orientation may fear these clients' judgments and therefore avoid disclosing their orientation when clients inquire without considering if the inquiry represents a CRB1 or CRB2.

FAP therapists who have the courage to admit the limits of their knowledge and experience, consider sexual variables in case conceptualizations and functional analyses, and strategically disclose personal information about their own sexuality are likely to encounter difficult therapeutic situations. In some instances their clients may respond with disappointment, hurt, or confusion, suggest that their therapists are homophobic, or argue that their analyses have been tainted by heterosexist bias. FAP therapists can approach these situations as therapeutic opportunities that may evoke CRBs (Rule 2) (see Chapter 1 in this volume for a summary of FAP's five rules). For example, consider this interaction between a therapist and her gay male client who is sexually active with multiple partners. This client's daily life problems include avoidance of emotional expression, avoidance of situations that evoke emotional pain, and lack of assertiveness.

Therapist:	*We've been working together for about 2 months now, trying to figure out how to increase your sense of purpose and fulfillment in life. You have this sense that something is missing, but you can't quite put your finger on it. I've noticed that during our sessions you focus mainly on frustrations with your family and at work. But you tend to not talk much about your romantic involvements. How do you think that fits into the picture?*
Client:	*I told you already, I don't think that's the problem.*
Therapist:	*I do remember you making a point of that in our first session. At the same time, I've noticed that we do a pretty good job of avoiding it altogether when, for a lot of people, finding a partner can be an important part of feeling fulfilled in life.*
Client:	*I can't believe I'm hearing this. You, too? Let me guess: Because I have my fair share of random hook-ups but don't have a serious relationship there's something wrong with me, right? [This is a potential CRB2 in terms of acknowledging some emotional pain rather than avoiding the issue altogether.]*

A therapist who is worried about being judged as homophobic might respond by leaving this charged territory, either retracting the question or quickly apologizing for posing such a faulty question. A productive alternative, however, is to view the interaction through the lens of clinically relevant behavior providing an opportunity for in vivo reinforcement:

Therapist:	*Tell me what just happened inside, Joel.*
Client:	*I can't believe it. Sorry, but that's just too classic and I didn't expect it from you.*
Therapist:	*I said something that really upset you, Joel, and I want to understand how that happened.*
Client:	*Well, I never said that my sex life was a problem for me but it seems like it's a problem for you. And then you implied that finding a partner is necessary in order to be fulfilled [client becomes tearful]. I've got an entire society telling me there's something wrong with how*

> *I am, and now you. [The client's assertiveness and specification of the evocative stimulus are both likely CRB2s.]*

The therapist might reinforce these CRB2 by further exploring and empathizing with the client's emotional response, attempting to develop deeper mutual understanding, strategically disclosing, asking her client to teach her more, or otherwise genuinely repairing the rupture. One example follows:

Therapist: *I see how much I've hurt you, Joel. I took a big risk in asking you about romantic relationships but chose to bring it up because I am 100% committed to getting to the heart of your dissatisfaction in life. And in that pursuit I don't want to leave any stone unturned. It sounds like by asking you that question I just got added to a long list of people in your life who have suggested that there is something wrong with how you do relationships.*

Client: *I'm so tired of it. That's why I tried to tell you in the beginning.*

Therapist: *There's a lot of history here and it makes sense that my bringing it up would stir up these feelings. And Joel, it took a lot of guts to tell me how hurt you were. You know that? [Reinforcing client's emotional disclosure]. What else, Joel? Is there anything you're holding back on saying to me? [This is Rule 2 – evoking CRB2.]*

Client: *Look, I've been in long-term monogamous relationships before, and at this point in my life I'm just not into it. The whole idea that you need a relationship to make you happy – that's so heterosexist and it's not why I started therapy.*

Therapist: *Ok, I'm stuck here. On one hand I am so moved at how honest and assertive you're being in telling me you don't want to focus on relationships in our therapy. I also want to be careful not to mistakenly apply society's value system on you when so much of our work depends on you being able to define your own values and goals [reinforcing client's CRB2 of assertiveness and direct communication]. On the other hand you've told me how hard it is to move into really emotional territory and I wonder if ignoring this issue is more about avoiding the emotions that come up here [evoking CRB].*

Client: *[sigh] It's not that I wouldn't ever want that relationship … I've tried – so hard. They don't work – or, I don't know – maybe I don't work [client becomes tearful once again].*

Therapist: *And you feel exhausted and discouraged just thinking about your efforts and experiences in the past [accurate empathy – reinforcing his CRB2]. When I brought up the question of relationships I bet I brought back all those feelings you're trying to get away from – the exhaustion the frustration, the fear of judgment. What else [evoking more disclosure]?*

Client: *I don't want to feel broken. I don't know if I want to do this [CRB2 in identifying the underlying private experience he has been avoiding].*

Although this conversation represents only one of countless ways the session might have unfolded, it demonstrates how a therapist who is willing to take the risk of proceeding into politically and personally charged territory can deepen the work and help her client identify a major block in discussing (and possibly, in forming) romantic relationships. As the conversation moves forward, the therapist would continue acknowledging the issue of heterosexist bias on her part in order to communicate to the client that she is aware of it and open to discussing it, and ultimately focused on the client's deepest values and life goals. While in this example the therapist worked to look beyond her client's accusation of heterosexist bias, in other cases in which such an accusation was itself a CRB2, the therapist would orient her responses around reinforcing the client's political analysis by expressing appreciation for the client's courage in pointing it out, openly acknowledging and exploring her bias, and/or making a genuine apology or repair for the rupture.

Shaping Therapist Behavior

Previous sections of this chapter have indicated a variety of domains in which therapists are encouraged to gain greater awareness of their own reinforcement histories, biases, private and public behaviors with regard to sexual minorities. The singular moments of awareness that have been evoked by reading this chapter, however, are not likely to lead to lasting observable improvement in therapist–client interactions. In order for such change to occur, therapists wishing to gain greater control of their heteronormative/homonegative biases would need to apply the same rules of behavior change to themselves as apply to FAP clients. Awareness is merely the first step – literally (Rule 1).

Rule 2 (evoke CRBs) is applied as FAP therapists maintain an ongoing practice of contacting their own controlling variables (discriminative stimuli) with respect to sexuality and sexual orientation, both in and out of session. In concrete terms this means FAP therapists will attempt to combat their own avoidance of LBG- or sexuality-related stimuli (e.g., forming close social connections with LGB individuals, consuming LGB media, participating in LGB cultural or political events). If their larger verbal community does not provide substantial access to such stimuli, FAP therapists are encouraged to move beyond their default environment to one which will provide more access to related stimuli and be more naturally evocative.

The mere exposure provided by following Rule 2 would be expected to decrease therapist bias to the extent that it allows for the modification of reflexive homophobic responses to LGB stimuli via classical conditioning. Rule 2's full potential, however, is attained with the introduction of Rule 3 (reinforce CRBs). By entering and engaging in communities with different sociopolitical contingencies that are more inclusive and reinforcing of LGB individuals, FAP therapists increase the likelihood that their own behaviors (implicit and explicit, public and private, verbal and affective) will be similarly shaped. Rule 3 also comes into play in session with LGB (and quite possibly heterosexual) clients, as well as in supervisory and consultative contexts in which less biased therapist behaviors with regard to sexuality have the opportunity to be naturally reinforced within the dyad or group.

Rule 4 (observe potentially reinforcing effects) is critical as it highlights the need for FAP therapists who are attempting to modify their biases to pay attention to the impact of their personal work on their own in-session behaviors with LGB clients (e.g., are they more likely to evoke relevant CRB and to be naturally reinforcing of CRB2s?) Furthermore, Rule 4 asks FAP therapists to observe the impact of their expanded behavioral repertoire on their clients. The new therapist behaviors resulting from therapists' personal work are intended to lead to more effective therapeutic relationships (e.g., closer, more intimate relationships with LGB clients, increased likelihood of evoking sexuality-related CRB and being naturally reinforcing of CRB2).

Therapist personal work with sexual bias can be expanded by including Rule 5 (interpretation and generalization) in the process. This rule would direct FAP therapists combating their heterosexual/homonegative bias to consider the antecedents and maintaining variables of this and other biases that may be part of the same functional class of behaviors. Gains made in the understanding of one's own heterosexism, for example, can translate into larger functional analyses that account for how environmental contingencies have shaped our sociopolitical leanings in ways that may inadvertently maintain oppressive practices in our clinical work. Rule 5 also takes this work beyond the clinical session, inviting FAP therapists to make the same "in-to-out parallels" we ask our clients to make when in-session experiences correspond to daily life events. That is, FAP therapists whose in-session repertoires are changed by their personal work can work to generalize these gains to their daily lives, creating a safer, and less oppressive cultural environment for LGB and other disempowered individuals and groups.

Conclusion

It is important to acknowledge that no data have been gathered in the FAP community to empirically examine the effectiveness of the therapist shaping strategies and practices described above. They are, rather, the result of personal and anecdotal experience that is largely consistent with behavioral principles, or have been directly deduced from FAP and behavior analytic theory. Single-subject work and publication of FAP case studies with LGB clients will be crucial to support and refine these ideas.

Considering the lack of empirical support for this particular application of FAP behavior change principles, and the considerable discomfort that is likely to be experienced if it is nevertheless undertaken, it will not be the average therapist who will carry out all the work described in this chapter. If you count yourself among those who will carry this torch, the potential professional and personal benefits may be substantial. Developing an understanding of experiences common to many sexual minorities is likely to result in more time for LGB clients to spend their session delving into what is most potent for them, rather than educating or arguing with their therapist. Learning how to construct case conceptualizations that consider clients' sexuality – without assuming its relevance – can help clarify appropriate treatment targets and related CRB. Examining your own identity, biases, and fears increases awareness, predictability, and control over related behavior. Direct shaping of therapist behavior affords the opportunity to expand one's own repertoire, becoming a more effective reinforcer for clients. By walking similar pathways of self-exploration as FAP clients are asked to do, FAP therapists can discover and distill their own voices and learn how to better reinforce their clients for unapologetically speaking their inner truths.

References

American Psychiatric Association. (1952). *Diagnostic and statistical manual of mental disorders* (DSM-I). Washington, DC: American Psychiatric Association.

American Psychiatric Association. (1980). *Diagnostic and statistical manual of mental disorders, third edition* (DSM-III). Washington, DC: American Psychiatric Association.

American Psychiatric Association. (1987). *Diagnostic and statistical manual of mental disorders, third revised edition* (DSM-III-R). Washington, DC: American Psychiatric Association.

American Psychological Association. (2000). Guidelines for psychotherapy with lesbian, gay, and bisexual clients. *American Psychologist, 55*(12), 1409–1421.

American Psychological Association. (2002). Ethical principles of psychologists and code of conduct. *American Psychologist, 57*(12), 1060–1073.

Bieschke, K. J., McClanahan, M., Tozer, E., Grzegorek, J. L., & Park, J. (2000). Programmatic research on the treatment of lesbian, gay, and bisexual clients: The past, the present, and the course of the future. In R. M. Perez, K. A. DeBord, & K. J. Bieschke (Eds.), *Handbook of counseling and psychotherapy with lesbian, gay, and bisexual clients* (pp. 309–335). Washington, DC: APA.

Blair, I. V. (2002). The malleability of automatic stereotypes and prejudice. *Personality and Social Psychology Review, 6*, 242–261.

Bronfenbrenner, U. (1979). *The ecology of human development: Experiments by nature and design.* Cambridge, MA: Harvard University Press.

Caitlin, R., & Futterman, D. (1997). *Lesbian and gay youth: Care and counseling.* Philadelphia, PA: Hanley & Belfus.

Cass, V. (1979). Homosexual identity formation: A theoretical model. *Journal of Homosexuality, 4*, 219–235.

Cochran, S. D., Sullivan, J. G., & Mays, V. M. (2003). Prevalence of mental disorders, psychological distress, and mental services use among lesbian, gay, and bisexual adults in the United States. *Journal of Consulting and Clinical Psychology, 71*(1), 53–61.

Dasgupta, N. (2004). Implicit ingroup favoritism, outgroup favoritism, and their behavioral manifestations. *Social Justice Research, 17*, 143–169.

Dohrenwend, B. P. (2000). The role of adversity and stress in psychopathology: Some evidence and its implications for theory and research. *Journal of Health and Social Behavior, 41*, 1–19.

Dovidio, J. F., Kawakami, K., & Beach, K. R. (2001). Implicit and explicit attitudes: Examination of the relationship between measures of intergroup bias. In R. Brown & S. L. Gaertner (Eds.), *Blackwell handbook of social psychology* (Vol. 4, pp. 175–197). Oxford, England: Blackwell.

Dworkin, S. H. (2001). Treating the bisexual client. *Journal of Clinical Psychology, 57*(5), 671–680.

Fassinger, R. E., & Miller, B. A. (1996). Validation of an inclusive model of sexual minority identity formation on a sample of gay men. *Journal of Homosexuality, 32*(2), 53–78.

Fazio, R. H., Jackson, J. R., Dunton, B. C., & Williams, C. J. (1995). Variability in automatic activation as an unobtrusive measure of racial attitudes: A bona fide pipeline? *Journal of Personality and Social Psychology, 69*, 1013–1027.

Fergusson, D. M., Horwood, J. L., & Beautrais, A. L. (1999). Is sexual orientation related to mental health problems and suicidality in young people? *Archives of General Psychiatry, 56*, 876–880.

Fishbein, M., & Ajzen, I. (1975). *Beliefs, attitudes, intentions and behavior*. Reading, MA: Addison-Wesley.

Garnets, L., Hancock, K., Cochran, S., Goodchilds, J., & Peplau, L. (1991). Issues in psychotherapy with lesbians and gay men: A survey of psychologists. *American Psychologist*, *46*, 964–972.

Gelso, C. J., Fassinger, R., Gomez, M. J., & Latts, M. G. (1995). Countertransference reactions to lesbian clients: The role of homophobia, counselor gender, and countertransference management. *Journal of Counseling Psychology*, *42*, 356–364.

Gilman, S. E., Cochran, S. D., Mays, V. M., Hughes, M., Ostrow, D., & Kesler, R. C. (2001). Risk of psychiatric disorders among individuals reporting same-sex sexual partners in the National Comorbidity Survey. *American Journal of Public Health*, *91*, 933–939.

Greenwald, A. G., & Banaji, M. R. (1995). Implicit social cognition: Attitudes, self-esteem, and stereotypes. *Psychological Review*, *102*(1), 4–27.

Hayes, J. A., & Gelso, C. J. (1993). Male counselors' discomfort with gay and HIV-infected clients. *Journal of Counseling Psychology*, *40*, 86–93.

Herrell, R., Goldberg, J., True, W. R., Ramakrishnam, V., Lyons, M., Eisen, S., & Tsuang, M. T. (1999). Sexual orientation and suicidality: A co-twin control study in adult men. *Archives of General Psychiatry*, *56*, 867–874.

Hooker, E. (1957). The adjustment of the male overt homosexual. *Journal of Projective Techniques*, *21*, 18–31.

Jones, M. A., & Gabriel, M. A. (1999). Utilization of psychotherapy by lesbians, gay men, and bisexuals: Findings from a nationwide survey. *American Journal of Orthopsychiatry*, *69*, 209–219.

Kinsey, A. C., Pomeroy, W. B., & Martin, C. E. (1948). *Sexual behavior in the human male*. Philadelphia, PA: W.B. Saunders Company.

Kinsey, A. C., Pomeroy, W. B., Martin, C. E., & Gebhard, P. H. (1953). *Sexual behavior in the human female*. Philadelphia, PA: W.B. Saunders Company.

Kohlenberg, R. J., & Tsai, M. (1991). *Functional analytic psychotherapy: Creating intense and curative therapeutic relationships*. New York: Plenum Press.

Meyer, I. H. (2003). Prejudice, social stress, and mental health in lesbian, gay, and bisexual populations: Conceptual issues and research evidence. *Psychological Bulletin*, *129*(5), 674–697.

Myers, J. E. (2000, October 1). Revisiting Cass' theory of sexual identity formation: A study of Lesbian development. *Journal of Mental Health Counseling*, *22*(4), 318–333.

Olson, M. A., & Fazio, R. H. (2001). Implicit attitude formation through classical conditioning. *Psychological Science*, *12*(5), 413–417.

Pettigrew, T. F., & Tropp, L. R. (2006). A meta-analytic test of intergroup contact theory. *Journal of Personality and Social Psychology*, *90*(5), 751–783.

Phillips, J. C., & Fischer, A. R. (1998). Graduate students' training experiences with gay, lesbian, and bisexual issues. *The Counseling Psychologist*, *26*, 712–734.

Rudman, L. A., Ashmore, R. D., & Gary, M. L. (2001). "Unlearning" automatic biases: The malleability of implicit prejudice and stereotypes. *Journal of Personality and Social Psychology*, *81*(5), 856–868.

Safren, S. A., & Heimberg, R. G. (1999). Depression, hopelessness, suicidality, and related factors in sexual minority and heterosexual adolescents. *Journal of Consulting and Clinical Psychology*, *67*(6), 859–866.

Safren, S. A., & Pantalone, D. W. (2006). Social anxiety and barriers to resilience among lesbian, gay, and bisexual adolescents. In A. M. Omoto & H. S. Kurtzman (Eds.), *Sexual orientation and mental health: Examining identity and development in lesbian, gay, and bisexual people* (pp. 55–71). Washington, DC: American Psychological Association.

Siever, M. D. (1994). Sexual orientation and gender as factors in sociocultural acquired vulnerability to body dissatisfaction and eating disorders. *Journal of Consulting and Clinical Psychology*, *62*, 252–260.

Troiden, R. R. (1979). Being homosexual: A model of gay identity acquisition. *Psychiatry, 42,* 362–373.

Tsai, M., Kohlenberg, R. J., Kanter, J. W., Kohlenberg, B., Follette, W. C., & Callaghan, G. M. (2008). *A guide to functional analytic psychotherapy: Awareness, courage, love and behaviorism.* New York: Springer.

Chapter 10
Transcultural FAP

**Luc Vandenberghe, Mavis Tsai, Luis Valero, Rafael Ferro,
Rachel R. Kerbauy, Regina C. Wielenska, Stig Helweg-Jørgensen,
Benjamin Schoendorff, Ethel Quayle, JoAnne Dahl, Akio Matsumoto,
Minoru Takahashi, Hiroto Okouchi, and Takashi Muto**

In discussing transcultural functional analytic psychotherapy (FAP), the treatment of clients from culturally diverse backgrounds, we draw upon not only the experiences of FAP therapists outside the United States (e.g., Carrascoso, 2003; Ferro, Valero, & Vives, 2006; López, Ferro, & Calvillo, 2002; Ferro, Valero, & López Bermúdez, 2009), but also the booming literature on cultural competence and multiculturalism. Decades of work in the latter area have spawned profound reflection (Sue & Zane, 1987; Sue & Sue, 2003; Fowers & Davidov, 2006), practical guidelines (American Psychological Association, 2003), and comprehensive strategies for adapting treatments to multicultural populations (Hays, 2001; Hwang, 2006; Hinton, 2006). As practitioners belonging to different cultures, we believe that the principles of FAP are broadly applicable across cultures and, in combination with ideas from the cultural competence literature, lead to strategies for therapists to work with clients from diverse backgrounds.

Cultural competence involves respecting, valuing, and integrating the sociocultural context of culturally diverse clients (López, 1997) and validating their perceptions on problems and solutions that may be at odds with mainstream perspectives. Therapeutic goals and interventions must be consistent with the client's values and life contexts. For this reason, it is fruitful to discuss both the client's norms and mainstream cultural norms whenever relevant during assessment and treatment planning (López, 1997; Tanaka-Matsumi, Higginbotham, & Chang, 2002; Sue & Sue, 2003; Okazaki & Tanaka-Matsumi, 2006).

In this chapter we will explore the importance of understanding how a client's cultural history, customs, traditions, and identity may affect not only his or her daily life problems, goals, assets, and strengths, but also what constitute clinically relevant

L. Vandenberghe (✉)
Pontifical Catholic University of Goiás, Goiânia, Brazil
e-mail: luc.m.vandenberghe@gmail.com

J.W. Kanter et al. (eds.), *The Practice of Functional Analytic Psychotherapy*,
DOI 10.1007/978-1-4419-5830-3_10, © Springer Science+Business Media, LLC 2010

behaviors. Then we will delve into therapist behaviors that can increase meaning, effectiveness, and intensity in transcultural FAP.

Relevant Personal and Cultural History

FAP case conceptualization (Kanter et al., 2008) calls for collecting information about important life experiences that account for the reinforcement of problem behaviors as well as why more useful interpersonal behavior was not reinforced and learned. This description makes it possible to see how behavior that may be self-defeating today had an adaptive function in the past, and it draws attention to consequences that may be currently maintaining these damaging repertoires.

When a client is from a different culture, it is essential that his or her cultural identity and level of acculturation be assessed as part of relevant history (Tanaka-Matsumi, Seiden, & Lam, 1996). Client experience might be influenced by being a member of a group that historically has struggled with the aversive consequences associated with marginalization, the stresses of immigration and adaptation, or even by collective dislocation as refugees. Helpless or self-defeating behaviors may emerge from such conditions. Behaviors that currently curtail the client's opportunities, like submissiveness or self-deprecation, may have been adaptive in times of oppression and exploitation. An example is a client from a traditionally discriminated-against group who readily lets important personal opportunities go by, upholds a predetermined fatalism, and makes excuses such as "People like us will never take care of ourselves – we will always depend on the rich."

Awareness of how a client's community has reinforced the practices and assumptions held by its members is called for, as well as knowledge of key historical events and environmental factors such as present economic or political conditions. Besides consulting objective information on the history and the social reality of the client's group, additional readings may also be illuminating. For example, a novel like *The Inheritance of Loss* by Desai (2006) or short stories such as those found in the collection *Unaccustomed Earth* by Lahiri (2008) are recommended. Set predominantly in the 1980s in northeast India, the characters in Desai's book struggle with feelings of cultural and familial alienation; loss of traditional values and ways of life; forces of modernization, discrimination, and oppression; shuttling between first and third worlds; experiencing pain of exile; desiring a better life; and questions of nationhood, modernity, and class. Lahiri's work abounds with the same themes and focuses on the choices of life directions and goals and the daily struggles of immigrants and their children in the context of clashes between values and traditions. Both books expose how trying to adapt to a dominant culture can lead people to develop self-defeating repertoires and how cultural and personal strengths are helpful in overcoming adverse conditions.

Carefully considering a client's relevant history is necessary for what Sue (1998) calls dynamic sizing, or flexibly incorporating into case conceptualization what is applicable about the client's culture of origin and nothing more. This allows the integration of relevant cultural issues in the case conceptualization while avoiding the perils of stereotyping.

Daily Life Problems and Goals

In FAP, a client's behavior is defined functionally in relation to the situation in which it occurs, what precipitates it, and the consequences that follow it. A functional understanding of the client's daily life problems is a prerequisite for selecting treatment goals and for identifying clinically relevant behaviors in-session. As a result, culture-specific antecedents and consequences of problem behaviors become visible as the therapist sets out to define the client's problems behaviorally.

There may be differences between the client's causal explanation of daily life problems and the therapist's functional analysis of those problems, and explicit negotiation may be needed regarding the cultural acceptability of the change techniques to be used (Tanaka-Matsumi et al., 1996). Consider the example of an unmarried young female client from rural northeastern Brazil who, after moving with the entire family to an urban area near to the federal capital, lived in perpetual conflict with her parents. Sometimes she would suddenly disappear for days after a fight, letting her parents "think about what she had said." Her therapist thought this woman had the skills and resources needed to live on her own, but when asked about this, the client refused to answer and kept bringing up new complaints. In the following two sessions she vacillated between agreeing with and rejecting the goal of becoming independent. Her therapist shared the confusion and weariness this evoked in him and wondered if his client also made it this difficult for her parents to understand what she wanted. When the client was asked about this, however, she ended the session, screaming at her therapist and walking out.

Despite not returning the therapist's phone calls, she returned for the next session. The therapist observed that the client used the same interpersonal strategies with him that she used in dealing ineffectively with the conflicts in her family and that this way therapy would also be ineffective. After insistent prompting, the client stated that she had expected her therapist to know that a woman from her region would only leave her parents for good reason, like when getting married or finding a job far away from home. The therapist asked her to look into the practices of her reference group and to identify alternative solutions. After some discussion, they agreed to target better skills for negotiating her needs and dealing with conflict.

In this case, the client explicitly stating her cultural preferences and openly re-negotiating treatment goals with the therapist were in vivo improvements related to her daily life goals. She was committed to her traditional role definition as an adult single daughter and preferred to develop behaviors that were valued in her traditional family culture. The intention, of course, is to work out a plan that is acceptable to all those directly involved in the treatment (Tanaka-Matsumi, Higginbotham, & Chang, 2002).

Assets and Strengths: Culture as a Therapeutic Aid

Being an effective FAP therapist requires an ability to respond selectively to people's positive characteristics, and this naturally highlights aspects of a client's culture that have positively influenced the client. As a member of a cultural group, the client may have acquired valuable communication skills, culture-specific problem-solving strategies, or other assets that can be therapeutic aids.

Strengths that clients present as part of their traditional heritage are not the only strengths to consider. In dealing with the challenges of living in two different cultures, people tend to acquire new skills. They may have become more flexible, open to different experiences, or better at observing people. These qualities also can be built upon when shaping more effective daily life repertoires.

In addition, minority membership may also offer the privilege of an effective social support network (Hays, 2001) which can be helpful during therapy. For example, take the case of a depressed client whose social isolation was related to the ways in which she discouraged and rejected people who cared for her. In session, she also initially punished her therapist's positive reactions toward her. As she and her therapist focused on her learning to accept and reinforce compassionate responses from the therapist, she began to allow others in her life to express more caring toward her. The generalization of this new behavior from therapy to daily life was greatly facilitated because she could tap into the intensely close-knit network of her social group.

Besides interpersonal support, natural and constructed resources may also be available in minority neighborhoods or ethnic communities that should be considered in therapy. These resources include ways of organizing living spaces, culture-specific provisions for meetings, recreation, and meditation or for culture-specific art (Hays, 2001).

Furthermore, a client's heritage can entail a broad variety of therapeutic aids. The arts and literature from a client's background may offer means to explore the client's behavior or to identify targets during assessment. In treatment, they can be used to elicit or evoke behavior. They can also be used by the therapist as a means of sharing his or her interpretations of clinically relevant behaviors with the client. For example, a client whose presenting problem was that she was sexually indiscriminate and monopolized initiative in relationships soon became openly seductive with her therapist. She agreed with him that she was wasting yet another opportunity as she had previously ruined several chances for friendships and co-worker relations. She stated she was willing to give up therapy for a sexual relationship as she was born that way and nothing would change her. Their treatment was stalled until her therapist used the analysis of a well-known character from the client's national literature to illustrate a clinical point. When the therapist proposed discussing the sensuous Gabriela from a novel by Amado (1958) who exemplified disbelief in personal change, she was surprised that, as a foreigner, the therapist had any knowledge about her national literature. She had read the book and seen a soap opera based on it. Although she argued she had little in common with Gabriela, this was the first time she gave attention to a theme her therapist introduced instead of ignoring or disqualifying any initiative or idea that was not hers as she was used to doing in daily life situations. This in vivo improvement marked a turning point in her therapy.

The Cultural Context of Clinically Relevant Behaviors (CRBs)

As stated throughout this book, FAP focuses on clinically relevant behaviors (CRBs): client in-session problem behaviors that are instances of their outside life behaviors are CRB1s, and in-session targets or improvements are CRB2s. When working with clients from diverse backgrounds, a major challenge for the therapist is to recognize the cultural contexts of their CRBs. Below are examples of potential CRB1s or in-session problem behaviors, along with possible cultural antecedents suggested by native Asian, European, and Latin American practitioners:

(1) A man who is suffering from depression is extremely passive, nonassertive, and obedient in therapy and wants his therapist to "fix" the problem. The background for this issue may vary immensely according to culture and the therapist must take this into account. For example, the treatment of psychological problems in Spain and various other countries may have strong ties with the medical profession. In several countries psychologists have only been included in the national health system in the last few decades, thus, clients generally arrive thinking the therapist will be very directive, will give instructions like a physician, and tell the client what to do. On the other hand, in Japanese culture, "amae" is a class of responses that manages others so one can be loved by and dependent upon them. Clients often expect or count on their therapists' goodwill and will ask their therapists to solve interpersonal problems for them rather than working on how the clients themselves might change. In addition, when clients come from a culture that emphasizes harmony and relatedness (e.g., certain Asian cultures) it is difficult for them to assert their personal wants and needs in therapy.

(2) A woman who is having difficulty developing close friendships struggles with revealing her feelings in therapy. If this client comes from a Spanish Mediterranean culture, her expression of feelings may seem awkward to a therapist of Anglo-Saxon background, who grew up in a community that focuses particularly on the personal-self but not on the social-self. It may be that the client's parents did not help their children speak about their private feelings in the same way. As a result, self-expression as handled by the therapist may not mesh with Spanish concepts where personal reference is usually done from the verb participle (e.g., "quiero," "tengo") so that "I" or "yo" has a more restricted linguistic role. Some Spanish therapists believe that a challenge for using FAP in treating Spanish people with interpersonal problems is that they do not talk directly in first person (e.g., "I want X"), but rather with an indirect, reflexive style (e.g., "X would be nice" or "X could be done").

The problem may also be related to cultural differences in the way intimacy is constructed. In Spanish culture, the concept of "intimate relationship" is strongly associated with a relationship between a couple or a sexual relationship and to a lesser degree a friendship. But to apply it to a professional relationship would seem strange. The therapist's adaptation may consist of presenting himself/herself as a personal adviser who is going to get personally involved in order to help the client as much as possible. If the client belongs to another culture, other differences may need to be considered. For instance, fear of intimacy as expressed in social phobia may have a specific history in Scandivania where a radical transformation took place from relatively homogeneous farming communities to more heterogeneous urban communities. Similar historical elements have been observed by a therapist in Ireland, who describes a tendency in her clients to avoid feelings, associated with the overuse of alcohol or prescription drugs and with eating disorders.

In French culture, criticism is sometimes more common than the sharing of positive opinions in relationships. In contrast to some other cultures, where individuals expressing negative emotions are seen as immature or inappropriate, French people often respond well to receiving criticisms, which may strengthen the practice of sharing negative feelings. This also may result, however, in low familiarity with one's own positive emotions for others and a relative lack of sensitivity to the positive emotions of others in relationships. It may be useful to invest time in helping some clients to identify their positive feelings as they arise in the relationship and to share them in ways that are likely to be naturally reinforced in the culture. Some clients also may profit from improving their perceptiveness of others' positive feelings toward them. An in vivo learning opportunity could occur when the therapist responds positively to client's behavior during the session. The therapist could then disclose these positive feelings, which may be both naturally reinforcing and evocative for clients to hear, or ask clients to share what feelings they believe they evoked in the therapist and why. Being able to reflect the therapist's feelings accurately will result in better attunement, make the therapist–client relationship more rewarding, and facilitate generalization to more connectivity in daily life relationships.

When culture defines intimacy in terms of specific activities, like physical contact, it will make it easier for clients to focus on the topography of the problem (i.e., what it looks like) than the function of the behavior (i.e., avoidance of distress). As a result, the relevance of intimacy, as a functional process, and the clients' difficulties with that process in their lives, may be easily overlooked by them.

(3) A woman is anguished by the caretaking demands of her elderly parents which interfere greatly with her own life and weeps in therapy when talking about the problem, but fervently defends her parents' needs. In cultures that are very family oriented (e.g., many South American or Asian sub-groups), clients may have learned to strongly value and protect their families no matter to what extent their problems are derived from their relatives' unfair demands and expectations.

(4) A man whose presenting problem is that he is having trouble getting a promotion at work has difficulty complying with therapy homework assignments. Again a culturally supported learning may be involved in this seemingly straightforward problem. Some Brazilian practitioners point at a cultural phenomenon called *jeitinho*, which loosely translated means "a not very strict way of doing things." This concept presupposes that an improvised intervention at a later moment will solve any problem, and previous organization or systematically following instructions is not needed to make things happen successfully. Doing homework would oppose the socially implicit contract that a solution will appear in the end.

    If the client is Danish, a suggestion of a Scandinavian practitioner would be that the law of *Jante*, which is famous in Denmark, may be relevant to his underachieving behavior. The law of *Jante* dictates social equality, and the client's difficulty in accepting homework assignments would roughly translate into "Do not think you are better than the rest. Do not think you know more than anybody else."

Being Naturally Reinforcing

Once behaviors are identified as problematic or as CRB1s, the therapist must be careful not to strengthen these classes of behavior. In some cases these in vivo problem behaviors may be conveniently collaborative (e.g., avoidance of discomfort for both therapist and client), but promoting them would dis-empower the client. Instead, it is important to naturally reinforce and to shape corresponding CRB2s or in vivo improvements. New behaviors generate new feelings, produce different consequences, and open space for many emotions during the change process. A therapist's naturally positive reactions emitted every time the client engages in a new behavior in the session increase the likelihood of it generalizing into daily life settings.

    In terms of natural reinforcement, the core mechanism of change in FAP is the therapist's spontaneous and contingent responding during the therapeutic interaction. Thus, qualities such as humility and therapeutic love form the foundation of the relationship and are emphasized in promoting change rather than rule-driven approaches that promote verbal control over behavior (e.g., following a protocol).

    Humility involves paying attention to areas in which one may hold biases, acknowledging inaccurate assumptions and working to replace them, openness to taking responsibility for mistakes, admitting that one's preferred methods or coping strategies may not be culturally adequate, and choosing options that will work in the client's milieu (López, 1997; Hays, 2001; Sue & Sue, 2003; Fowers & Davidov, 2006).

    Therapeutic love means that therapists will act for the good of the client even when this is difficult, such as seeing the client at an inconvenient time or reducing the client's fee (if such requests are CRB2s). Sue and Zane's (1987) notion of "gifts," which highlights that it is crucial that the therapist offer something of value to the client, is relevant here. From the first session on, therapeutically loving therapists "give" by pointing out new perspectives on a client's problems, by observing and reinforcing a personal asset that the client was not aware of or not using, or by lending a book that may help. Giving one's dedication, energy, inspiration, and creativity to its fullest out of caring for the client positions the therapist to nurture and strengthen CRB2s throughout the course of treatment.

Shaping a wide response class in clients' repertoires facilitates generalization to many other situations. Often, a client's culture becomes a guide for progress in unsuspected ways, even when the client's problems occur in dealings with members of the mainstream culture. In fact, FAP's functional orientation often permits strategies that are part of a client's heritage to take on new meaning. For instance, consider the client who agrees with her therapist that learning to express her needs is a goal for therapy and the mainstream culture prefers that people do so in clear, direct language, but the client's culture prescribes hinting and metaphor. The therapist can help this client to develop more sensitivity to the context of the interaction and to conversational cues and feedback and then, in turn, to express needs by effective hints and metaphors. There will be plenty of in vivo opportunities for this type of learning to happen in the therapeutic relationship as the client attempts to make her needs clear to a member of the mainstream culture.

In the example above in which a client's CRB1 is not complying with homework assignments, the therapist can avoid a therapeutic rupture by acknowledging that the careful monitoring of events and behaviors can be nearly impossible for clients from certain cultures in which spontaneity is valued. In shaping data collection behavior, the therapist then can get a detailed verbal report, including an exhaustive description of context and the emotional expressions and feelings that were experienced. Then, with the client's help, the data can be organized in columns according to subject, and although frequency data are less reliable, one is able to get a vivid description of behaviors and emotions.

Sometimes behaviors that would be good targets for development in a therapist's view may be rejected by a client because of religious prohibitions. While the therapist typically will want to respect these prohibitions, there is the possibility that doubts expressed by the client are clinically relevant avoidance. As Paradis, Cukor, and Friedman (2006) suggest, consultation with the client's own religious guide (e.g., rabbi, priest, minister, or shaman) could clear up doubts about the legitimacy of a facet of treatment. When a rejection appears to be a CRB1, the FAP therapist needs to share this with the client. Approaching the event as an in vivo learning opportunity, the therapist can block avoidance behavior and evoke more facilitative behavior by asking the client to propose and discuss adequate alternatives.

Overall, in working with CRB1s that have cultural antecedents, while the objective is not to adapt clients into the mainstream, neither should therapists talk clients into returning to their roots when they prefer mainstream solutions. Clients can be delicately guided to discover how to blend their own desires while addressing the customs and traditions of both cultures.

Decreasing and Making Use of Therapist Mistakes

An important theme in the multicultural literature is the warning against mistakes that will harm rapport, such as using inappropriate language or stereotypes (Sue & Lam, 2002). Many of those mistakes fall under the heading of micro-aggressions, namely brief, everyday exchanges that send denigrating messages because the person on the receiving end belongs to a minority (Sue et al., 2007). Such mistakes may communicate that the therapist is prejudiced or will not be able to understand the client's experiences, prompting the client to withhold important disclosures or to drop out of therapy altogether.

Literature on rapport building is obligatory reading for therapists who intend to work with populations with whom they have little experience. Such suggestions, for instance, are included in texts on cognitive behavior therapy with Bosnian fugitives (Schulz, Huber, & Resick, 2006), Native Americans (De Coteau, Anderson, & Hope, 2006), and Orthodox Jews (Paradis, Cukor, & Friedman, 2006). Using such information stereotypically, however, can also turn into a micro-aggression, so the warning generally included in these texts to heed is that the individual client's identity must be taken seriously. Therapists must be aware that the level of acculturation varies highly among members of the same group and that every culture in itself is diverse and evolving. Using strategies in stereotyped ways would violate the multicultural principle of treating people as individuals instead of as representatives of a certain group (American Psychological Association, 2003). In addition, it would reduce therapists' genuine contact with what is happening between them and their clients, substantially hindering FAP.

In FAP, the therapist–client relationship is not just a frame for applying treatment, but can be the treatment itself. Providing a FAP rationale sets the stage for crucial in-session activity in the shaping of more effective daily life repertoires (Tsai, Kohlenberg, Kanter, & Waltz, 2008). The client is cued to share his or her thoughts and feelings about the therapist's behavior, making the therapist–client relationship a space for learning. Setting the scene for discussing the relationship does not imply that mistakes can be made freely and cleared up without causing harm. In reality, detrimental effects of therapist mistakes may be exacerbated exactly because person-to-person interaction is the nexus of the treatment rationale.

Despite a therapist's best efforts, mistakes will occur in any therapy and are more likely to occur with clients from different cultures. These errors provide an opportunity for the therapist to encourage clients to express their feelings and views and to let their therapists know when they make mistakes. For clients who are reluctant to give negative feedback, criticizing a therapist constitutes a CRB2. Because CRB2s can cause discomfort, therapists who have not conceptualized such criticism as in vivo progress would be at risk for inadvertently punishing such improvements. The only natural way to strengthen these new assertive behaviors is to provide the reinforcing consequences of making changes in the direction that the client requests. When mistakes occur, therapists must unambiguously take responsibility and be willing to rectify them. It is important for therapists to ascertain whether their mistake signals a need to work on a therapeutic skill deficit or to reduce rigid rule-following as when they mindlessly act according to information about the client's group in a way that is not appropriate to the client or situation. It may also be a cue for addressing issues like lack of information or lack of experience in interacting with a particular cultural group. A mistake non-defensively discussed and analyzed with a focus on the client's needs likely will be a positive turning point in the therapist–client relationship. When therapists address their mistakes with concern and with willingness to learn and to make amends, this creates further opportunities for the client not only to grow closer to the therapist, but to develop relationship-building behaviors that can generalize to daily life relationships.

Increasing Therapist Self-Awareness

Cultivating self-awareness is a prerequisite for doing FAP, but it is also a way to decrease making mistakes in transcultural therapy. In observing the effects of their contingent responding, it is important for therapists to note that observation is not free of cultural bias. Therapists with little cross-cultural experience may be unaware of how much their way of seeing is shaped by their milieu.

The multicultural literature urges an awareness of the influences of the therapist's culture (American Psychological Association, 2003; Sue & Sue, 2003). Endorsement by one's social group of a certain behavior only makes the assumption concerning the meaning or effect of that behavior obvious to those that hold it. For example, a therapist's expressions of closeness or amplification of feelings may be too intense or overwhelming for clients who come from cultures that do not promote a focus on discussions of feelings.

At least three solutions are available to raise therapist awareness. First, in-session interactions must be compared diligently to the client's daily life interactions and must be used to focus awareness on how the therapist influences the client's behavior. This is a standard interaction in FAP, but it deserves extra caution in transcultural dyads to prevent the repeat of interactions that are negative for the client. For example, what behavior instigated by the client's boss evoked a particular response from a client? In what aspect was the therapist's behavior similar? Or, what does the client's spouse (who is from a different culture) do that helps to maintain the client's problem behavior at home? Finally, what does this have in common with the therapist's response that seems to have strengthened the client's CRB1?

Second, therapists can improve their self-awareness by using the opportunity provided by working with a culturally diverse client to do a critical examination of their own enculturation. This will help them detect when exactly their communication style, preferences, and views are at variance with the client's needs and what changes they need to make to these behaviors. To understand how their group membership can make their views and commitments different from those of their clients, they must dig into historical conditions that shaped the practices and preferences held in their milieu. This includes how economic and political conditions faced by their group affect the way that they relate to other groups' practices and values.

One extension of this exercise should lead the therapist to seek an understanding of how historical conditions influenced the emergence of therapy as a cultural practice, and that may be quite different from the problem-solving and change practices that evolved in the client's culture.

A third strategy to promote therapist self-awareness can be described as cultivating appreciative distancing from one's own heritage. As Launghani (2005) pointed out, people are flexible enough to transcend to a certain degree the boundaries of their culture without losing the benefits of its strengths. But often, some effort is necessary to stay aware of the stream of experiences that make up one's history and that influence how one will face the client in-session. Formal or informal mindfulness exercises (e.g., Kabat-Zinn, 2005) may be helpful for this purpose.

Such distancing refers to being able to experience oneself as having preferences, assumptions, and values as tools at one's disposition, instead of defining one's self in terms of these. Thus, "I came, because of such-and-such experiences during my training or education, to value x for this-or-that purpose" puts the preference for "x" into a better perspective, and at a larger distance from "I" than would "I stand for x." This distancing keeps therapists from mindlessly using the assumptions they might identify with as if they were the only possibility. It is less threatening to question one's own practices when one is aware that they are part of an ongoing process and do not make up the essence of one's "I." Also, blind spots are easier to admit to and examine from this perspective. Most importantly, appreciative distancing allows a context-sensitive use of the therapist's cultural strengths and professional expertise.

Conclusion

Our experience as FAP therapists from different cultures suggests that FAP techniques and principles are universal to the extent that they rely on the functional analysis of the circumstances of behavior and its consequences. Awareness of how outside life problems can show up in vivo; the evoking, shaping, and natural contingent reinforcement of CRB2s or target behaviors; and helping clients understand the nature of functional relationships can be applied to any therapeutic relationship. In fact, any therapeutic relationship automatically starts from a multicultural perspective because therapy is the interaction between two individuals representing two unique micro-cultures. Every client is a micro-culture, carrying deeply rooted cultural, social, generational, and reinforcement histories, highly different from the therapist's.

FAP not only concurs with the multicultural literature that stipulates clinicians actively promote inclusion, racial equity, social justice, and pro-social change (Sue & Sue, 2003; American Psychological Association, 2003), but further advocates that the building blocks of these ideals begin within the therapeutic relationship (Rabin, Tsai, & Kohlenberg, 1996). Therapists can advance such values by embracing the richness of varied cultures, by helping clients address conflicting needs that stem from bi-cultural tensions, and by taking into account the personal strengths and assets associated with clients' cultural histories. In addition, therapists need to be vigilant for our own cultural biases to avoid presuppositions about a client's cultural profile and judgmental expressions. Instead, we should observe, ask questions, listen deeply, and read and consult about the history and social conditions of the client's cultural group to supplement our knowledge. When clients experience power to create change within the therapeutic relationship, that power to effect change can generalize into their social and family relationships and ultimately into their communities.

References

Amado, J. (1958). *Gabriela. Cravo e Canela*. São Paulo: Martins Fontes.

American Psychological Association. (2003). Guidelines on multicultural education, training, research, practice and organizational change for psychologists. *American Psychologist, 58,* 377–402.

Carrascoso, F. J. (2003). Jealousy: A case of application of Functional Analytic Psychotherapy. *Psychology in Spain, 7,* 88–98.

De Coteau, T., Anderson, J., & Hope, D. (2006). Adapting manualized treatments: Treating anxiety disorders among Native Americans. *Cognitive and Behavioral Practice, 13,* 304–309.

Desai, K. (2006). *The inheritance of loss*. New York: Grove Press.

Ferro, R., Valero, L., & López Bermúdez, M. A. (2009). La conceptualización de casos clínicos desde la Psicoterapia Analítica Funcional [The conceptualization of clinical cases through Functional Analytic Psychotherapy]. *Papeles del Psicólogo, 30(3),* 3–10.

Ferro, R., Valero, L., & Vives, M. C. (2006). Application of Functional Analytic Psychotherapy: Clinical analysis of a patient with depressive disorder. *The Behaviour Analyst Today, 7,* 1–18.

Fowers, B. J., & Davidov, B. J. (2006). The virtue of multiculturalism. Personal transformation, character and openness to the other. *American Psychologist, 61,* 581–594.

Hays, P. A. (2001). *Addressing cultural complexities in practice: A framework for clinicians and counselors*. Washington, DC: American Psychological Association.

Hinton, D. E. (Ed.). (2006). Special issue culturally sensitive CBT. *Cognitive and Behavioral Practice, 13(4)*.

Hwang, W.-C. (2006). The psychotherapy adaptation and modification framework. Adaptation to Asian Americans. *American Psychologist, 61,* 702–715.

Kabat-Zinn, J. (2005). *Coming to our senses: Healing ourselves and the world through mindfulness*. New York: Hyperion.

Kanter, J. W., Weeks, C. E., Bonow, J. T., Landes, S. J., Callaghan, G. M., & Follette, W. C. (2008). Assessment and case conceptualization. In M. Tsai, R. J. Kohlenberg, J. W. Kanter, B. Kohlenberg, W. C. Follette, & G. M. Callaghan (Eds.), *A guide to functional analytic psychotherapy: Awareness, courage, love and behaviorism* (pp. 37–60). New York: Springer.

Lahiri, J. (2008). *Unaccustomed earth*. New York: Knopf.

Laungani, P. (2005). Building multi-cultural counselling bridges: The Holy Grail or a poisoned chalice? *Counselling Psychology Quarterly, 18,* 247–259.

López Bermúdez, M. A., Ferro, R., & Calvillo, M. (2002). Una aplicación de la Psicoterapia Analítica Funcional en un trastorno de angustia sin agorafobia. [*An application of FAP in a case of panic disorder without agoraphobia*]. *Análisis y Modificación de Conducta, 28,* 553–583.

López, S. R. (1997). Cultural competence in psychotherapy. A guide for clinicians and their supervisors. In C. E. Watkins (Ed.), *Handbook of psychotherapy supervision* (pp. 570–588). New York: Wiley.

Okazaki, S., & Tanaka-Matsumi, J. (2006). Cultural considerations in cognitive-behavioral assessment. In P. A. Hays & G. Y. Iwamasa (Eds.), *Culturally responsive cognitive-behavioral therapy. Assissment, practice and supervision* (pp. 247–266). Washington, DC: American Psychological Association.

Paradis, C. M., Cukor, D., & Friedman, S. (2006). Cognitive-behavioral therapy with Orthodox Jews. In P. A. Hays & G. Y. Iwamasa (Eds.), *Culturally responsive cognitive-behavioral therapy. Assissment, practice and supervision* (pp. 161–176). Washington, DC: American Psychological Association.

Rabin, C., Tsaui, M., & Kohlenberg, R. J. (1996). Targeting sex-role and power issues ith a functional analytic approach: Gender patterns in behavioral marital therapy. *Journal of Feminist Family Therapy, 8*, 1–24.

Schulz, P. M., Huber, L. C., & Resick, P. A. (2006). Practical adaptations of Cognitive processing therapy with Bosnian refugees. Implications for adapting practice to a multicultural clientele. *Cognitive and Behavioral Practice, 13*, 302–321.

Sue, S. (1998). In search of cultural competence in psychotherapy and counseling. *American Psychologist, 53*, 440–448.

Sue, D. W., Capodilupo, C. M., Torino, G. C., Bucceri, J. M., Holder, A. M. B., Nadal, K. L., & Esquilin, M. (2007). Racial microaggressions in everyday life. Implications for clinical practice. *American Psychologist, 62*, 271–286.

Sue, S., & Lam, A. G. (2002). Cultural and demographic diversity. In J. Norcross (Ed.), *Psychotherapy relationships that work* (pp. 401–421). New York: Oxford University Press.

Sue, D. W., & Sue, D. (2003). *Counseling the culturally diverse: Theory and practice* (4th ed.). New York: Wiley.

Sue, S., & Zane, N. (1987). The role of culture and cultural techniques in psychotherapy: A critique and reformulation. *American Psychologist, 42*, 37–45.

Tanaka-Matsumi, J., Higginbotham, H. N., & Chang, R. (2002). Cognitive-behavioral approaches to counseling across cultures: A functional analytic approach for clinical applications. In P. B. Pedersen, W. J. Lonner, J. G. Draguns, & J. E. Timble (Eds.), *Counseling across cultures* (5th ed., pp. 337–354). Thousand Oaks, CA: Sage.

Tanaka-Matsumi, J., Seiden, D., & Lam, K. (1996). The Culturally Informed Functional Assessment (CIFA) interview: A strategy for cross-cultural behavioral practice. *Cognitive and Behavioral Practice, 3*, 215–233.

Tsai, M., Kohlenberg, R. J., Kanter, J. W., & Parker, C. R. (2008). Therapeutic technique: The five rules. In M. Tsai, R. J. Kohlenberg, J. W. Kanter, B. Kohlenberg, W. C. Follette, & G. M. Callaghan (Eds.), *A guide to functional analytic psychotherapy: Awareness, courage, love and behaviourism* (pp. 37–60). New York: Springer.

Chapter 11
FAP Strategies and Ideas for Working with Adolescents

Reo W. Newring, Chauncey R. Parker, and Kirk A.B. Newring

> *It would be absurd to deny that there are such things as childhood and adolescence, at least in our society, but we need to bear in mind the historical, cultural and social nature of the categories, if only to remain alert to the many different ways in which childhood and adolescence are understood and experienced within a society.*
>
> (Gordon, 2000, p. 342)

For a therapy that concerns itself with function over topography, devoting a chapter to functional analytic psychotherapy (FAP) and adolescents presents some challenges. In this chapter we begin with a discussion of adolescence, and why it matters when engaging in FAP. Following that exploration we turn our attention to the important procedural aspects of assessment and on-going case conceptualization with this challenging population. The heart of this chapter is the practice of FAP with adolescents, which lends itself to a discussion of the problems and pratfalls we have experienced in this endeavor. Near the end of this chapter, we turn to the behavior of the therapist, and how that impacts FAP. We conclude with a review of some of the unique ethical considerations when conducting FAP with adolescents and a case example.

What does it add to a functional analysis to specify that you are working with an *adolescent*? When conducting a functional analysis, we are looking for functional relationships among stimuli, behavior, and consequences. Furthermore, we are vigilant that we have developed a hypothesis that is constantly revised based on data reported by the client (feelings, thinking, and other behavior) or observed by the therapist (e.g., affect, voice tone, tics, posture). Conducting analyses with adolescents is often made more challenging by the conditions and events unique to that developmental group. Some of these conditions are external, such as changes in the social, family, and school contexts. Some are internal, such as hormonal, physical, affective, and existential changes (a full review of these changes is beyond the scope of this chapter; consult a textbook such as Berk, 2005, for a review). Sometimes

R.W. Newring (✉)
Children's Behavioral Health, Children's Hospital and Medical Center, Omaha, NE, USA
e-mail: reo.newring@gmail.com

J.W. Kanter et al. (eds.), *The Practice of Functional Analytic Psychotherapy*,
DOI 10.1007/978-1-4419-5830-3_11, © Springer Science+Business Media, LLC 2010

environment can even be a belief system, or a way of believing or perceiving what is valid or valued. These factors may affect therapy in several ways: first, defining clinically relevant behavior (CRB) and differentiating them from "normal" behavior becomes difficult; second, what is evocative of CRB may change; third, reinforcing and punishing properties of stimuli may change; fourth, changing self-awareness may impact the ability to verbalize rules (i.e., as the adolescent changes her mind about who she is and what she wants, she may have increased or decreased ability or motivation to express herself and communicate these changes); and last, generalization becomes very difficult, as the landscape in which the adolescent is expected to change (i.e., daily life) is ever-changing.

The concept of "adolescence" is a relatively recent socio-cultural construction. The category *adolescent* can alert a therapist to the probability of certain conditions not usually found in other developmentally-based terms (i.e., adult, infant, child, elder), but there is no certainty about what it adds to a functional analysis. Some adolescents are highly articulate, responsible, expressive, self-aware, independent, and insightful, more so than many adult clients. However, a majority of adolescents are quite different to work with than younger children, mid-life adults, and elders. Their environment includes many conditions and events not found in other developmental groups. Adolescence may be effectively conceptualized as a culture, with a shared language and belief system. Viewing adolescence from a cross-cultural perspective might assist the clinician to engage and form a therapeutic relationship with the adolescent client (see Chapter 10 by Vandenberghe et al., this volume, for a discussion of FAP and culture). Adolescents might also view themselves as between one or more cultures – a gang culture, a family culture, a peer culture, and a treatment culture – each with its own values, language, and customs. However, the relatively transitory nature of adolescence suggests that perceived cultural stability is lacking in adolescent cultures.

A dictionary definition (Merriam-Webster's Online Dictionary, 2009) of *adolescent* states that adolescence is the period between puberty and maturity, a somewhat nebulous category. In essence, it is a transitional period that includes a number of drastic changes in their world (i.e., physiological and developmental changes that influence how they experience themselves and the world around them, as well as affecting how others respond to them). Additionally, adolescents face social demands such as subordination to the rules and authority of caretakers, negotiating status within peer groups, and developing autonomy.

As for FAP and adolescence, FAP is both a contextual and pragmatic psychotherapy rooted in five rules (Kohlenberg & Tsai, 1991). FAP posits that the adolescent's behaviors are controlled by the variables of which they are a function. These behaviors occur in a special and dynamic context: adolescence. FAP provides some basic rules on what to do; however, the legal, ethical, and developmental differences between adolescents and others warrant a full discussion of these concerns and contexts.

Until individuals reach the age of majority, that is, they no longer are considered a minor, they live under the care and influence of a guardian and they can be legally sanctioned and coerced into complying with the guardianship. One of the changes that most youth experience is transition from the care, protection, and control of guardianship to emancipation and responsibility. The following paragraphs address a number of domains to consider as contributing to: (a) other contingencies including the influence of parents and guardians, the influence of siblings and other relatives, social influences of friends and teachers, and the influence of music and other media; and (b) motivational operations (establishing *and* abolishing, see Laraway, Snycerski, Michael, & Poling, 2003; Michael, 2000) that modify the effects of various contingencies.

Parenting and Adolescence

One of the primary factors influencing the behavior of adolescents is the parenting approach of the guardian(s). Although not based on a functional analysis, Baumrind's (1971, 1991) model of parenting styles (i.e., authoritarian, authoritative, permissive, and uninvolved) is a helpful framework for evaluating how the guardian affects interpersonal interactions and other environmental contingencies. Often, when adolescents are withdrawn, shutdown, angry, depressed, or a combination of these, it is primarily in response to the conditions exerted by the guardian (i.e., this is learned behavior that has served the adolescent in interactions with the guardian, and when overlearned, may be the focus of clinical intervention). Sometimes guardians are so rigid in their view that the problem lies completely with the adolescent, or they are so disengaged from parenting, that they are unwilling or unable to engage in the therapy process to alter their parenting style. When this is the case, the therapeutic task is restricted to working with the adolescent to tolerate the conditions associated with the guardian and to aim for clarifying and living in accordance with life values that are meaningful to the adolescent. If guardians are open to working with the therapist to alter their parenting style, it can be helpful for them to learn about how their behavior functions in interactions with the therapist and the adolescent.

The most prominent therapeutic challenges frequently encountered with adolescents tend to show up in one or two ways: (1) the adolescent does not give detailed or accurate descriptions of his/her own psychological and emotional experience (private experience) of events in the environment, or the effects of behavior; or (2) the guardian sees the adolescent as solely responsible for the presenting problem and his/her parenting style tends to be either harsh authoritarian with coercion and aversive consequences as the primary contingency, or highly permissive, paying little attention to the adolescent. While families experiencing the other parenting styles do occasionally come to our clinical attention, for whatever reason, the two listed above constitute the majority of our referrals.

In the first case, adolescents disclose little information for a variety of reasons. They might be protective of the parent and therefore are reluctant to reveal details of the guardian's harsh or inappropriate behavior (i.e., physical abuse or substance abuse). Some enter therapy with a defensive stance based on believing that there is not a problem, or that there is nothing a therapist can do to fix the problem. Some adolescents are referred for therapy as a result of having their trust and boundaries violated by an adult or other caregiver; in severe cases this can involve physical or sexual abuse. Sometimes, an adolescent has learned that emotional avoidance is the most effective strategy for coping, and is unwilling to discuss or in any way turn toward the problem topic. An adolescent may not voice complaints about how the home is running – especially if that adolescent is "running" the home, typically getting what he or she wants, and "winning" in conflicts with adults. Some adolescents wish to present themselves in a positive light, so they downplay the problem, or their part in it.

FAP Case Conceptualizations with Adolescents

Some challenges that a FAP therapist may encounter include: identifying the primary client(s), clarifying the identified daily life problem(s) and problematic beliefs, increasing client commitment and engagement with therapy (which may be an example of CRB), having influence when clients are less than fully engaged and committed to therapy, identifying CRB1s (problem behaviors that occur in-session) and CRB2s (in-session improvements), identifying strategies for reinforcing CRB2s and if necessary, contingencies for extinguishing or punishing CRB1s, training and shaping caregivers to use effective contingencies, and finally, addressing special challenges to being an engaged and caring in vivo therapist.

In adult outpatient psychotherapy, the presenting problem and the commitment of the client might be unclear, but who the treatment is aimed at is obvious: the presenting adult. Adolescent cases are not so clear. The adolescent might be the identified client according to the guardian, but the true problem can be the behavior of the guardian such as parenting practices, substance abuse, or other clinical issues. Several different scenarios may confront a therapist. The problem behavior might be with the adolescent, the presenting guardian, or an additional person involved with the adolescent (the guardian's partner, another parent who has shared custody or visitation, a birth parent in an adoption family, another child in the family, other treatment providers such as doctors, legal service providers such as caseworkers and judges, or others in the adolescent's life such as peers or teachers). The adolescent might agree with the adults' conceptualization of the problem, disagree that there is a problem at all, identify different problems, or might attribute the problem to a guardian or sibling. If an adult has referred the adolescent to therapy, the adolescent may have identified some problems in the relationship with that adult. In each of these cases the individual(s) whose behavior is the problem may or may not be receptive and willing to engage in therapy.

Now that we have addressed the questions of who to treat and what treatment goals are, we need to specify particular classes of behavior as treatment targets (CRBs). It is important to assess baseline frequency, intensity, and skill levels of behavior. When shaping behavior, as with any client, you must start with behavior that is already in the adolescent's repertoire. Typically, for any client presenting to therapy, CRB1s are at full strength, whereas CRB2s are much weaker or less likely. What behaviors belonging to the improvement class does the adolescent already engage in? Another consideration, when clarifying CRB, is that adolescents are typically faced with two equally difficult and competing areas of growth: increasing autonomy, and learning how to relate with others (Havas & Bonnar, 1999). It is important to determine which direction is more consistent with goals (or if both are equally consistent), without relying solely on the values of the therapist or the guardians.

It is important to define – and redefine over the course of therapy – both the interpersonal goals, and what functional classes of behavior constitute an improvement. The therapist should also consider the shaping capability of the client, or the amount of behavioral change a client will display, as well as how much of an effect therapist consequences have on client behavior (intended or otherwise). It might be helpful to remind yourself as a clinician that every interaction with an adolescent is a learning interaction. The adolescent will learn something about you: how you respond, how you express your values, and whether your actions and words are perceived as consistent.

All of these factors will help determine what magnitude of approximations to reinforce. How changeable is the client? How obvious are the changes, as they occur? How quickly do they occur? How much therapist behavior does it take to evoke CRB? Some clients show improvement very slowly: perhaps it will take an emotionally unexpressive adolescent (per parental report) five sessions to smile at the therapist. That smile may seem small when compared with more grandiose behaviors displayed by other youth, but for some clients, this will be the biggest change you, as a therapist, see in therapy.

A FAP therapist working with adolescents may struggle to adapt the case conceptualization, and the case conceptualization form, to reflect the CRBs to look for with each client from whom the therapist hopes to see behavior change. Creating separate case conceptualizations for each family member or looking for CRBs that might be relevant for all members of the family may help in this task.

FAP Assessment and the Adolescent

The FIAT (Functional Ideographic Assessment Template; Callaghan, 2006a) is a behaviorally based assessment system that places client responding into classes of behavior based on function of responding. When using the FIAT, function is tied to interpersonal effectiveness and distress. While the FIAT was designed primarily for use with an adult outpatient clientele, there are no theoretical bases for excluding this instrument when performing functional assessment of an adolescent client's presenting problems. This assessment tool can help identify treatment targets that clients might not bring up or acknowledge spontaneously.

In addition to a structured approach, each member of the adolescent's constellation of guardianship can be consulted for establishing treatment objectives. Regardless of the accuracy of each party's perspective, treatment targets must be established and agreed upon. In every case, the challenge is to come up with goals that all parties (parents, adolescents, others, and you) can agree on. The parent, guardian, or referral source may have difficulty accepting and agreeing to therapy goals that involve anything other than changing an adolescent's behavior and attitudes, such as addressing deficits in parenting abilities. It may be important to highlight areas that are not working to the adolescent's satisfaction. An approach to getting the client to generate goals that the therapist agrees with might involve queries about how the adolescent wants his or her relationship with those family members to look in the future and use those relationship goals as a starting point. An adolescent may be able to agree with therapy goals such as improving communication with adults, improving relationships with adults, and developing and improving coping skills for dealing with adults and other difficulties in the adolescent's life. As with adult clients, there may be a benefit to casting the goals in a win–win framework, insofar as the client's goals and interests are linked with goals and outcomes desired by the parent (or therapist, or all of the above). With an adolescent who has requested therapy or is there of his or her own volition, there may be less difficulty in coming to agreement about the goals of treatment.

Occasionally a referral issue can involve traumatic events such as assault, severe injury, or death of a significant friend or relative. In these cases, the adolescent may need the service of addressing the physical and emotional sequelae and the guardian may need service for tolerating the adolescent's distress. Such a situation may require a release of information for consultation and referral to another provider, and depending upon the rules, regulations, and statutes in the jurisdiction, such referrals may require the consent of the legal guardian.

The Practice of FAP with Adolescents

If you, as a reader, are coming from a more traditional behavior therapy model, you might be struggling with some of these concepts. One thing FAP adds to that model is an understanding that clinical problems will likely come with the client into the room. Therefore, we can get a direct sample and we can respond directly and contingently to problems and improvements. In answer to the question, "Who do we FAP?", we reply, "Anyone with whom it might be effective." For example, you might see a FAP therapist evoking CRB in a parent: "So, what does it feel like bringing Johnny to see a shrink?" Paying attention to, drawing out, judiciously extinguishing, or reinforcing anything happening in the moment that is relevant to target behavior is FAP. A traditional behavior therapist who is not FAP-focused might be listening to the accounts and considering contingencies only at the site of the described behavior (e.g., in the home or school); whereas a FAP therapist will also assess, evoke, and consequate behavior in the session. From a FAP standpoint, any instance of in-session behavior in the same functional class as an identified problem behavior may be a CRB, and can be addressed as such, provided that it relates to agreed-upon treatment goals.

One example of this challenge occurred recently when the first author (RN) had a telephone conversation with the father of a 16-year-old male. Her client, the adolescent, had described his father to RN as a domineering, verbal bully who kept talking until he got his way. The client described walking away from arguments, because he felt that he could not "win" in a verbal altercation. In RN's conversation with the father, he repeatedly stated his opinions, argued with or denied every one of hers, and rejected all of RN's attempts to address his concerns, until she stopped trying and just agreed with him. In other words, he engaged in behavior of the same function with RN, in the therapeutic context (CRB1), that he engaged in with his son in daily life. During this telephone conversation, RN had an opportunity to observe the father's CRB1 of bullying others, to evoke CRB in the father by presenting a dissenting opinion, to consequate his behavior, and to notice her effect on his behavior. In this case, his behavior had more effect on RN than hers on him.

Not all caretakers believe that the child needs to do all of the changing; some caretakers might be well aware that they need to do things differently but are at a loss for what to do. Some general (not FAP-specific) interventions that might be helpful are education about families, adolescents, and parenting, and feedback about the impact of caretaker behavior on the child. FAP interventions might include feedback about the impact of their behavior on the therapist (as an example of their impact on others including their child), and contingent responding (i.e., reinforcement or punishment) by the therapist to efforts that the parents make in a desired direction, or to shift blame and responsibility away from themselves. Again, the adolescent's behavior is controlled by the variables of which it is a function; altering the variables in the adolescent's world may lead to appreciable and desired change in the adolescent's behavior.

To refresh the reader, the five FAP Rules are as follows:
(1) Watch for CRBs
(2) Evoke CRBs
(3) Reinforce CRB2s
(4) Notice the effect of the therapist behavior on client CRBs
(5) Give interpretations of variables that affect client behavior

FAP is an inherently flexible system because it is based on principles with a small set of rules to guide therapist behavior. This framework of principles allows for tremendous creativity in session. The second author (CP) has learned that he needs a chair with wheels because it allows him to easily move around the room to see what is evoked by different proximities to the client. With most clients, it is easy to demonstrate what one's feelings are by moving very close to them or very far from them (very small rooms can be a drawback). Moving in very close usually elicits moderate to strong discomfort in the client and one can use this experience to discuss several points: for example, feelings as a physical experience, the urge to withdraw from or push away discomfort, and willingness to be with discomfort. From a FAP perspective, each of these interventions might be considered an example of evoking CRBs in clients (Rule 2), or possibly reinforcing or punishing (Rule 3) the client behavior that occurred just before (watch for a change in client behavior in the future, Rule 4).

When there are multiple targets of treatment it can be helpful to prioritize what to emphasize first. The treatment hierarchy developed by Linehan (1993) and refined by Schmidt et al. (2002) for use in the residential programs of the Juvenile Rehabilitation Administration in Washington State is a useful tool for ranking treatment targets. In order of clinical need, the hierarchy aims first at self-harm and suicidal behaviors, then aggressive behaviors. Next is treatment interfering behavior (other than self-harm and aggression), and finally, behaviors that interfere with quality of life (e.g., substance abuse, criminal behavior, ineffective work or school behaviors, problematic interpersonal behaviors) are addressed. These behaviors might be seen and need to be addressed in the adolescent, the parents, or both (Miller, Glinski, Woodberry, Mitchell, & Indik, 2002). For example, RN recently worked with a 14-year-old girl who presented to her clinic with the problem of self-harm (cutting). In working with her, RN realized that the function of the cutting was not to kill herself; rather, it was a dual function emotion-regulation and attention-getting behavior, as it functioned to draw mom away from dad and toward the client. However, the possible risk for self-harm warranted addressing that behavior before addressing the other parental concerns of substance abuse (smoking cigarettes regularly) and disrespect (fighting with dad). In this case, the FAP approach was guided by the above, with the functional analysis of the target behavior providing hypotheses for CRB.

As a reminder, the establishing and abolishing properties of the therapy context, and the reinforcing and punishing aspects of therapist behavior, are highly variable in the context of adolescence. For example, consider the parent who is attempting to use concert tickets to motivate a certain behavior. It may very well be that by the time the concert comes to town, that ticket is no longer the hot commodity it was 3 months ago. Such is one of the challenges with working with an adolescent: the power of arbitrary reinforcers is variable. However, our experience has been that the natural consequences of a consistent, caring and therapeutic relationship with an adult can have a profoundly reinforcing impact.

Once you have identified some in-session target behaviors and improvements, it is necessary to identify stimuli whose occurrence will strengthen those behaviors. But what is reinforcing to adolescents? It depends, of course, on their histories. For some of our clients, our laughter and joking are reinforcers. When we laugh with them, they are more likely to engage in the behavior that brought on our laughter. For some, it is access to music or the computer or drawing. For some, it may be sitting in a room with an adult who listens without yelling, lecturing, or criticizing. We have found that playing catch with a football, playing video games (and getting "owned" by the adolescent!), and going on walks can function to reinforce target behavior. Flexibility is the key – while some clients experience a sense of mastery with video games, some, like their therapist, did not.

Recently, RN asked one of her clients to complete a questionnaire about how therapy was going, what he wanted to see more of and less of. He shared information with RN via this format that he had never said aloud, and she felt closer to him than ever before. Her natural inclination was to smile at him, lean toward him, and make a great deal of eye contact; however, he had told her explicitly in his answers that he preferred less eye contact, more writing (less talking), and more space to come up with his own answers. Since processing this information, most of their interventions, both within and outside of sessions, have been conducted in written form, and RN works hard not to stare at him or push him. He, in turn, shares more information with her than before, comes regularly to therapy, and expresses that the interventions are more helpful.

The next area of concern involves noticing the effect of the therapist on the client (Rule 4). How can you tell improvement from what an adolescent does to avoid or escape therapy? Some clients develop adult language in the therapy room, verbalize their part in their problems, talk in therapy about our relationship and the similarities between it and other relationships in their lives, and adjust their behavior based on adult feedback. In other words, the topography (and maybe even the function, at least in session) resembles therapeutic success. Is this actual success? Does it matter?

We have observed the incredulous looks of parents when their adolescent made a clumsy effort at the DEAR MAN skill (Describe situation, Express feelings/opinions, Assert request/wishes, Reinforce response, Mindful, Appear confident, Negotiate) from Dialectical Behavior Therapy. Even if the youth were able to present the skill in a fluent and facile manner, the behavior was so different from what the parents experienced in the past, the parents' natural response (i.e., suspicion or perplexed doubt that the adolescent was genuine) did not in anyway reinforce the skill. While the skill demonstration did not lead to the youth getting his or her request met, it did function in a way to open a new line of communication for the youth with the parents and counselor. So it goes with FAP.

Clearly, one metric of therapeutic success or failure is the behavior of the client outside of the therapeutic milieu (i.e., generalization). A first step might be getting the adolescent to negotiate with the guardian or parent after the therapist has shaped such negotiations in session with the therapist. After that, the therapist might assess whether the adolescent is improving in other significant relationships with adults. If not, it is important to teach the adolescent how to assess the problem, and get the client to engage in behaviors that work with the therapist, outside of the therapy room. One potential problem with that metric of success is the difficulty in getting the environment to reinforce the client's successive approximations. Another potential problem is that sometimes, adult responses or contingencies are less powerful than other influences the adolescent encounters (e.g., social, sexual, or sensory experiences such as euphoric drug experiences).

A number of relationship variables warrant attention. Most importantly, if the therapist is not reinforcing in some way, the adolescent's behavior will not change.

Thus, the therapist must matter to the client – or at least what the therapist says or does must have an effect somehow. Some adolescents present to therapy sullen and resentful, uninterested in what yet another adult is going to tell them about what they are doing wrong. How does the therapist develop the relationship so that the adolescent's behavior can change? The more the therapist *tries* to matter to the adolescent, the less he or she actually will. Adolescents are typically sensitive to authenticity, and inauthenticity. Being sincere and consistent are imperative. Someone once said that an adolescent "can smell a lie"; saying things that you do not mean, making promises without keeping them, and changing allegiances all likely will damage the fragile therapeutic relationship. The therapist must remember to functionally reinforce client behavior in the strictest sense – rather than providing verbal praise that the therapist thinks should be meaningful, he or she must determine what actually changes the client's behavior. Things that are important to adults may not impact the adolescent. In addition, if the adolescent does not matter to the therapist, this will likely be reciprocated. If a teen senses that the therapist does not care, or cares more about taking care of parent or referral source needs, or therapist needs (i.e., wanting to be liked by clients, feel successful), the client is unlikely to work for therapeutic change.

How to matter to an adolescent in five easy steps
  (1) Don't try to matter
  (2) Be sincere
  (3) Be consistent
  (4) Be functional (respond in a way that matters to your client, not in a way that matters to you)
  (5) Care (i.e., the adolescent matters to you)

Problems and Issues Likely to Present in FAP with Adolescents

Parent/Child

Issues may arise in the area of the relationship between a parent and child. From the perspective of the parent, this may be looked at as an issue of the child having a poor attitude, not taking responsibility, or lacking respect. From the adolescent's perspective, the parent may have unreasonable expectations, be a poor role model, or fail to take on parental responsibilities (forcing the adolescent to parent the parent). Conflicts arise over divorce, custody, remarriage, blending homes, and a host of other situations and experiences.

In session, the client may be sullen and defiant, refusing to share his or her views, do homework, or even speak. Some youth will sit with their arms crossed, watch the clock, and text their friends (or family members in the lobby) for the duration of the session. On the other side of the adult-pleasing spectrum, an adolescent may be too ready to do any task assigned by the therapist, regardless of the applicability to the problem. Some clients will complete all homework and agree with every statement made by the therapist without ever providing actual feedback about what is helpful.

The therapist may engage in behavior that evokes or occasions "the problem." An inquiry might lead to what about the therapist presentation evoked such a response and an examination of how the adolescent's response impacts the therapist. From there, the youth and therapist might be able to collaborate on what an improvement would look like and how it would work.

Self-Discovery

Most adolescents are engaging in the task of figuring out who they are. This may be in reaction to people such as family or friends ("I'm nothing like her"), or a more self-reflective, self-directed process. If the person the adolescent is becoming is markedly different from the parent, from the perspective of either, then that adolescent may be referred to therapy. Sometimes this takes the form of adolescents requesting therapy because they are having difficulty figuring out who they are, or who they want to be, or how to tell their parents who they are. These issues may present in therapy as over-identification with the therapist, rejection of everything the therapist seems to be, or both. Less extreme behaviors may also present, such as taking a psychology class. One therapeutic challenge, common to many approaches, is responding when pressed to "take sides" in parent/child or family therapy. Our experience has been that taking the side of the adolescent's health is often a side that all parties can support.

Values

Likewise, adolescents are figuring out what is important to them, what is important to others, and how to negotiate differences and communication. The challenges can show up in a variety of contexts, such as religion and spirituality, educational and occupational goals, values about crime and punishment, and the importance of family, to name only a few.

Substance Abuse

Typically, concerned adults refer these cases. An adolescent may or may not agree that there is a problem; may cite parental deficits or role modeling as the problem; or may identify a different area as the source of difficulty. This topic must be treated delicately due to the legal, ethical, and practical considerations and obligations that arise (this topic is discussed more fully below). Disclosure may arise as a topic of discussion, as the adolescent tries to identify on issues he or she considers important where the therapist stands. A common therapy pratfall is focusing on the topography of substance abuse at the expense of its function. Is the substance abusing youth engaging in the behavior as a means of escape or avoidance, and of what? In FAP, we would expect that if we therapeutically "take away" the response of the substance abuse, unless there is a healthy and effective alternative to meet that need, something else (i.e., extinction burst/response variability) may step forward in the youth's repertoire.

Sexuality, Sexual Identity, and Gender Identity

In our work with juveniles convicted of sexual misbehavior (KN, CP), we have had clients, both boys and girls, express concerns about their sexuality, their sexual misbehavior, and their experience of sexual victimization. This can be an especially precarious position for the therapist, as it is difficult to address aspects of sexuality from a value-free stance. For such value-laden topics, consultation, supervision, and a therapist case conceptualization may prove helpful (see Chapter 13 by Newring & Wheeler, this volume, for a more in-depth discussion on the use of FAP in treating sexual misbehavior and sexual violence).

Disorders of Childhood (Learning Disorders, Attention-Deficit and Disruptive Behavior Disorders, Elimination Disorders)

Frequent referral concerns are, "Our child is out of control," "She has a bad attitude and is defiant," and "He is very angry." Some of these adolescents are self-referred, but most will come in at a guardian's insistence. In our experience, few adolescents want to follow more rules or talk about enuresis. However, most adolescents would like to be more effective agents in their worlds.

Depression and Anxiety

As Bart Simpson once said, "making teenagers depressed is like shooting fish in a barrel" (Archer, 1996). Gaynor and Lawrence (2002) applied interpersonal interventions strongly related to FAP in a group setting with adolescents struggling with depression. They reported promising results, both on the use of FAP with depressed adolescents and FAP in a group setting.

Therapist 1s and 2s When Working with Adolescents

On the other side of the relationship coin, the therapist must care about the client, and doing so often requires therapists to become aware of their own problematic behaviors that occur in session (Therapist 1s or T1s) and in-session improvements

(Therapist 2s or T2s). For RN, this has involved coping with frustration, helplessness, disappointment, and disillusionment without reacting like every other adult in the adolescent's life. She finds herself reacting to her clients' actions, to the reactions of other adults in the clients' lives, and to her own actions when she was an adolescent. Gordon's (2000) point is well-taken: "Working with people from this age group, one must be prepared to be touched, often unpleasantly, by memories of one's own adolescence and youth, to be reminded of one's own stupidities, vanities, and cruelties . . ." (p. 350). In order to do effective therapy, it is important for therapists to watch for their own judgments, unwillingness, impatience, and avoidance (T1s). Therapists must strive to be non-judgmental, and push for change when appropriate, at a pace that is suitable (T2s). It is imperative that therapists be aware of their effect on clients, and watch for therapist clinically relevant behavior. Several clients have taught RN that at times she needs to get out of her regular desk chair, set her note pad aside, and "just talk with them". She has seen this change in her behavior decrease the pressure on clients, which in turn decreases their anxiety and increases their openness to disclosure and engagement in therapy.

FAP is explicit in attending to how the therapist's clinically relevant behaviors impact the treatment process (Tsai et al., 2008). Therapists working with adolescents will likely engage in a host of T1s and T2s. Depending upon the client, therapist, and relationship history, the balance of acceptance and realism might form a T1-T2 dyad. For another setting, a balance of empathy and opaque, verbalized self-defense might be a T1-T2 dyad. Just as case conceptualization is important for working with clients, the therapist case conceptualization is important as well, as it will help clinicians monitor the impact of their behavior on the client (see Callaghan, 2006b).

FAP and Adolescents: When Ethics, Laws, and Best Practices Collide!

In therapy with many adolescents, confidentiality and the limits thereof may be a pressing concern for the adolescent (see Behnke & Warner, 2002, for a review). Parents, by law, have access to treatment content in many states. The age and other criteria at which adolescents obtain the right of consent and confidentiality varies between states and is important for therapists to know. Clinically speaking, adolescence is generally a time of becoming independent and autonomous; reporting requirements complicate this process. Laws, clinical judgment, and the American Psychological Association and state ethical codes may suggest conflicting directions when a therapist is faced with the request to tell a parent what their child said in session (Pitcairn & Phillips, 2005). As Behnke and Warner state, "while it is clinically and ethically indicated to make clear how the relationship is structured and how information will be shared, a psychologist *cannot promise* a minor that information will be kept from a parent who has legal custody" (emphasis in original, p. 4).

The resulting lack of trust may be a source of difficulty in forming a relationship with an adolescent. A therapist who can keep a secret will be more trusted in most cases by a youth, but there are problems with confidentiality when adults such as legal guardians have access to the child's treatment records. Issues such as drug or alcohol use, illegal activities, and sexual relationships particularly pose problems because they may be considered as belonging to a functional class of self-harm behavior. In our efforts within residential agency-based care, we have often encountered therapeutic conundrums in which the contingent and functional therapeutic response is overridden by an agency rule or care standard (e.g., all acts of self-injury trigger the "policy" even when the adolescent has stated that such claims have the sole purpose of getting out of a math test; or a youth who sings along with Roberta Flack's "Killing Me Softly" spends the next two hours in meetings signing contracts against self-harm). We take a very conservative stance, as when we view these behaviors as self-harm, we will report the behavior to an adult in charge of the client's care in addition to responding to them in a functional and contingent manner consistent with the case conceptualization. As Behnke and Warner (2002) suggest, we discuss the limitations of confidentiality with both the adolescent and with the legal guardians at the outset of therapy, and clarify and restate them as the clinical and developmental picture changes.

Education at the outset may prevent rifts in therapeutic rapport later in therapy (Society for Adolescent Medicine, 2004). This area is governed less by idiographic treatment needs than by laws and regulations. Notably, the rules and regulations vary by jurisdiction, and are subject to change with the passage of legislation and time, and as culture and societal standards change. It is in the therapist's best interest to adhere to ethical standards and to keep abreast of the limits of confidentiality, reporting requirements, and consent requirements for their practice.

Some topics are less difficult for an adolescent to share with a parent. Frequently, RN will sit with a client and a parent together, and either ask the client to tell his or her parent the treatment issue (if this will evoke CRBs or goal behavior), or ask for permission to tell the parent (modeling) with the adolescent in the room, so that if she does not say it right, she can be corrected (assuming that correcting the therapist or practicing restating would be a CRB2 for that youth). In this manner, the adult can have access to what therapy is about, and how it is done.

Interventions such as educating, parent training, and problem-solving are not specific to FAP unless they involve direct contingent responding to in-session occurrences of problem or goal behaviors. For instance, helping a parent come up with a way to handle grades would not be considered a FAP intervention. Giving a parent direct feedback on his or her communication style, and the effect of that style on you as a therapist, would be a FAP intervention (if communication style is interfering with the parent–child relationship and has been identified as a problem in daily life).

We have also faced the therapeutic challenge of multiple levels of guardianship, in our work in juvenile rehabilitation and residential care settings. We have each worked with clients who were wards of the state while maintaining relationships with their birth parent(s), and at the same time, were the charges of adult staff during their stay. This presents the opportunity for the adolescent to have different objectives than the biological parent, both of whom may have different objectives than the care providers (treatment staff), who may also have different objectives than the legal guardian (guardian ad litem or caseworker), who may also have different treatment objectives than the therapist! Why would a therapist enter into such a tangled therapeutic web? A primary reason is that a therapist can have an intensely powerful impact during a crucial period of formative development in a young person's life.

Case Example: Laura

To illustrate some of the points in this chapter, RN will discuss the case of Laura,[1] an 18-year-old Caucasian female. Laura was referred to therapy just after turning 17 due to substance use (alcohol and methamphetamines), academic difficulties, running away, and poor family relationships. Treatment goals, as specified by her guardians, were to process thoughts and feelings around drug use, teach appropriate coping skills, decrease symptoms of depression, and improve family relationships – all within the context of individual therapy. They started with weekly sessions for approximately 1 year, and then moved to twice-monthly sessions, as her high school graduation neared.

Therapy did not begin comfortably. Laura presented to sessions initially with passive compliance (CRB1), agreeing on the surface with everything in her treatment files and telling RN what her diagnoses and issues were. She kept therapy very shallow and became defensive (CRB1, pushing others away) when RN tried to talk about any of the problems that Laura had experienced prior to treatment such as her drug use, family relationships, or ex-boyfriend. On the good days, she was friendly and talkative, if only on a shallow level. If anything had gone wrong for her earlier in the day, she would be resistant and hostile, and make little eye contact and no conversation (CRB 1, Rule 1). During one of these sessions, out of frustration, RN gave up on talking and took out a deck of cards (Rule 2). The intent was to try to connect with Laura somehow; the result, Laura later confided (CRB2), was that she felt that she had been given permission to take her time at building trust, and was not being punished for having a bad day (Rule 3). During the next session, RN talked with Laura about how frustrating her lack of communication had been and the fact that Laura had almost gotten "kicked out" of therapy that day (Rule 5). Laura appeared surprised by RN's reactions to her and to her honesty about those reactions; she responded by opening up a bit more (CRB 2; Rule 4).

Another important turning point occurred in therapy over the topic of family relationships and drug use. Laura was reluctant to discuss her family or their problems, as most revolved around poor decision-making, drug use and abuse, and harsh legal and social consequences of their actions. RN noticed that Laura became

---

[1] In an effort to ensure confidentiality, the name has been changed and facility-specific references have been modified.

defensive whenever she was asked questions about what could be considered the faults or weaknesses of her family members (CRB1; Rules 1 and 2). The first time Laura told RN some information about them (CRB2), RN brought up her own family, some of the poor choices that they had made, and the way those choices had affected her relationship with them (Rule 3, T2). Laura responded to what she considered a display of trust by becoming more willing to talk about imperfections in her loved ones, and how they affected her (CRB2, Rule 4). Likewise, after Laura had talked at length about her mother in therapy (CRB2), RN introduced Laura to her own mother (with guardian permission; Rule 3).

Laura had graduated high school and had been sober for 18 months at the time therapy was terminated. Her coping, judgment, and insight had improved significantly. Her depression had remitted. She left therapy a more trusting person, especially with authority figures (including her mother). She was better able to speak openly and honestly with people whom she cared about. She was honest with herself about the faults and weaknesses displayed by the people she loved, more understanding and empathic with those people, and careful about keeping her expectations realistic. She was better able to accept the feedback of others, make decisions about how she wanted to impact others, and then act effectively on her decisions.

FAP can be a challenge with any client, as it requires a flexible and dynamic case conceptualization, as well as a flexible and dynamic therapeutic stance. Conducting FAP with adolescents is a complex and variable task. The population is so diverse that no rule universally applies, other than, "It depends." Therapy may involve difficulty clarifying the identified client, target behaviors, and treatment goals. The therapist may struggle with establishing therapeutic rapport, or providing reinforcement. Assessing progress in treatment also may be difficult. In our work with adolescents, we have encountered challenges, endured frustrations, and experienced powerful reinforcement. While each adolescent is an individual with his or her own strengths and struggles, we offer this chapter to assist in your efforts in collaborating with these youth.

References

Archer, W. (Director) (1996, May 19). Homerpalooza. In J. L. Brooks, M. Groening, & A. Jean (Executive Producers), *The Simpsons*. Beverly Hills, CA: 20th Century Fox Television.

Baumrind, D. (1971). Current patterns of parental authority. *Developmental Psychology Monographs, 4*, 1–103.

Baumrind, D. (1991). The influence of parenting style on adolescent competence and substance use. *Journal of Early Adolescence, 11*(1), 56–95.

Behnke, S. H., & Warner, E. (2002). *Confidentiality in the treatment of adolescents. APA Monitor.* Retrieved January 07, 2007, from http://www.apa.org/monitor/mar02/confidentiality.html

Berk, L. E. (2005). *Child development* (7th ed.). Old Tappan, NJ: Allyn & Bacon.

Callaghan, G. M. (2006a). The Functional Idiographic Assessment Template (FIAT) System: For use with interpersonally-based interventions including Functional Analytic Psychotherapy (FAP) and FAP-enhanced treatments. *The Behavior Analyst Today, 7*, 357–398.

Callaghan, G. M. (2006b). Functional Assessment of Skills for Interpersonal Therapists: The FASIT System: For the assessment of therapist behavior for interpersonally-based interventions including Functional Analytic Psychotherapy (FAP) or FAP-enhanced treatments. *The Behavior Analyst Today*, 7, 399–433.

Gaynor, S. T., & Lawrence, P. S. (2002). Complementing CBT for depressed adolescents with Learning Through In Vivo Experience (LIVE): Conceptual analysis, treatment description, and feasibility study. *Behavioural and Cognitive Therapy*, 30, 79–101.

Gordon, P. (2000). Play for time: A psychotherapist's experience of counseling young people. *Psychodynamic Counseling*, 6(3), 339–357.

Havas, E., & Bonnar, D. (1999). Therapy with adolescents and families: The limits of parenting. *The American Journal of Family Therapy*, 27, 121–135.

Kohlenberg, R. J., & Tsai, M. (1991). *Functional analytic psychotherapy: Creating intense and curative therapeutic relationships*. New York: Plenum.

Laraway, S., Snycerski, S., Michael, J., & Poling, A. (2003). Motivating operations and terms to describe them: Some further refinements. *Journal of Applied Behavior Analysis*, 36, 407–414.

Linehan, M. M. (1993). *Cognitive-behavioral treatment of borderline personality disorder*. New York: Guilford Press.

Merriam-Webster's Online Dictionary. (2009). Merriam-Webster, Inc.: Springfield, MA. Retrieved October 3, 2009, from http://www.merriam-webster.com/dictionary/adolescence

Michael, J. (2000). Implications and refinements of the establishing operation concept. *Journal of Applied Behavior Analysis*, 33, 401–410.

Miller, A. L., Glinski, J., Woodberry, K. A., Mitchell, A. G., & Indik, J. (2002). Family therapy and dialectical behavior therapy with adolescents: Part I: Proposing a clinical synthesis. *American Journal of Psychotherapy*, 56(4), 568–584.

Pitcairn, M. S. L., & Phillips, K. A. (2005). *Ethics, laws, and adolescents: Confidentiality, reporting, and conflict*. Accessed on October 15, 2007, from http://www.counselingoutfitters. com/vistas/vistas05/Vistas05.art14.pdf

Schmidt, H., Baltrusis, R., Beach, B., Brunson, K., Byars, M., German, N., et al. (2002). *Integrated treatment model report*. Olympia, WA: Washington State Juvenile Rehabilitation Administration.

Society for Adolescent Medicine. (2004). Confidential health care for adolescents: Position paper of the Society for Adolescent Medicine. *Journal of Adolescent Health*, 35(1), 1–8.

Tsai, M., Kohlenberg, R. J., Kanter, J. W., Kohlenberg, B., Follette, W. C., & Callaghan, G. M. (2008). *A guide to functional analytic psychotherapy: Awareness, courage, love and behaviorism*. New York: Springer.

Chapter 12
The Application of FAP to Persons with Serious Mental Illness

**Thane A. Dykstra, Kimberly A. Shontz, Carl V. Indovina,
and Daniel J. Moran**

The prevalence of schizophrenia is similar to epilepsy and diabetes mellitus, showing a lifetime morbidity of about 1–1.5% of the general population (Anderson, Reiss, & Hogarty, 1986; Gottesman, 1991). According to these estimates, between four and six million people in the United States will at some point in their lifetimes experience an episode of schizophrenia (Anderson, Reiss, & Hogarty, 1986). While advancements in psychopharmacology have assisted in alleviating distressing symptoms associated with the disorder, a significant level of residual symptoms often remain that may vary in intensity over time and across individuals. The course of the disorder can be characterized by intermittent relapses marked by periods of re-hospitalization (Anderson, Reiss, & Hogarty, 1986; Kopelowicz & Liberman, 1998). Even among persons who are medication compliant, relapse rates may exceed 20% per year (Gorman, 1996).

Given the degree of distress and morbidity often suffered by individuals diagnosed with schizophrenia, continued efforts for improving clinical outcomes are justified. Unfortunately, the effectiveness of psychotherapy for individuals diagnosed with psychotic disorders has historically and erroneously been viewed as dubious. In 1905, Freud assisted in establishing this uncertainty when he wrote, "Psychosis, states of confusion and deeply rooted depression are not suited for psychoanalysis; at least not for the method as it has been practiced at present" (p. 264). Since that time, psychotherapy for psychosis has been relegated to a status of ancillary importance (Eells, 2000). Psychotherapeutic interventions have been prescribed mostly for modest goals, such as providing support or ensuring medication compliance (Eells, 2000).

Many exciting lines of research, however, suggest psychotherapy can play an important role in improving prognosis for individuals with psychotic disorders. For example, early researchers found that token economies could impact symptoms of amotivation (Atthowe & Krasner, 1968). In addition, researchers (Leff, Kuipers, Eberlein-Vries, & Sturgeon, 1982) demonstrated that treatments designed

T.A. Dykstra (✉)
Behavioral Health Services, Trinity Services, Inc., Joliet, IL, USA
e-mail: tdykstra@trinity-services.org

J.W. Kanter et al. (eds.), *The Practice of Functional Analytic Psychotherapy*,
DOI 10.1007/978-1-4419-5830-3_12, © Springer Science+Business Media, LLC 2010

to reduce the level of expressed emotion (EE) exhibited in family environments reduced risk of relapse. More recently Turkington, Kingdon, and Turner (2002) provided evidence that cognitive behavioral therapy may assist in reducing residual psychotic symptoms. Finally, Acceptance and Commitment Therapy (ACT, Hayes, Strosahl, & Wilson, 1999) has been shown to reduce relapse rates for individuals diagnosed with psychotic disorders (Bach & Hayes, 2002; Bach, Gaudiano, Pankey, Herbert, & Hayes, 2005; Gaudiano & Herbert, 2006).

These lines of research justify exploring the usefulness of Functional Analytic Psychotherapy (FAP) in treating serious mental illness. FAP is a therapy appropriate for individuals experiencing diffuse and pervasive patterns of interpersonal difficulties (Kohlenberg & Tsai, 1991; Tsai et al., 2008). This approach provides a framework for understanding client–therapist interactions and for intervening to assist the client[1] in developing new or more adaptive interpersonal repertoires. FAP interventions are performed in the context of a genuine and caring therapeutic relationship and are guided by radical behavioral principles.

Much of the research cited above has focused on treatment strategies that assist persons with serious mental illness by addressing interpersonal variables. Behavior therapists have improved interpersonal functioning of individuals with serious mental illness with skills training (Wallace & Liberman, 1985). Vaughn and Leff (1976) studied expressed emotion (EE) and demonstrated that clients residing with families exhibiting high levels of EE, such as interpersonal criticism and over-involvement, showed a significantly greater risk of relapse. These findings led to the development of treatments designed to address variables associated with EE, such as frequency of critical comments in familial interactions. These interventions have shown a significant impact on relapse rates (Anderson, Reiss, & Hogarty, 1986; Leff et al., 1982).

Before proceeding with a discussion of the application of the five fundamental rules of FAP to persons with serious mental illness, it may be helpful to provide a brief overview of the treatment setting in which the authors have worked extensively with persons with serious mental illness.

---

[1] The term "client" is used throughout this chapter to identify persons receiving services from mental health providers. The authors have chosen to use this identifier instead of "consumer" (which has gained wide-spread use) for several reasons, including the fact that the former term is preferred by the majority of individuals with whom the authors work. Second, the term "consumer" conveys a somewhat passive tone (it seems preferable to be a "producer") and does not reflect the extent to which persons with serious mental illness play a vital role in their own recovery process and contribute to the welfare of others. Finally, for many persons with serious mental illness, there are often too few services and supports to choose from or consume. We acknowledge that labels can have a harmful impact, and hope that this explanation of language is helpful.

Trinity Services, Inc.

The authors provide therapeutic supports to persons with serious mental illness within the Behavioral Health program of Trinity Services, Inc., located in Joliet, Illinois. The program provides residential supports to approximately 120 individuals. In addition, psychosocial rehabilitation (PSR) programs are available to individuals to address such issues as symptom management, life skills, and recovery. The programs provide structured milieus, daily psycho-education groups, and individual therapy. Generally, clients attend the PSRs 5 days per week for 6 hours a day. As clients progress, they often transfer from the PSR settings to vocational or educational settings. An outpatient clinic is also available for clients who do not require the level of service intensity provided in a PSR program. In addition, the Behavioral Health program operates a nightclub, the Roxy, which provides opportunities for socialization and skill generalization.

Trinity's Behavioral Health program is unique in its emphasis on functional contextual interventions (cf. Hayes, 1993). Specifically, all staff and students receive extensive intramural training in FAP, DBT (Dialectical Behavior Therapy; Linehan, 1993), and ACT.

The primary focus of the present chapter is to highlight the application of FAP to persons with serious mental illness in the context of individual psychotherapy sessions. It should be noted, however, that the FAP framework also has proven helpful in structuring Trinity's treatment milieus and guiding therapist interactions with clients outside of the therapy rooms. The milieu-based application of FAP, Functional Analytic Rehabilitation (FAR), has been described by Holmes, Dykstra, Diwan, and River (2003). One tenet of FAR is that intensive treatment programs for persons with serious mental illness should be functionally similar to social environments within the broader community. In part, this is accomplished by incorporating level systems within the PSR programs. The point is emphasized to clients that level systems create a hierarchy that mirrors those found in natural settings such as the work place. Attending to responsibilities yields movement up the level system and can lead to greater privileges and increased expectations.

FAR also emphasizes the importance of observing and responding to clinically relevant behaviors (CRBs) during non-structured time periods that occur even in intensive treatment programs (e.g., time between groups, lunch). These less formal interactions are seen to be as important as behavior emitted during groups or individual treatment sessions. These interactions can be tricky in that all staff working in a milieu must be aware of and skillfully respond to each client's relevant CRBs. FAP and FAR facilitate this process.

It is acknowledged that Trinity's programs utilize arbitrary reinforcement procedures. This occurs chiefly through the use of level systems, token economies (point systems), and idiosyncratic incentives. When possible, arbitrary reinforcers are gradually faded during the course of treatment.

Prerequisites for Using FAP for Persons with Serious Mental Illness

Before proceeding with a discussion of how the five FAP rules are relevant to persons with serious mental illness, it is important to emphasize that FAP intervention strategies should only be employed in the context of an established or developing therapeutic relationship. From a pragmatic perspective this makes sense given that the social contingencies used by therapists are likely to be most effective when the therapist has become meaningful to the client. When working with clients who have less obvious interpersonal issues, the initial rapport building phase of therapy is useful in helping the therapist formulate hypotheses regarding potential client CRBs. For some individuals with serious mental illness, CRBs may be so salient that the clinician may rush to address them before a relationship has been established. This may result in a therapeutic roadblock that results in frustration (for both the client and therapist) and premature termination of treatment.

Some persons with serious mental illness have histories which include poor relationships with mental health professionals. Other individuals may even find limited and superficial interpersonal interactions to be anxiety provoking and aversive. In such circumstances, it may take considerable time for the client to tolerate therapy sessions of standard duration. When working with clients who find social interactions to be unpleasant, it may be helpful for the therapist to begin by negotiating such issues as session length and location. Some individuals find standard therapy rooms to be confining and frightening, and respond better (even temporarily) in non-stimulating, more open locations such as conference rooms, meeting rooms, or small break rooms where sessions might be held over coffee. Several clients have expressed gratitude to therapists for helping them feel more comfortable during initial sessions.

On some occasions, particular clients were unable to engage in reciprocal interactions as the result of extreme symptoms or impoverished social repertoires. Under these circumstances, the therapist may make the discrimination that work in the area of skills building is necessary as a prerequisite to more standard individual therapy sessions. Not all clinicians have an interest in or knowledge of skill building protocols developed for persons with serious mental illness. In such cases, the therapist may decide that it is in the client's best interests to be referred to another clinician or treatment program that is better able to address the client's needs.

A final caveat is that the purpose of the present chapter is to highlight the beneficial impact that the FAP approach may play in helping persons with serious mental illness in their recovery process. As will be discussed, especially with regard to FAP's Rule 4 (observe potential reinforcing effects of therapist behavior, see below), psychotic behavior is not viewed to have a unique function because of its unusual form or response to psychotropic medications. Consequences (including responses by the therapist) are also seen to play a significant role in the occurrence of "psychotic" behavior. Although little emphasis is placed on pharmacological treatments in this chapter, the authors acknowledge that medication may be essential for persons living with mental illness. FAP is not seen as an alternative to consultation with a psychiatrist. Indeed, during the course of therapy, issues of medication compliance and frustration with side effects are common topics that clients bring into session. At times, these topics evoke strong CRB1s (i.e., clinically relevant behaviors that are in-session problems) when clients disagree with others including professionals about the need for medications (despite evidence in the moment that not taking medications is leading to harmful consequences). Increased abilities for trusting others, resolving conflict and developing meaningful relationships with others are but a few of the behavioral repertoires that may be shaped via FAP.

Application of the Five Basic Rules in Treatment

The remainder of the chapter will review the five basic rules of FAP while highlighting special considerations that may be helpful in working with this clinical population. Discussion will include areas of skill development that the authors frequently incorporate in their work with persons with a serious mental illness.

Rule 1 – Watch for CRBs

CRBs can vary widely across clients. Although this may seem obvious to a FAP clinician, diagnostic labels such as schizophrenia often evoke thoughts or images of persons who are acutely psychotic. For instance, the natural association may be of a person who is unkempt or disheveled, talks in an incoherent manner, or is in a paranoid state believing that the mafia is out to get him. Such beliefs are based upon societal misconceptions and stigma and the notion that persons with serious mental illness are chronically symptomatic. The vast majority of persons with serious mental illness function well and they do not require custodial care (Anderson, Reiss, & Hogarty, 1986; Kopelowicz & Liberman, 1998). Often acute psychotic symptoms are managed effectively by psychotropic medications, may vary as a function of stress, and may be managed without the need for hospitalization. Further, each person with a serious mental illness is unique with regard to his/her life experiences (including symptoms), personal preferences, life goals, and ability and desire to develop and maintain interpersonal relationships. It is evident therefore that persons with serious mental illness will vary considerably with regard to the presentation of CRBs.

With this in mind it may be helpful to highlight behavioral topographies that the authors most commonly have encountered in their work with persons with serious mental illness, beginning with the more obvious CRB1s.

Psychotic behavior. The intrusion of odd behaviors and delusional thought content is easily recognized by clinicians as a CRB1. Despite this fact, clinicians often struggle with managing this general category of behavior within session. At times they may view the occurrence of psychotic behavior as a sign that the client is in a fragile state and that any signals from the therapist that the client's experience is in any way unusual might evoke further decompensation. Further, other clinicians have the misperception that psychotic behavior does not respond to therapeutic interventions, but requires the attention of a psychiatrist and a change of medication. The following example illustrates this point.

One of the authors was approached by a senior therapist who indicated that a male client on her caseload needed to go to the hospital because "he had lost touch with reality." When queried, the therapist explained that during the previous week she had loaned the client $5.00 for bus fare. The client had promised to repay the loan on Monday. When the therapist asked about the money on Monday, however, the client indicated that he was not able to get to the bank. On the present day, the therapist noticed that the client was eating food from a carry-out restaurant. Thinking that the client had gone to the bank, she asked if he had the money owed to her. The client reached into his wallet and pretended to hand the therapist "invisible" money. The therapist's intervention was to approach the supervisor regarding hospitalization.

In this situation the clinician responded in an ineffective manner on the basis of her own anxiety and likely would have reinforced symptomatic behavior via an escape/avoidance contingency. Although the client was adamant that he had paid real money, hospitalization was averted and he spontaneously repaid the therapist with visible money the following week.

Certainly the persistence of delusions may frustrate clinicians' attempts to manage this category of CRB1. Many of our junior therapists report being frustrated on occasion with their inability to help clients respond more effectively to delusional thoughts and persistent psychotic verbalizations. This issue will be discussed further in the section below regarding Rule 4.

Obvious but unreported symptoms. Many individuals with serious mental illness show within-session signs that they are experiencing intrusive private experiences (e.g., incongruent affect, orienting to auditory and visual hallucinations, guarded or suspicious demeanor, or extreme withdrawal), but do not acknowledge these symptoms when asked by the therapist. Although not reported, these private experiences prevent the individual from forming close relationships with others including the therapist. The clinician's task is to maintain rapport with the client while promoting increased self-disclosure.

Exclusive focus on problems and symptoms. It is expected that considerable time in session is spent discussing problems and symptoms that clients experience. For many persons with serious mental illness, however, this content area is so pervasive that it becomes part of their personal identity. Although the monitoring of symptoms and medication side effects may be useful, focusing on this content does little to promote social relationships and intimacy (except perhaps with one's psychiatrist). This was evident during a recent interaction when a client introduced himself to a therapist visiting the program by stating "Hi, I'm Jack … So, what medications do you take?" A similar interpersonal dynamic occurs with a subset of clients who, because they are in a state of constant crisis, become aversive to others.

Negative symptoms. Negative symptoms (behavioral deficits such as lack of motivation, social withdrawal, and inability to experience pleasure) are considered to be a prominent issue for persons who experience disorders such as schizophrenia. These symptoms also tend to be less responsive to psychotropic medications (Anderson, Reiss, & Hogarty, 1986; Smith, Liberman, & Kopelowicz, 2000). Consistent with this category of CRB1s, persons with serious mental illness may have difficulty formulating and following through on the steps necessary to attain personal goals. In this regard, attendance and completion of homework assignments also may become recurrent areas of focus during treatment. In the most extreme cases, it may be helpful for clinicians to implement arbitrary reinforcement systems (even temporarily) to overcome these obstacles. The effectiveness of these procedures is facilitated by the clinician's knowledge of the person with whom they are working. For example, one individual in the Trinity program was unwilling to meet with her individual therapist or attend group therapy sessions. In order to promote participation in these activities, spicy chips, tomatoes, and pickles were provided on a transitional basis. Because of the persistence of the negative symptoms, it is important for the clinician to be especially observant of the slightest improvements in goal-directed behavior.

Impoverished social repertoire. Social skills deficits have been widely documented for persons with serious mental illness. These deficits include an inability to initiate, sustain, or end conversations effectively; difficulty in reading and interpreting the social cues of others; and specific repertoire deficits such as eye contact, volume and tone of voice, and expression of emotion (Bellack, Mueser, Gingrich, & Agresta, 1997). From a FAP perspective, it is possible to address these areas in the context of individual therapy sessions. In situations where profound skills deficits exist, it may be helpful to supplement individual therapy with evidence-based social skills training programs. Generally these programs are conducted in small groups and utilize modeling, behavioral rehearsal, and role-play.

Reluctance to accept diagnosis as a CRB1. For clinicians who frequently work with persons with serious mental illness, the issue of clients not accepting their diagnosis (e.g., schizophrenia, bipolar disorder) may be viewed as a CRB1. In part this may occur because clinicians believe that clients who understand and accept their diagnostic labels will be more likely to honestly report symptoms of their disorder and pursue helpful lifestyle choices such as participation in treatment and compliance with medications. It should be noted, however, that acceptance of diagnosis has not been positively related to treatment outcome (Corrigan & Lundin, 2001; Doherty, 1975).

The fact that individuals with serious mental illness may be reluctant to accept their diagnostic label is hardly surprising given the tremendous social stigma associated with particular diagnoses such as schizophrenia. This issue may be compounded in larger treatment settings where individuals may be exposed to others experiencing acute psychosis or debilitation as a result of their own mental illness. This leads to the natural observation, "I'm not as bad off as those people."

Tension in the client–therapist relationship may develop when the clinician over-emphasizes the diagnosis and insists upon the client's acceptance of the label. It is important for clinicians to "meet clients where they are" and incorporate their under-standing of the illness and the tacts (see Kohlenberg & Tsai, 1991 for a discussion of tacts) they utilize to describe symptoms. Issues such as medication compliance can be addressed by discussing how they function when they are not taking their medi-cations. Noticing and rating an increase in symptoms may be helpful to encourage the client to discuss specific lifestyle changes that have been effective in the past. Reviewing the identified values and goals of the client in the context of a commit-ment to treatment and effective action without focusing on the diagnostic label may decrease resistance and promote hopefulness.

Observing CRB2s (i.e., clinically relevant behaviors that are in-session improve-ments). When working with persons with a serious mental illness, it is easy to overlook CRB2s that occur in session. For some clients, willingness to openly dis-cuss their symptoms takes considerable courage and should be reinforced. For an individual experiencing paranoid thoughts, simply developing a trusting relation-ship with a therapist can be a monumental improvement and a step toward trusting others.

Clinicians also want to be attentive to client mands (i.e., imprecisely known as requests) that occur in session. Many individuals with serious mental illness have lived in environments that extinguished or punished expression of one's wants and needs. Institutional settings are notorious for this pattern of unresponsiveness to residents. When individuals move out of these settings this pattern often persists. Working in a comprehensive treatment setting, the authors have noted how infre-quently clients make requests to participate in community activities, visit friends, or purchase personal items that would enhance quality of life.

Clinicians must also be careful not to extinguish client tacts on the assumption the client is expressing delusional content. The next case presentation illustrates how one of the authors worked with a client who often reported engaging in physical aggression toward others when angry or frustrated, even though historically, these reports were not supported by fact.

Doug came to my office and reported that while in the lunchroom he became very upset and angry with two of his peers, kicking one and punching the other. I responded to Doug by saying "I know at times when you get really upset with people, you feel like you want to punch or kick them. But I've never known you to follow through on those thoughts." My thought was that if this had occurred, a fellow staff member would have reported the incident to me. Doug left my office and returned to the lunchroom. Within two minutes, a staff member came to my office and relayed to me the incident just as it was described by Doug. I immediately left my office to find Doug to apologize for not believing him and to reinforce his CRB2 of accurately tacting the situation and seeking my assistance to effectively resolve the conflict. During our discussion Doug was able to share that he felt invalidated by my initial response. I also took advantage of the opportunity to discuss similar reports that Doug had made in the past that were not based on fact and how these made it less likely for me to respond appropriately to his needs in this situation.

Rule 2 – Evoke CRBs

The struggle for clinicians working with clients who present with more acute or persistent symptoms tends to be the effective *management* of CRB1s rather than *evoking* CRB1s. At times, CRB1s may occur at such frequency that clinicians feel overwhelmed and incapable of assisting the client. This may be particularly true when clients present with prominent delusions or when their speech is so loosely organized that meaningful sustained conversation seems impossible. As previously indicated, clinicians sometimes feel incapacitated by the fear that addressing this issue in session might lead to further exacerbation of symptoms. Consequently, clinicians may engage in therapeutically ineffective behaviors such as passively listening to client reports of delusional content or keeping topics of conversation at a superficial level that avoids the manifestation of symptoms. In some cases, clinicians may find it difficult to engage clients in regular therapy sessions. This may be particularly the case for clients who have a history of negative experiences with health care settings and the staff who work there.

With regard to this latter point, it may be helpful for clinicians to employ strategies mentioned earlier in the chapter and conduct initial therapy sessions outside of traditional therapy rooms. In our own programs, "resistant" clients have often been willing to meet with their therapists outside at the picnic table or over a cup of coffee at a local café. These positive contacts often promote willingness to meet in more traditional therapy settings.

For other clients, social interaction may be so aversive that typical session durations are frightening such that they evoke client avoidance. In such circumstances, it may be helpful to begin with sessions of shorter duration with a goal of having more sustained sessions over time. It cannot be overstated that some persons with serious mental illness are aware that social situations including meeting with their therapist are anxiety provoking and that they feel they do not know what to say. Accommodation may go a long way in promoting development of the therapeutic relationship.

For clients who present with significant disorganized thinking or who spend considerable time in session with speech characterized by delusional content, it may be helpful for the therapist to highly structure sessions and promote skill acquisition. The alternative of passivity (letting clients engage in their usual patterns of CRB1s) runs the risk of inadvertently reinforcing ineffective client responses. For clinicians not accustomed to working with individuals who experience delusional thought patterns, the clinicians may be so fascinated by the content of the thoughts that they listen attentively across a number of sessions and inadvertently reinforce psychotic talk. If therapeutic rapport is well-established, however, this hardly can be seen as in the client's best interest. The authors have noted this pattern on several occasions with beginning therapists in the context of supervision. One example of this dynamic occurred when a clinician spent much time in session listening to a client interpret personal messages that he was receiving from license plates on automobiles. The client would bring lists of the plate numbers to session so that he could recount with precision (and unfortunately, at great length) messages that he had received during the week. A second individual appeared to fascinate several clinicians with his accounts of boxing with evil spirits.

For clients with repertoires that prevent meaningful sustained conversations, it may be helpful to incorporate empirically supported social skills protocols to develop a foundation for productive interactions with the therapist. On several occasions the authors have sought to shape sustained verbal reports by introducing topics of conversation and providing feedback regarding client participation in these tasks. The therapist might, for instance, introduce a topic (of interest to the client, brief newspaper article, etc.) and use a timer to provide structure to the exercise. In such circumstances, a therapist generally records the number of intrusions and lengthens exercises as improvement occurs. It is helpful, of course, to provide the client with a rationale for why these exercises may be helpful. Similar within-session activities may be helpful for clients whose speech may be dominated by delusional content.

Given that delusions by definition are not highly amenable to change, this category of CRB1s may be frustrating to clinicians. In addition to structuring sessions to minimize their occurrence, it is recommended that therapists deemphasize the content of the thoughts and focus on how the client's response to the delusion has worked for him or her in the past. Generally with prompting, clients are able to recognize adverse consequences including criticism from others and hospitalization. The incorporation of mindfulness exercises also promotes the ability to notice thoughts without examining their content or truthfulness. For some clients this groundwork has generalized to the ability to effectively respond to intrusive or delusional thought patterns. For clients who struggle with paranoid or suspicious thoughts, it may be helpful for the clinician to set a context for expecting similar thoughts to emerge in the client–therapist relationship. Based on the client's history, the clinician should provide an expectation that "It's likely that you might experience similar concerns about me. I hope you will share these experiences with me if it occurs." When the client describes a situation in his or her daily life in which someone is viewed as not safe or trustworthy, it should be hypothesized that this dynamic may also be occurring within the therapeutic relationship. Acknowledgment of similar feelings toward the therapist lends itself to standard FAP interventions such as the therapist exploring the function of the admission of these unsafe feelings and having a genuine interaction with the client regarding the impact of the disclosure.

A final recommendation for evoking CRBs is to take advantage of therapist stimulus properties that might naturally set the occasion for this category of behavior. If a female client tends to struggle with interpersonal relationships with men, it makes sense from a FAP perspective that she might benefit most from contact with a male therapist. When a client's history includes bizarre or frightening responses to men, however, treatment teams or clinicians may be reluctant to follow this guideline. In one situation, a female client became obsessed with a male staff member (not her therapist) and was delusional to the point that she believed she was married to him. This led her to accuse female peers and staff members of sleeping with her "husband." One of the male authors felt this individual would benefit from therapy with him. The treatment team expressed great concern regarding the therapist's welfare. As expected, a series of CRB1s emerged rather quickly. One included the client gaining access to the therapist's coat and wearing it in the therapeutic milieu. Over time, however, the client's highly unusual and interfering responses were extinguished and an effective interpersonal repertoire was developed and reinforced. This progress would have been less likely in the context of a relationship with a female therapist.

Rule 3 – Reinforce CRB2s

The concept of recovery for people with serious mental illness is essential to positive outcomes in the treatment setting. If a clinician is working under the assumption that people with serious mental illness require custodial care and are incapable of significant behavior change, it will be more difficult for the clinician to identify and reinforce CRB2s and act in the client's best interest. People with serious mental illness want to live meaningful lives, making the work of defining a valued life direction and goal-setting imperative in the process of recovery. Bach and Moran (2008) suggest "[c]lients with serious mental illness or intellectual deficits do not lack values; instead they have been denied the opportunity to explore values, often by well meaning mental health professionals. For instance, many clients are *told* their treatment goals instead of *setting their own* treatment goals" (p. 104, italics original). For clinicians who lack in this understanding or who have difficulty believing in the capacity for change, it likely will be difficult to recognize the occurrence of client CRB2s. This being said, it is especially important for therapists to match expectations with the clients' current repertoires. A clinician's frustration and impatience with the slow-pace and necessity for basic skill building can further impede this process. Recognizing CRB2s especially can be difficult when the client's repertoire is very limited or when the clinician does not have a history with the client. The following case example provides an illustration.

Each year in our psychosocial rehabilitation programs, one client is recognized for "outstanding achievement and dedication to self-improvement." Cindy was nominated for this award by her therapist. The visual, auditory, and tactile hallucinations that Cindy experienced were among some of the most extreme observed by the staff. After having been in treatment for 4 years, Cindy began to provide sustained eye contact, reciprocate the greetings of others, present direct mands that were more than five words in length, and started to tact private experiences. However, because of her somewhat isolative behavior, newer staff members could not understand why Cindy was nominated. Veteran staff recognized that Cindy was indeed most deserving of this recognition. When Cindy was presented the award in front of 150 people, she was asked if she wanted to say a few words. Cindy indicated that she did, took the microphone, and wished everyone a merry Christmas, further substantiating the validity of her award. Cindy provides a wonderful example regarding the importance of taking into account the client's pre-existing repertoire when assessing treatment gains or outcomes.

When a client presents with the negative symptoms of schizophrenia or an impoverished social repertoire (i.e., difficulty reading and interpreting the social cues of others), it is especially important for clinicians to amplify their feelings in response to CRB2s. Although there is a risk of the reinforcement becoming arbitrary, the response to CRB2s with this population may need to be more intentional within session. This includes both the private experience of the therapist and the naturally reinforcing responses that may go unnoticed by the client. They might miss an encouraging tone, approving smile, head nod, look of interest on the clinician's face, or other overt body language that would reinforce a CRB2 within session. The clinician may have to explicitly point out and explain his or her responses to the client such as "I am smiling at you right now because it made me happy that you made a direct request to use the phone after this session. You have been working on making direct requests instead of getting angry with people because they don't know what you want."

Of course, it is also important to check in with the client to ensure that they are reading the non-verbal social cues of the therapist correctly (Rule 4). For a person with extreme paranoia, smiling and nodding your head may be misinterpreted as mocking or sarcastic. The aforementioned suggestions for naturally reinforcing the client's CRB2 also hint at providing a statement of a functional relationship between the social reinforcer and the client's behavior (Rule 5) and the way that natural reinforcers need to be monitored by the clinician to notice their effects on the client (Rule 4). The robust FAP interaction will often demonstrate that the client is responding to several rules at once.

A trap that clinicians, direct care staff, and family members may fall into is to "do" for the client as opposed to allowing the client to "do" for himself or herself. This is especially a risk in residential programs. "Doing for" the client robs the client of opportunities for contact with natural reinforcement occurring as the result of growth and self-fulfillment of goals. Too often the clients have had the experience of being cared for instead of contributing to their environment, which eliminates opportunities for them to demonstrate CRB2s that can be reinforced.

Many people with serious mental illness live in a social flatland with few incentives to change. Limited natural contingencies exist for gaining access to increased levels of freedom and independent living. As a result, rule-governed behavior associated with immediate contingencies and survival in the current conditions emerge (Holmes, Dykstra, Diwan, & River, 2003). For this reason, the use of arbitrary or atypical reinforcers (tokens, points) in a milieu-based program may be considered to increase participation in treatment and group attendance. A milieu-based program also lends itself to the development of CRB2s that may not otherwise be available to the client. A program structure that encourages clients to facilitate groups, coach peers to use effective skills, and participate in a workforce allows for the generalization of skills and the development of goal-directed CRB2s.

Reminding oneself that the relationship exists for the benefit of the client can be helpful when working with a person with a cyclic disability. It can be exhausting and disappointing when a client appears to be making progress one week and returns the next in a state of decompensation or amotivation. The clinician must identify and reinforce CRB2s specific to the repertoire available to the client in the present moment and adjust how the reinforcer is delivered to ensure that it has the desired effect as a behavior change strategy.

Rule 4 – Observe the Potential Reinforcing Effects of Therapist Behavior in Relation to Client CRBs

FAP emphasizes the importance that consequences play with regard to future prob-abilities of behavior in similar contexts. This rule highlights the value of observing functional relationships that occur in the interactions between clients and therapists. Moreover, it is important to note that both the client's and the therapist's responses are mutually influenced (reinforced, extinguished, and punished) by one another during the course of a therapy session. This fact is important given that highly symp-tomatic behavior by clients may shape ineffective therapist behavior with regard to helping the client develop a repertoire that will lead to more positive social or per-sonal outcomes. When working with a client whose speech is bizarre and highly disorganized, a therapist's attempts to prompt CRB2s by redirecting conversation may be extinguished when the client does not respond in the intended manner. If the therapist "gives up" and comes to develop a tolerance for bizarre speech (thereby not following Rule 4), then CRB2s will not occur and little will be accomplished in benefiting the client.

In situations where the client has a long history of engaging in problematic behavior, the clinician should expect, while observing Rule 4, that limited attempts of redirection will have a minimal impact on client responding. When working with a client who has disorganized or tangential speech, it is not feasible to expect that such a response pattern can be overcome by simple redirection. When a therapist is mindful of Rule 4, the effects of redirection will be observed, and it may become important to utilize more intensive and sustained therapeutic interventions for this clinically relevant behavior.

In natural environments, psychotic talk often is reinforced by escape/avoidance contingencies. In the presence of psychotic talk in a therapeutic milieu, novice clinicians and peers may be likely to cease social interactions. The reinforcing effect may be great for a client predisposed to find social interactions aversive. Novice clinicians also may remove behavioral expectations (participation in activ-ities) when clients present with symptomatic behaviors. In other cases, attention may reinforce symptomatic behavior. Such might be the case when clinicians or others listen intently to speech with a highly delusional (albeit fascinating) content. The intentive listening, with corresponding verbal and non-verbal cues that sug-gest the clients should continue with their story, is likely to reinforce the delusional story-telling. Within our own program, peers frequently have been observed to pro-mote (and likely reinforce) grandiose ideas expressed by clients. In one instance, a group of clients in one of our psychosocial rehabilitation programs gave a rousing and sustained cheer based on the claims of one individual that he had won the lottery and was going to purchase the agency. His peers certainly contributed to the social reinforcement of the delusional behavior, further underscoring the need for clinicians to be mindful of their own potential to reinforce problem behavior with attention.

Even tangible items may reinforce psychotic behavior. During one staffing a parent handed a client a pack of cigarettes, saying "Why don't you just go out and smoke for a while." This interaction occurred after the client made frequent and loud disruptive comments during the meeting. By not interceding, the clinician failed to follow Rule 4.

It is imperative that therapists remain vigilant to the influence that their own responses may play in the occurrence of psychotic behavior. In an illustrative example, the authors worked with a male client, Fernando, whose verbal repertoire was limited almost exclusively to illogical and sexual phrases. This behavior was so pervasive and interfering that a formal functional assessment was conducted (Dixon, Benedict, & Larsen, 2001) which showed a strong attention function (strengthened by comments such as "You know you should not say things like that"). This points to the fact that even redirection may serve to reinforce psychotic talk. When an intervention consisting of the differential reinforcement of alternative behavior (DRA) was implemented, significant reduction of inappropriate behaviors occurred. In the years following this intervention, treatment gains have been maintained and Fernando's verbal repertoire has become much more functional (as noted by spontaneous and goal-directed speech).

Clinicians also should be sensitive to the fact that a client's behavior may punish their own attempts to maintain a therapeutic frame during session. This is a real risk when a client is exhibiting negative symptoms. CRB1s such as lack of motivation, poor follow-through on homework assignments and social withdrawal can be punishing (and extinguishing) to a therapist's attempts to engage the client as a partner in treatment. Therapists may begin to feel like they are "pulling teeth" or like they are doing "all the work" in session. Potentially, the therapist's attempts to engage the client can begin to decrease over time. This may serve to reinforce the client's attempts to retreat from social interaction. The therapist must be mindful of this pitfall and maintain the goal of client engagement.

Rule 5 – Give Interpretations of Variables that Affect Client Behavior

In work with individuals experiencing serious mental illness, adherence to Rule 5 can be an important part of the plan for relapse prevention. Kohlenberg and Tsai (1991) indicate that interpretations of variables that impact the client's behavior can assist in enhancing the salience of controlling variables. This increased salience can lend a sense of predictability (better understanding of cause–effect relationships) to the client's world. For example, a client may learn to identify that a conflict with her mother is often followed by an increase in auditory hallucinations. Typically, relapse prevention efforts assist clients in identifying environmental stimuli that are associated with changes in symptom severity. Awareness of these functional relationships may facilitate a client to take compensatory action to prevent a downward spiral.

Frequently, increases in symptoms appear during times of increased stress. Therefore, events such as a conflict with a roommate or a new job might precipitate an increase in symptoms. The vigilant clinician will recognize the early warning signs of decompensation and be ready to assist the client in both developing an understanding of how stress-provoking situations may impact the course of their illness, and helping implement effective coping skills.

Interpretations do not have to be limited to the domain of client symptoms, but may be extended to more general patterns of social responding as well. One of the authors recently attended a holiday party that was held for clients in our program, and the following exchange occurred.

While talking to a woman about her recent transition from a group home to an apartment, a second client (Karen) approached the author and proceeded to make a number of statements about her own progress in treatment. The author maintained the conversation with the first client and noticed that Karen had walked away, rather than waiting to talk. When the author went into the kitchen to bring out some snacks, Karen approached him in a loud tone saying "I heard what you said about me!" Karen again repeated her statement, "I know what you said." The author explained that Karen was mistaken if she heard him say anything negative about her. To this Karen replied, "I know what you're thinking." The author responded, "I'd be curious what you think that I am thinking right now." Karen responded, "You think that I'm attention seeking" (an interpretation of similar behavior patterns likely shared with Karen by others). The author responded, "Actually, what I'm thinking is that your feelings were hurt when you tried to talk to me in the other room. I was in the middle of talking to someone and didn't stop my conversation to speak with you. I think this made you feel angry, and possibly jealous. It seems like you want me to know that you're angry at me and it is easier for you to bring up a 'good' reason to be upset with me – such as, if I said something bad about you, instead of what is really bothering you."

During this interaction where the clinician was providing statements of important social environment–behavior relationships, Karen was not in any way psychotic or delusional. She quickly apologized to the author and time was spent further discussing the behavior pattern. The author was quite direct in providing his interpretation of the factors that influenced the client's confrontational response. In retrospect, this route may have been taken because the client's anger seemed likely to prevent her from analyzing her own behavior. Interestingly, the interpretation had the immediate effect of decreasing her anger. This example also illustrates the generalization of FAP rules outside of formal therapy settings.

Skills Training and Other Strategies

For clinicians working with persons with serious mental illness, it is important to be aware of "skills building" approaches that may be supplemented by FAP. Two areas that merit special consideration are social skills training and the management of symptoms. In programs such as our own, skills building is often introduced and practiced in group settings with additional focus in individual therapy sessions. Social skills groups promote effective interpersonal interactions (Bellack, Mueser, Gingrich, & Agresta, 1997). Social repertoires often deteriorate after the onset of serious mental illness and may decline further as the client spends time in mental health settings where ineffective social responses are modeled and reinforced.

A common problem faced by clients is the difficulty interpreting subtle social cues. This may be demonstrated by such problems as discerning that someone is unavailable to talk because they are on the phone. Clients may also be challenged in choosing topics of conversation that are appropriate to the interpersonal context (Wallace, English, & Blackwell, 1990). Clients exhibiting serious mental illness have also been noted to have difficulty effectively asserting needs and resolving conflict (Bellack, Mueser, Gingrich, & Agresta, 1997).

Social skills groups often focus on such topics as conversation skills, assertiveness, and conflict management. Typically, clinicians use didactic teaching, role-plays, and homework assignments to facilitate mastery of such skills and this can be supplemented by FAP strategies that focus on evoking and shaping skilled behavior in session. Skills may be shaped by individual therapists in session, and then homework assignments may involve practice of skills between group sessions. As the client's repertoire improves, the therapist can assist the client in the acquisition of new skills and their application to on-going interpersonal relationships. For example, after assisting the client in developing increased awareness of the steps for appropriate manding, the therapist will have an easier time assisting the client in making direct requests in-session.

Symptom management also is important for clinicians who frequently work with clients who have serious mental illness (Eckman, Liberman, Wirshing, Lelord, & Hatcher, 1988). Approximately 75% of persons with serious mental illness who are medication compliant continue to experience psychotic symptoms (Breier, Schreiber, Dyer, & Pickar, 1991). Given that symptoms often are perceived as aversive, many clients are quite sensitive to their occurrence and are vigilant in their monitoring of "warning signs." Other clients seem unaware or hesitant to report symptoms even when their occurrence is salient to the clinician and has an impact on the client–therapist interactions (e.g., thoughts that may be distressing, but not recognized by the client as being delusional). At times, application of the basic FAP rules may be helpful with regard to how clients respond to intrusive private experiences. When symptoms have an apparent function (e.g., facilitating the avoidance of social interactions), FAP therapists may attempt to block this pattern of responding or may help the client understand factors present in the moment that impact symptoms. The therapist may also, in the moment, help the client utilize identified coping skills that reduce distress versus engaging in actions that result in further distress (e.g., yelling or becoming withdrawn).

In addition to these more straightforward FAP interventions, the authors have also incorporated techniques and strategies from other contextual-behavioral frameworks in the management of symptoms. For example, the distress tolerance skills module of Dialectical Behavior Therapy (Linehan, 1993) has been a helpful resource to help individuals identify and practice coping skills that prove useful in alleviating the intensity and duration of disturbing symptoms. The key is working with clients to practice the use of skills, and learning which are most helpful, rather than talking about skills on an intellectual basis. A common pitfall in our milieu-based programs is for clinicians to reinforce client verbalizations that include the word "coping skills" (e.g., "I should use a coping skill now, huh?") rather than helping clients implement skills in times of distress. Put differently, therapists may reinforce descriptions of potential CRB2s rather than actual CRB2s. In most circumstances, it is helpful to work with clients to regularly practice specific skills during times of non-distress. When motivation or follow-through is an issue, in vivo practice of skills during session is essential.

For many clients who *are* medication compliant, symptoms may still occur on a frequent basis (Kopelowicz & Liberman, 1998). Despite the persistence of symptoms, many of these individuals are able to lead healthy and productive lifestyles (Eckman et al., 1988). This is an important point because clinicians who are not aware of this phenomenon may unknowingly promote the unrealistic treatment agenda of eliminating symptoms, thus presenting a barrier to the recovery process. For some clients, education regarding the commonality of persistent symptoms may alleviate distress caused by thoughts that they are doing something wrong or the notion that they are "unstable." Family members and loved ones also benefit from education that the presence of symptoms is not incompatible with the pursuit of personal goals and values.

For clients who struggle with persistent symptoms, it often has been helpful to incorporate material from Acceptance and Commitment Therapy (ACT; Hayes, Strosahl, & Wilson, 1999), particularly strategies targeting the futility of changing or eliminating intrusive thoughts. Although it is beyond the scope of the present chapter to discuss the useful applications of ACT, exercises such as *Mary had a Little ...* or *What are the Numbers?* have been quite helpful. For one client who struggled terribly in her attempt to rid herself of terrifying and shameful thoughts and images (eating family members in a cannibalistic manner), the generalization of such exercises to her own private experiences was in her words "life saving." A case study demonstrating the combined use of ACT and FAP interventions for a person with psychotic symptoms has been presented by Baruch, Kanter, Busch, and Juskiewicz (2009).

In conclusion, rehabilitating individuals experiencing serious mental illness requires a multi-faceted treatment. The FAP approach to developing an intense and curative relationship with clients is apropos to working with individuals with serious mental illness, and can be well integrated into milieu-based interventions. Each of the five rules can be considered an important part of developing a therapeutic relationship with clients diagnosed with psychosis and other related disorders. The Trinity Services PSR programs have had successful clinical results by incorporating contextual psychology components into skills groups, milieu-based interactions, and individual therapy sessions which are all imbued with the principles, practice, and promise of FAP.

References

Anderson, C. M., Reiss, D. J., & Hogarty, G. E. (1986). *Schizophrenia and the family*. New York: Guilford Press.

Atthowe, J. M., & Krasner, L. (1968). Preliminary report on the application of contingent reinforcement procedures (Token economy) on a "chronic" psychiatric ward. *Journal of Abnormal Psychology, 73*(1), 37–43.

Bach, P., Gaudiano, B. A., Pankey, J., Herbert, J. D., & Hayes, S. C. (2005). Acceptance, mindfulness, values, and psychosis: Applying Acceptance and Commitment Therapy (ACT) to the chronically mentally ill. In R. A. Baer (Ed.), *Mindfulness-based treatment approaches: Clinician's guide to evidence base and applications* (pp. 94–116). Burlington, MA: Elsevier.

Bach, P., & Hayes, S. C. (2002). The use of acceptance and commitment therapy to prevent the rehospitalization of psychotic patients: A randomized controlled trial. *Journal of Consulting and Clinical Psychology, 70*(5), 1129–1139.

Bach, P., & Moran, D. J. (2008). *ACT in practice: Case conceptualization in acceptance and commitment therapy*. Oakland, CA: New Harbinger Press.

Baruch, D. E., Kanter, J. W., Busch, A. B., & Juskiewicz, K. (2009). Enhancing the therapy relationship in acceptance and commitment therapy for psychotic symptoms. *Clinical Case Studies, 8*, 241–257.

Bellack, A. S., Mueser, K. T., Gingerich, S., & Agresta, J. (1997). *Social skills training for schizophrenia: A step-by-step guide*. New York: Guilford Press.

Brier, A., Schreiber, J. L., Dyer, J., & Pickar, D. (1991). National Institute of Mental Health longitudinal study of chronic schizophrenia: Prognosis and predictors of outcome. *Archives of General Psychiatry, 48*, 239–246.

Corrigan, P., & Lundin, R. (2001). *Don't call me nuts: Coping with the stigma of mental illness*. Tinley Park, IL: Recovery Press.

Dixon, M. R., Benedict, H., & Larsen, T. (2001). Functional analysis and treatment of inappropriate verbal behavior. *Journal of Applied Behavior Analysis, 34*, 361–363.

Doherty, E. G. (1975). Labeling effects in psychiatric hospitalization. A study of diverging patterns of inpatients self-labeling processes. *Archives of General Psychiatry, 32*, 562–568.

Eckman, T., Liberman, R. P., Wirshing, W., Lelord, F., & Hatcher, V. (1988). *Symptom management trainer's manual*. Los Angeles, CA: UCLA Department of Psychiatry.

Eells, T. D. (2000). Psychotherapy of schizophrenia. *Journal of Psychotherapy Practice and Research, 9*, 250–254.

Freud, S. (1905/1953). On Psychotherapy. In J. Strachey (Ed. & Trans.), *The standard ed. of the complete psychological works of Sigmund Freud* (Vol. 7, pp. 255–268). London, England: Hogarth Press. (Original work published 1905).

Gaudiano, B. A., & Herbert, J. D. (2006). Acute treatment of inpatients with psychotic symptoms using acceptance and commitment therapy: Pilot results. *Behaviour Research & Therapy, 44*(3), 415–437.

Gorman, J. M. (1996). *The new psychiatry*. New York: St. Martin's Press.

Gottesman, I. I. (1991). *Schizophrenia genesis: The origins of madness*. New York: Freeman.

Hayes, S. C. (1993). Analytic goals and the varieties of scientific contextualism. In S. C. Hayes, L. J. Hayes, H. W. Reese, & T. R. Sarbin (Eds.), *Varieties of scientific contextualism* (pp. 11–27). Reno, NV: Context Press.

Hayes, S. C., Strosahl, K., & Wilson, K. G. (1999). *Acceptance and commitment therapy: An experiential approach to behavior change*. New York: Guilford Press.

Holmes, E. P., Dykstra, T. A., Diwan, S., & River, P. (2003). Functional analytic rehabilitation: A contextual behavior approach to chronic distress. *The Behavior Analyst Today*, *4*(1), 34–46.

Kohlenberg, R. J., & Tsai, M. (1991). *Functional analytic psychotherapy: Creating intense and curative therapeutic relationships*. New York: Plenum Publishing Corp.

Kopelowicz, A., & Liberman, R. P. (1998). Psychosocial treatments for schizophrenia. In P. E. Nathan & J. M. Gorman (Eds.), *Treatments that work* (pp. 190–221). London: Oxford University Press.

Leff, J. P., Kuipers, L., Berkowitz, R., Eberlein-Vries, R., & Sturgeon, P. (1982). A controlled trial of social intervention in the families of schizophrenic patients. *British Journal of Psychiatry*, *141*, 121–134.

Linehan, M. M. (1993). *Cognitive behavioral treatment of borderline personality disorder*. New York: Guilford Press.

Smith, T. E., Liberman, R. P., & Kopelowicz, A. (2000). Schizophrenic disorders: Rehabilitation. In H. Helmchen, F. A. Henn, H. Lauter, and N. Sartorius (Eds.), *Current concepts in psychiatry* (pp. 1–42). Heidelberg: Springer.

Tsai, M., Kohlenberg, R. J., Kanter, J. W., Kohlenberg, B., Follette, W. C., & Callaghan, G. M. (2008). *A guide to functional analytic psychotherapy: Awareness, courage, love, and behaviorism*. New York: Springer.

Turkington, D., Kingdon, D., & Turner, T. (2002). Effectiveness of brief cognitive behavioral therapy intervention in treatment of schizophrenia. *British Journal of Psychiatry*, *180*, 523–527.

Vaughn, C. E., & Leff, J. P. (1976). The influence of family and social factors on the course of psychiatric illness. *British Journal of Psychiatry*, *129*, 125–137.

Wallace, C. J., English, S. B., & Blackwell, G. A. (1990). *Basic conversation skills trainer's manual*. Los Angeles, CA: UCLA Department of Psychiatry.

Wallace, C. J., & Liberman, R. P. (1985). Social skills training for patients with schizophrenia: A controlled clinical trial. *Psychiatry Research*, *15*(3), 239–247.

Chapter 13
FAP with People Convicted of Sexual Offenses

Kirk A.B. Newring and Jennifer G. Wheeler

The history of sex offense treatment parallels the history of treatment within the broader field of psychology. When psychoanalytic theories and approaches were popular, clinicians offered psychoanalytic approaches to address sexual offense behavior. When institutionalization was the norm for treating significant behavioral problems, hospital-based "sexual psychopath" treatment programs were employed to treat sexual offense behavior. When behavioral approaches increased in popularity, clinicians increasingly employed behavioral approaches to target sexually problematic behavior (Kohlenberg, 1974a, 1974b). When cognitive psychology vied for the psychological spotlight, again, sex offense treatment emphasized cognitive approaches. In the mid-1980s, Relapse Prevention (RP) emerged as a viable approach to treatment for sexual offense behavior. Within two decades, RP reigned as the "gold standard" for treating sexual offense behavior (Newring, Loverich, Harris, & Wheeler, 2009). For the last decade, RP has been regarded as the most popular cognitive-behavioral approach to treating sexual offending (Laws, Hudson, & Ward, 2000).

The application of RP to sexual offending involved a transfer of theory and techniques from the addictions field to treatment for sexual offense behavior. However, in transferring the RP model from addictive behavior to sexual offense behavior, the original RP model was modified in several important ways. One important change to the RP model for sexual offenses was the use of RP as a primary treatment approach. Although RP may be useful for identifying problematic thoughts and behaviors and possible points of intervention in a client's sexual offense "cycle," it was not intended to be the primary approach to change those aspects of an offender's lifestyle that result in sexual offending (i.e., limited coping skills, deficits in self-regulation, criminogenic thinking styles, and/or interpersonal skill deficits). The purpose of RP never was to be the agent of behavioral change in addicted persons, but rather, to assist them in their efforts to maintain the successful sobriety they had already achieved. Accordingly, a broad concern has been raised that in its current

K.A.B. Newring (✉)
Forensic Behavioral Health, Papillion, NE, USA; Nebraska Wesleyan University, Lincoln, NE, USA
e-mail: newring@gmail.com

J.W. Kanter et al. (eds.), *The Practice of Functional Analytic Psychotherapy*,
DOI 10.1007/978-1-4419-5830-3_13, © Springer Science+Business Media, LLC 2010

form, RP is an insufficient approach to the treatment of sexual offense behavior. Specifically, it has been observed that a primary treatment approach is needed to eliminate the cognitive and behavioral problems that support sexual offense behavior, and that RP might be a useful adjunct treatment to help maintain the successful gains made in primary treatment (see Wheeler, George, & Stoner, 2005).

New Directions in Treatment for Sexually Offensive Behavior

Positive and collaborative approaches. In the last several years, a movement has been undertaken to improve upon the noted limitations of RP as a primary treatment for sexual offending. In practice, RP for sexual offending typically involves a focus on avoidance-based interventions (e.g., do not go certain places, do not allow certain thoughts or feelings to persist), using a confrontational therapeutic approach. More recently, these typical confrontation-based and risk-centered treatment approaches have been challenged (Marshall et al., 2005). While acknowledging the need to identify and manage risk for the individual offender, these new approaches offer a strength-based approach in which a therapeutic alliance provides the context in which good lives are fostered. For example, Marshall et al. (2005) assert that working collaboratively with the offenders toward these goals will enhance treatment compliance and maximize treatment effects. They also assert that offender self-esteem and hopefulness need to be early treatment targets, as deficits in those areas can impede treatment progress.

In another example of this paradigm shift in sex offense treatment, a typical RP intervention for sexual offense behavior is modified to include an emphasis on approach goals (Mann, Webster, Schofield, & Marshall, 2004). This approach-based intervention was designed to be consistent with the Good Lives approach (Ward & Hudson, 2000; Ward & Stewart, 2002). The Good Lives and Self-Regulation (c.f. Webster, 2005) models posit that sexual offending occurs for a reason and within a context. Furthermore, there is some empirical evidence to support that approach-goals may be more salient factors in clients' risk to sexually re-offend (Hudson, Ward, & Marshall, 1992; Ward, Hudson, & Marshall, 1994; Wheeler, 2003).

The motivation for sexual behavior often can be linked to a common human need, or needs, such as affiliation, mastery, competence, or efficaciousness. Many offenders may lack the agency to be interpersonally effective in sexual encounters with same-aged peers. In order to fulfill an otherwise normative human need to affiliate and feel competent, individuals who lack skills for engaging in prosocial sexual relationships may resort to sexual relationships that are characterized by coercion, exploitation, manipulation, or even force. Thus, the "goods" in the Good Lives model are those motivators, either establishing operations, antecedents, or consequences, common across clients (and people) which lead to maladaptive behaviors to obtain said goods (e.g., intimacy, agency, competence).

Synthesizing the Mann et al. (2004) and Marshall et al. (2005) works provides an example of an approach goal consistent with the Good Lives model that can be addressed collaboratively – modification or suppression of deviant arousal versus enhancement of healthy sexual functioning. By focusing on what to increase, it is argued that the treatment participant will have a clear plan of what to do and how to do it, rather than a somewhat nebulous concept of what to avoid or not to do. The shift in "what to do" has also led to a shift in "how to do it."

As stated in the Marshall et al. (2005) article title, "working positively" calls for a shift in the therapeutic stance in which sex offense treatment is provided. Marshall (2005) calls for an inclusion of the research on therapeutic change to the field of sex offense treatment. Marshall recommends that sex offense treatment providers display "empathy and warmth in a context where they provide encouragement and some degree of directiveness" (p. 134). Marshall also recommends therapists demonstrate flexibility and adapt their style and focus to the needs of the patient over the needs of a treatment protocol or manual.

Dynamic risk factors. The last decade of research on sexual offense behavior has resulted in significant gains in our understanding of numerous personality and lifestyle variables associated with sexual recidivism risk. The term "dynamic risk factor" (DRF) refers to those aspects of an offender's behavior or environment that are associated with increased likelihood to re-offend, and that are potentially subject to change. Accordingly, if a stable dynamic factor can be reduced in treatment, this may affect longer-term change in an individual's re-offense risk. Although research on dynamic factors is an ongoing process, these preliminary findings provide a basic framework for integrating dynamic risk factors into extant approaches to sex offense treatment. Currently, available data indicate that dynamic risk factors for sexual offense recidivism appear to be associated with one of two broad categories: (a) a pathological orientation toward love and sex, or "erotopathic risk-needs" (Wheeler, George, & Stephens, 2005; Wheeler, George, & Stoner, 2005), or (b) a generally antisocial orientation (Hanson & Morton-Bourgon, 2004; Hanson & Bussiere, 1998; Hanson & Harris, 2001; Hudson, Wales, Bakker, & Ward, 2002; Quinsey, Lalumiere, Rice, & Harris, 1995; Roberts, Doren, & Thornton, 2002).

"Erotopathic risk-needs" refer to the dynamic risk factors that are associated with the development and maintenance of maladaptive sexual behaviors and romantic relationships. For example, a client's erotopathic risk-needs would include thoughts, emotions, relationships, or other behaviors that support the development and maintenance of emotionally detached, abusive relationships and avoidance of relationships and interactions that threaten his detachment; a preference for "relationships" with partners whom he can control (e.g., with minors, or through the use of force), and avoidance of partners who challenge his control. For clients with dynamic risk factors in this area, treatment should focus on building behavioral skills and activities to develop and maintain satisfying and prosocial intimate/sexual relationships that could serve to curtail future acts of sexual offending. Again, from an applied behavior analytic perspective, this approach is consistent with a differential reinforcement of alternative (or incompatible) behavior that achieves the same or similar acquisition of "good" at a more palatable social cost for the treatment participant and society.

The second broad category of dynamic risk factors, or "antisocial risk needs" (Wheeler, George, & Stephens, 2005; Wheeler, George, & Stoner, 2005), refers to the dynamic risk factors that are associated with the development and maintenance of a chaotic, irresponsible, defiant, or otherwise antisocial lifestyle. For example, antisocial risk-needs would include thoughts, emotions, relationships, or other behaviors that support a generally unstable lifestyle (e.g., unsteady employment, antisocial peers); facilitate and indulge the use of deception, manipulation, and secrecy (e.g., criminal activity, psychopathic personality traits); foster resentment of others and a sense of entitlement and self-indulgence (e.g., hostility, persecution); support non-compliance with rules and authority; and provide reinforcement for behavioral disinhibition (e.g., substance use, aggression, violence). For clients with dynamic risk factors in this area, treatment should focus on building behavioral skills and activities to develop and maintain a satisfying and prosocial lifestyle, which could serve to curtail future acts of sexual offending. From an applied behavior analytic perspective, this approach is consistent with a differential reinforcement of alternative (or incompatible) behavior that achieves the same or similar acquisition of good (a la Good Lives) at a more palatable social cost for the treatment participant and society.

FAP as a Useful Approach to Treat Sexual Offense Behavior

Consistent with the collaborative, positive, and ideographic approach emphasized by Marshall (2005) and Marshall et al. (2005), Functional Analytic Psychotherapy (FAP; Kohlenberg & Tsai, 1991; Tsai et al., 2008) offers an effective approach to identify and target clients' dynamic risk-needs in the context of sex offense treatment. In the FAP model, clients' needs are identified and operationalized into behaviorally specific treatment targets (clinically relevant behaviors or CRBs), with interventions designed to increase desired behavior, reduce undesired behavior, and promote generalization beyond the therapy room.

As many of the identified dynamic risk domains relevant for sexual offense recidivism are related to behavior and expressed attitudes, behavioral approaches appear most applicable in addressing these risks. Furthermore, most dynamic risk factors for sexual offense recidivism are rooted in interpersonal domains (i.e., romantic, sexual, and/or social relationships), so an interpersonal psychotherapeutic approach is consistent with addressing these risks. Given these contingencies, FAP is well-suited for clinical use with this population. While it unlikely for a client to engage in outside life topographically similar problematic sexual behaviors (O1s) or improvements (O2s) in session, it is quite likely that the client will engage in functionally similar in-session problematic behaviors (CRB1s) and in-session improvements (CRB2s) when those behaviors are similarly occasioned. For example, when faced with distressing interpersonal conflict "in the world," a client may to coping though masturbation, impersonal sex, use or pornography or other topographically similar sexualized problem solving (O1 and O2); in the therapeutic context, the demands may inhibit an overtly sexual coping response, yet may evoke a response that works similarly, such as sexualized talk, directed conversation toward a previous sexually inappropriate act (CRB1 or CRB2), that would function in the same sexually self-soothing manner as would more overtly sexual behavior.

FAP's focus on the assessment and conceptualization of functional classes maps on well to the risk areas outlined in dynamic risk assessments for sexual offense behavior. FAP's emphasis on the clinically relevant examples of the behavior, including topographical and functional, speaks toward the probabilistically more frequent functional analogues to sexual misbehavior in therapy, relative to the probabilistically less frequent overt exemplars of sexual misbehavior. By combining the functional equivalents (FAP) with the most relevant treatment domains (assessed dynamic risk related to sexual recidivism), the inclusion of FAP in treating sexual offense behavior is ideal for the interpersonally based dynamic risks for the individual offender. Using FAP terminology, these areas of dynamic risk-needs may capture functional classes of behavioral excesses of deficits, or exemplars of these risk areas may speak toward classes of CRBs. In sex offense treatment, CRBs should be related to identified risk-needs, and identified risk factors, if present, should be related to CRBs. Accordingly, FAP rules can be applied to guide the clinician in noticing, evoking, and reinforcing clinically relevant client behavior related to the client's risk for sexual re-offense. As a reminder, the FAP rules are:

Rule 1: Watch for clinically relevant behaviors (CRBs). In FAP, CRBs are noted as instances of the problem or target behavior (CRB1), instances of improvements related to the problem or target behavior (CRB2), or behavior (verbal or otherwise) about a CRB1 or CRB2 without being an instance of a CRB1 or CRB2 in and of itself (CRB3). The following section provides general guidelines for instances of clinically relevant behavior associated with relevant areas of dynamic risk related to sexual offense recidivism.

Rule 2: Evoke CRBs. FAP therapists may attempt to evoke improvements, or work to create the *opportunity* for the client to demonstrate improvement. For a behavior to be reinforced, the behavior needs to occur. For clinically relevant and low frequency behavior, the clinician may need to create opportunities for the client to demonstrate improvements. Ideally, such evocations will be natural and sincere.

Rule 3: Naturally reinforce CRB2s. As many of the dynamic risks for sexual offense behavior are related to interpersonal behaviors, skills, or interactions, the therapeutic relationship is a prime context in which salient reinforcement and punishment can be delivered on clinically relevant behavior. As a reminder, the intention of the therapist or the topography of the behavior does not determine its reinforcing properties (e.g., praise is only reinforcing when it functions to reinforce a specific behavior contingently). What determines the reinforcing properties is the observed impact of the therapist-delivered response.

Rule 4: Notice the therapist's effect on the client. Related to Rule 3 above, clinicians are to notice their impact on the client, not just their intended impact on the client. As a therapist, one may have many stimulus properties for clients – be attractive, remind them of a prosecutor or judge, have similarities to a former sexual partner, be the first one to demonstrate a consistent and caring disposition, be the first person in their life who matters to them, and who they allow themselves to care about. The impact therapists have on their clients may change over time, and may change in accordance with the level of attachment and intimacy developed between the therapeutic dyad. The therapist might be intending to reinforce or punish an exemplar of a class of behavior – whether or not this effect occurs is for the therapist to observe.

Rule 5: Provide functional interpretations of client behavior. To promote the generalization of CRB2s from the therapy room to the world in which the client lives, functional interpretations assist the client in shifting from rule-governed approaches (e.g., avoid parks, avoid schools) to function-governed approaches (e.g., approach relationship-enhancing discussions, discuss emotions with the support team to foster communication).

There are important differences between working with persons convicted of sexual offenses and non-offending clients. To highlight some of these differences, we offer the following FAP principles for working with persons convicted of sexual offenses:

> Principle 1: The client and therapist must matter to each other for FAP to work in reducing risk to sexually re-offend.
>
> Principle 2: Functional assessment informs treatment practices, and dynamic risk assessment informs functional assessment.
>
> Principle 3: Reinforcement of prosocial behavior and punishment of anti-social/deviant behavior are functional not topographical. Shaping involves reinforcement and extinction.
>
> Principle 4: Just because the problem is about sex doesn't mean that treatment is always about sex.
>
> Principle 5: Even though treatment is not always about sex, it may still be addressing a problem that is about sex.

Assessing Dynamic Risk-Needs

Therapists who provide treatment for sexual offense behavior must be familiar with the dynamic risk-need areas, and how these might present themselves in a treatment setting. One of the most popular dynamic risk assessment instruments for sexual offense behavior is the SONAR/Stable 2000/Stable 2007 (Hanson & Harris, 2002; Hanson, Harris, Scott, & Helmus, 2007). This instrument was originally developed for the purposes of providing community supervisors with a structured method for evaluating and identifying factors about the offender's community lifestyle that indicate when he is at increased risk to re-offend. With some additional modification, this instrument is readily adapted for use in treatment settings (see Wheeler & Covell, 2007), to identify offenders' treatment needs, and appropriate targets for intervention.

In addition to the use of formal assessment instruments such as the Stable 2007, observable indicators of dynamic risk may occur regularly – in the living area, during recreational activities, and of course, in treatment sessions. Effective treatment depends on a therapist's ability to recognize when and how an offender's immediate problem behavior is related to his or her chronic dynamic risk-needs. This will be a relatively straightforward task when the problem behavior is sexual in nature, and somewhat more challenging when the problem behavior is not overtly sexual. It is important to remember that many dynamic risk factors are not sexual per se, but they do contribute to the offender's overall risk to engage in harmful, illegal sexual activity (e.g., traits associated with psychological or narcissistic personality disorders). These are indicators of underlying dynamic risk factors to be targeted in treatment.

A clear conceptualization of the client's relevant dynamic risk factors for sexual re-offense and FAP Rules 1–5 can guide the clinician working collaboratively with the person convicted of sexual offense behavior. The dynamic risk areas can help generate the case conceptualization.

The FIAT (Functional Ideographic Assessment Template; Callaghan, 2006a) is a behaviorally based assessment system that breaks client responding into classes of behavior based on function of responding. When using the FIAT, function is tied to interpersonal effectiveness and distress. The FIAT and dynamic risk assessment measures such as the Stable 2007 can be integrated meaningfully. Further, some aspects of the dynamic risk assessment measures may be better suited for other approaches (e.g., Dialectical Behavior Therapy for specific behavioral skills training; Wheeler, George, & Stoner, 2005; Acceptance and Commitment Therapy for concerns rooted in matters conceptualized as cognitive fusion or emotional avoidance; Penix, Sbraga, & Brunswig, 2003). For people convicted of sexual offense, the Stable 2007 can be a useful tool to assist in the identification and prioritization of treatment targets. However, it is important to consider that other tools are available to help guide the assessment of dynamic risk-needs in this clientele (e.g., Level of Service Inventory-Revised; Psychopathy Checklist-Revised; see Wheeler, George, & Stephens, 2005; Wheeler & Covell, 2007), and future research may identify additional dynamic risk-needs. For the purposes of illustrating the general process of applying FAP to target dynamic risk-needs, the following section provides a brief summary of the dynamic risk factors outlined in the Stable 2000 and 2007, including behavioral indicators of these risk-needs as O1s and O2s in daily life and as CRB1s and CRB2s in the treatment setting.[1] While we acknowledge the seeming hypocrisy of providing topographical examples for functional problems, we intend the descriptions below to provide some examples of how sex offense specific CRBs may present themselves in the therapy process.

---

[1] Where indicated, descriptions of behavioral indicators are quoted directly from the SONAR Stable 2000 manual. Additional treatment specific indicators are adapted from Wheeler and Covell (2007).

Significant social influences. The basic construct from the Stable 2007 is: "The nature of an offender's social network is one of the most well-established predictors of criminal behavior. A direct way of assessing social influences is to list everyone in the offender's life that is not paid to be with them. Then, make a judgment as to whether each person is a positive, negative, or neutral influence . . ." To understand the importance of this domain and develop appropriate treatment interventions, it is important to understand what prevents the offender from developing and maintaining more prosocial peer relationships and why he affiliates with antisocial peers and family members. For this section and those following we have provided a list of some of the possible outside (O1s and O2s) and clinically relevant (CRB1s and CRB2s) indicators of this need area:

- O1s and O2s. O1s might include a history of forming unstable or conflictual peer relationships; engaging in violence, aggression or other behavioral extremes that people do not like (e.g., self-harm, stealing, lying, "mooching"); affiliating with peers who define themselves by their antisociality (e.g., biker gang, street gang). O2s might include making and maintaining prosocial peer groups (e.g., healthy social networking, volunteering).
- CRB1s and CRB2s. CRB1s might include verbal or physical aggression (or other behavioral extremes) directed at the therapist, staff, or other group members; engaging in frequent conflict or "power struggles" with therapist, staff, or group members; exhibiting a spotty attendance record; failing to form adaptive relationships with other group members; affiliating with more "antisocial" group members; engaging in verbal or other behavior supporting drug use/trafficking; continuing to use drugs while in treatment; rejecting more "prosocial" group members, therapist, and staff; rejecting prosocial activities (e.g., employment; school; athletics; hobbies); engaging in verbal or other behavior supporting use of antisocial/criminal means to achieve material gains; rejecting legitimate employment. Possible CRB2s include demonstrating appropriate turn-taking in group, making appropriate solicitations for assistance from staff and peers.
- FAP Moves: For this and each of the following sections, the FAP moves involve using the FAP rules in a manner consistent with the approaches advised by Marshall (2005). From a warm and compassionate stance, address CRBs as they speak to relevant dynamic risk related to sexual recidivism risk. Identify and respond to the CRBs in a collaborative manner consistent with identification and reinforcing of approach-goals.

Capacity for relationship stability. The basic construct is: "Does the offender currently [have] an intimate partner [in the community] in a relationship without obvious problems?" For clinical purposes, consider what factors historically have been associated with his lack of stable romantic partnerships, as well as barriers he currently faces to developing a romantic relationship. Behavioral indicators of this need area include:

- O1s and O2s. O1s include a history of forming highly unstable or conflictual romantic relationships; exhibiting infidelity, jealousy, mistrust, or a combination of these in romantic relationships; avoiding stable, committed romantic relationships. O2s include developing and maintaining effective and functional romantic relationships.

- CRB1s and CRB2s. Potential CRB1s include engaging in verbal behavior indicating mistrust of partner, meaningful peers, and therapist; exhibiting jealousy of partner's or therapist's relationships with others; using verbal behavior that perpetuates conflict-stance (versus resolution-stance) in romantic partnership; using verbal behavior that supports infidelity; rejecting fidelity in romantic relationships; using verbal behavior that impairs his ability to have an adaptive relationship (e.g., expresses hostility toward women). CRB2s include demonstrating behaviors consistent with healthy intimacy-enhancing disclosures about self and relationships.

Emotional identification with children (only for offenders with victims age 13 or younger). The basic construct is: "Child molesters may be attracted to children based on feeling emotionally close or intimate with them. Parents typically feel close to their children, but their roles are clearly differentiated. In contrast, child molesters may feel that children are their peers or equals and may feel that they can relate to children more easily than to adults. . . . consider not only attitudes and values, but also leisure and work activities suggestive of a child-oriented lifestyle." Behavioral indicators may include the following:

- O1s and O2s. O1s include a history of engaging in employment, social, and leisure activities in child-oriented settings; dressing or acting in ways that are appealing to children; lacking adult peer relationships. O2s include developing and maintaining hobbies and employment in adult-themed or adult-appropriate settings (e.g., darts, billiards, bridge clubs).
- CRB1s and CRB2s. CRB1s include engaging in verbal behavior supporting children as peers; dressing, acting in ways that are appealing to children; engaging in child-oriented activities and hobbies; engaging in child-focused conversations or themes; exhibiting distress when discussing adult-themed responsibilities or values; displaying inappropriate interest in conversations involving group members' or therapist's children or childhood. CRB2s include showing interest in adult-themed responsibilities and discussions; demonstrating distress tolerance when discussing mature content.

Hostility towards women. The basic construct is: "Both rapists and child molesters may have deficits in their capacity to form warm, constructive relationships with women. These deficits can be expressed as sexist attitudes, hostility toward women, or an inability to consider women as people worthy of trust and respect. Offenders with deficits in this category may have sexual or personal relationships with women, but these relationships are adversarial and conflicted." Behavioral indicators may include:

- O1s and O2s. O1s include a history of engaging in violence toward women; using dominance as part of sexual pleasure; engaging in sexual harassment;

displaying evidence of gender discrimination; failing to form and maintain non-sexualized relationships with female peers. O2s include developing appropriate and functional relationships with female peers, supervisors, group members, and therapists; identifying the controlling variables related to these improvements.

• CRB1s and CRB2s. CRB1s include using verbal behavior that supports hostility toward women; exhibiting adversarial sexual beliefs; endorsing sexual dominance of men over women; displaying overt hostility directed at female peers, therapist, and staff; sexualizing or objectifying women; exhibiting rigid attitudes about female sexuality, sexual behaviors, and the "proper" way for a woman to behave with regard to her sexuality. CRB2s include forming and maintaining appropriate and healthy interactions with female peers and therapists; engaging in appropriate discussions of male and female sexuality.

General social rejection/loneliness. The basic construct is: "The general capacity to make friends and feel close to others (secure adult attachment). Clients deficient on this dimension would feel lonely and socially rejected. Offenders without deficits would feel emotionally close to friends and family." Behavioral indicators may include the following:

• O1s and O2s. O1s include a history of isolating from social interaction and relationships; endorsing symptoms of phobias associated with social behavior; engaging in leisure activities that do not require social contact (e.g., television, reading, video games, collecting); lacking adult peers; withdrawing, distancing, alienating from family members. O2s include demonstrating affiliative and socially enhancing efforts in social settings.

• CRB1s and CRB2s. CRB1s include failing to engage in interpersonal interactions with other group members before, after, during group; exhibiting limited eye contact; speaking infrequently in group; exhibiting inappropriate verbal or other behavior; directing conversation to topics that have little relevance or interest to others; maintaining bad hygiene. CRB2s include demonstrating increased attempts (and successes) at interpersonal interactions with peers and therapists.

Lack of concern for others. The basic construct is: "Offenders who have little consideration for the feelings of others and act according to their own self-interest. They may be indifferent to the suffering of [others they have hurt/harmed] or feign shallow displays of regret. They may have little or no remorse. Interactions with others would be characterized as unfeeling, ruthless, or indifferent. This callousness is not just restricted to their reaction to their victims or adversaries, but would be present in many social interactions. Although they may have some friends, associates, and acquaintances, they would not be expected to have warm, caring, relationships.... The offender has to show a lack of attachment/lack of feeling for virtually all relationships." Behavioral indicators may include the following:

• O1s and O2s. O1s include failing to form and maintain long-standing, warm, caring relationships; forming social relationships that are superficial and possibly exploitative in nature. O2s include demonstrating altruistic efforts (or reasonable approximations) such as volunteering without a contracted or social pay-off (e.g., community service, impression management).

- CRB1s and CRB2s. CRB1s include engaging in harmful or hurtful verbal behavior directed at therapist, staff, or group members (e.g., teasing, mocking, harassing); engaging in verbal or other behavior that supports discrimination or prejudicial attitudes or behaviors; stealing, lying, exploiting others; lacking interest in the successes of others. CRB2s include exhibiting treatment-consistent and peer-supportive behavior in session; demonstrating interest in healthy relationship boundaries with peers and therapist.

Impulsivity. The basic construct is: "Does the offender engage in impulsive behavior that has a high likelihood of negative consequences? For this item, consider the extent to which the offender is easily bored, seeks thrills and has little regard for personal safety or the safety of others. This behavior must be exhibited in several settings and not just represented by a history of sexual offending." Behavioral indicators may include the following:

- O1s and O2s: Possible O1s include a history of driving recklessly; abusing substances; partying; accepting bets and dares; quitting jobs with no other job in sight; changing residences; engaging in unsafe work practices; starting fights with men much bigger than himself. Possible O2s include demonstrating follow-through on assumed responsibilities, acting in manner consistent with "a boring life is a healthier life for me."
- CRB1s and CRB2s: CRB1s include exhibiting sudden, unexpected movement activity in session; using inappropriate or out-of-context verbal behavior; abruptly leaving a session; attending a session under the influence of drugs or alcohol; "stirring the pot" in session to keep things exciting or to deflect focus from self; exhibiting treatment interfering behavior or deflecting tangential verbal behavior; displaying revelry in other's discussions of impulsive behavior. CRB2s might include showing distress tolerance skills when bored, displaying an ability to support peers when group focus is on others, maintaining group focus.

Poor problem solving skills. The basic construct is: "Offenders are at an increased risk for recidivism if they have difficulty accurately identifying and solving problems. They may fail to accurately identify the problems they have, propose unrealistic solutions (or none at all) ... fail to recognize the consequences of their actions." Behavioral indicators may include the following:

- O1s and O2s: Examples of O1s include a history of leaving a job or residence without another job or residence to go to; failing to get psychotropic medications refilled before running out. O2s include demonstrating short-term and long-term planning and follow-through consistent with healthy values and treatment-consistent expectations.

- CRB1s and CRB2s: CRB1s include failing to state problems clearly and specifically; failing to generate possible solutions without evaluating or rejecting them; demonstrating an inability to weigh the pros and cons of potential outcomes; displaying difficulty selecting effective solutions. CRB2s include showing a clear grasp of pros and cons to in-session and outside challenges, exhibiting an ability to marshal effective resources to enhance likelihood of goal acquisition.

Negative emotionality (hostility). The basic construct is: "Negative emotionality is a tendency towards feeling hostile, victimized, and resentful and feeling vulnerable to emotional collapse when stressed. Although possibly linked to real grievances, the offender's emotional response is excessive. Rather than attempting to cope constructively, the offender ruminates on the negative events and feelings and may appear to be 'getting into it.' Efforts to provide helpful suggestions are dismissed or belittled." Behavioral indicators may include the following:

- O1s and O2s: O1s include a history of displaying emotional "collapse" when distressed; engaging in aggressive acting out or other explosive expression of emotions. O2s might be demonstrating healthy coping when facing emotional stressors, making use of supports when appropriate.
- CRB1s and CRB2s: CRB1s include displaying verbal behavior that indicates hostility, suspicion, grievance; aggressive behavior; using verbal behavior that indicates rumination, rehearsing negative emotions; reporting attitudes such as "the world owes me something" or is "out to get me"; exhibiting explosive expression of emotions. CRB2s include demonstrating in vivo use of positive emotionality, using coping skills, and verbal enlistment of social supports appropriately.

Sex drive/sex preoccupation. The basic construct is: "In contrast to romantic attraction or infatuation, sexual pre-occupation focuses on recurrent sexual thoughts and behavior that are not directed to a current romantic partner. The degree of casual or impersonal sexual activity may interfere with other prosocial goals … or be perceived as intrusive or excessive by the offender. However, high levels of sexual preoccupation should be considered problematic even if the offender sees little wrong with his behavior …" Behavioral indicators may include the following:

- O1s and O2s. O1s include masturbating excessively; regularly using prostitutes, strip bars, massage parlors, phone-sex; engaging in sex-oriented internet use, such as sexually explicit sites, chat rooms; collecting and/or trading pornography (videos, magazines); having 30 or more lifetime sex partners; working at an "adult" bookstore; a child molester buying toys to facilitate sexual contact with children. O2s include discussing age-appropriate and healthy sexual outlets; identifying and discussing controlling variables (functional analysis) regarding precursors and consequences of healthy sexual behavior.
- CRB1s and CRB2s. CRB1s include displaying excessive sexual content in typical conversations; exhibiting preoccupation with own or other's sex crimes; verbally reporting disturbing sexual thoughts; introducing sexual themes or discussions

out of context. CRB2s include indicating healthy and respectful acknowledgement of sexual urges and desires; acquiring and demonstrating effective proactive and reactive interventions when aware of sexual preoccupation.

Sex as coping. The basic construct is: "When faced with life stress or negative emotions, some sex offenders start thinking sexual thoughts or engage in sexual behavior in efforts to manage their emotions. The sexual thoughts may be normal or deviant." Behavioral indicators may include the following:

- O1s and O2s. O1s include a history of seeking impersonal sex or masturbating when experiencing negative emotional states. O2s include developing and practicing stress inoculation efforts (especially if involving FAP-consistent peer supports).
- CRB1s and CRB2s. CRB1s include failing to employ adaptive coping responses when distressed; increasing frequency of sexualized discussions when distressed. CRB2s include demonstrating healthy coping skills when experiencing stressors in the moment during groups or sessions.

Deviant sexual preference. The basic construct is: "These interests could include sexual interest in [pre- or peri-pubescent] children, non-consenting adults [or minors], voyeurism, exhibitionism, cross-dressing, and fetishism." Behavioral indicators may include the following:

- O1s and O2s: O1s include a pattern of engaging in sexual activity with pre-pubescent children; using force during sex; demonstrating paraphilic interests and/or activities. O2s include developing healthy sexual values and behaviors.
- CRB1s and CRB2s: CRB1s include exhibiting verbal behavior that indicates sexual interest in pre-pubescent children; discussing use of force during sex; engaging in paraphilic activity; denying any sexual urges and interests; increasing frequency of discussion of fetishes during times of distress. CRB2s include discussing healthy sexual appetites and practices; engaging in open discussion of sexual interests and ongoing functional analysis of sexual practices when prompted by therapist.

Cooperation with supervision. The basic construct is: "Whether you feel that the offender is working with you or working against you … In addition, the offender may… not [be] taking the conditions of his supervision seriously …" From a clinical perspective, the offender fails to comply with instructions, conform to group norms, or make expected progress, despite clear and consistent information about treatment expectations and attempts to adapt to his individual needs. Behavioral indicators may include the following:

- O1s and O2s: O1s include a history of obtaining violations/infractions while on supervision/parole or while incarcerated; a history of failing or dropping-out of treatment. O2s include attending required meetings (e.g., with parole officer).

- CRB1s and CRB2s: CRB1s include often arriving late; failing to attend scheduled appointments; frequent requests to reschedule; breaking treatment rules/conditions; testing known risk factors or not avoiding high-risk situations; being silent or failing to disclose in group and/or individual sessions; verbalizing negative attitudes about treatment, therapists, and group members; trying to "play the system" (e.g., superficially participating, but exhibiting no genuine effort); trying to be "buddy-buddy" with staff; asking for special favors; lies or deceives therapist and staff or other group members; manipulating staff [e.g., "staff splitting"]. CRB2s include cooperating with peers and therapists, adhering to group norms, boundaries, rules, and expectations.

Clinically Relevant Behavior and Acute Risk to Re-offend

Acute dynamic risk factors are those aspects of the client's personality and/or lifestyle that are potentially more labile, and may be present within days, hours, or even minutes preceding a sexual offense. When present during a treatment session, these behaviors are clinically relevant not only for long-term progress monitoring, but also as potential indicators of a more imminent risk to re-offend sexually, violently, or both violently and sexually.

Victim access. The basic construct is: This item assesses "opportunities for contact, grooming, interaction with potential victims, and whether the offender appears to be changing or arranging his or her life so that they "naturally" contact members of their preferred victim group."

- O1s and O2s: O1s include engaging in activities or hobbies that increase opportunities for him to be around children or women, beyond what would be expected in the course of his normal daily life or routine; arranging or failing to avoid repeated opportunities to meet and engage with targets of preference; appearance or evidence of intentional access to victims; grooming or stalking behavior. O2s include engaging in healthy activities that do not increase his risk to re-offend in the short-term.
- CRB1s and CRB2s: CRB1s include exhibiting verbal behavior that supports activities or hobbies that increase opportunities to be around children or women; dressing, speaking, or acting in ways that would make him more attractive or interesting to children or women; displaying evidence he is hiding or lying about access to victims; increasing frequency or intensity of discussions related to this risk factor. CRB2s include demonstrating appropriate adult-focused activities or environments when in their daily activities (including group therapy).

Hostility. "This construct has two factors: (a) irrational and reckless defiance and (b) general hostility towards women. The overall level of characterological hostility is important to consider – some people are more hostile than others. You are looking for that which goes beyond their baseline level."

- O1s and O2s: O1s include declining or ridiculing suggestions just because they were made by a certain person in his life (e.g., partner, employer, parole officer); acting against his own best interests just to express this defiance; getting into verbal or physical altercations; engaging in verbal altercations and hostility differentially directed toward women. O2s include showing warmth and empathy toward self, peers, and others with whom he interacts.
- CRB1s and CRB2s: CRB1s include declining or ridiculing suggestions just because they were made by therapist or staff or particular group members; acting against his own best interests just to express this defiance; being unable to see things from another person's perspective (especially a woman's); engaging in veiled or direct threats; displaying angry rumination; exhibiting paranoia; planning retribution or revenge. CRB2s include being able to act in accordance with values while acknowledging competing interests (e.g., being effective when wanting to be right); effectively managing emotions with men and women; appropriately disclosing struggles in session and soliciting feedback from peers and therapist.

Sexual preoccupations. The basic construct is: "The extent to which the individual is focused on sexual matters and sees them as a central part of their life – possibly tying them into everyday coping mechanisms."

- O1s and O2s: O1s include using sexual thoughts or behavior to handle distress; increasing behaviors related to sex (e.g., frequenting adult bookstores, strip clubs, peep shows, internet porn); masturbating once a day or more. O2s include using healthy adult sexuality appropriately; using treatment-consistent interventions when facing stressors.
- CRB1s and CRB2s: CRB1s might include increasing sexual thoughts or behaviors; exhibiting verbal behavior that suggests sex is assuming increased importance or relevance in day-to-day functioning; verbally perseverating on sexual themes; reporting increased sexual urges and acting out; focusing on "sexual tension"; reporting an increase in self-costs for sexual behavior (e.g., harm, expense, missed opportunities, or activities). CRB2s include using appropriate non-sexual coping in group; acknowledging, processing, and engaging in appropriate functional analysis in-group or in-session.

Rejection of supervision. "The basic concept is whether you feel the offender is working with you or working against you."

- O1s and O2s: O1s include engaging in the behaviors below with other supervisors or authority figures (e.g., parole officer, employer, and parents). O2s include demonstrating cooperation with all aspects of healthy living continuum (e.g., spouse, church, and employer).
- CRB1s and CRB2s: CRB1s might include appearing silent, withdrawn; displaying reluctance to disclose information; missing appointments, appearing actively hostile to therapist and staff or group members; testing limits of supervision

or treatment conditions or breaching them, asking therapist and staff to bend or break the rules of treatment or supervision, being found to be in possession of dangerous items (e.g., weapons, contraband). CRB2s include enlisting and effectively using supervision from peers and therapist.

Emotional collapse. The basic construct is: "In contrast to normal negative affect, (having a bad day) offenders during emotional collapse are unable to maintain normal routines and may feel out of control of their thoughts and overwhelmed by their emotions."

- O1s and O2s: O1s include exhibiting significant changes in routine in an effort to cope (e.g., watching more TV than usual), engaging in maladaptive behaviors in an effort to "self-soothe," (e.g., substance use, self-harm, gambling, aggressive verbal or physical behavior), behavioral efforts to "restore power" in a relationship; acting impulsively (e.g., driving recklessly, quitting a job, leaving a relationship). O2s include using treatment-consistent coping skills when faced with stressors.
- CRB1s and CRB2s: CRB1s include exhibiting evidence of negative mood state beyond that which is reasonable given life circumstances; displaying flattened affect, poor eye contact, bad hygiene, psychomotor agitation or retardation, or other symptoms of mood disturbance; engaging in aggressive or assaultive verbal behavior directed at therapist, staff, or group members; verbally perseverating or ruminating; making statements that offense behavior would improve their emotional state or that they would be "better off" in jail; exhibiting evidence of paranoia. CRB2s include making self-reports of hopefulness, displaying positive emotions, engaging in behavior and actions consistent with an enriched emotional environment.

Collapse of social supports. The basic construct is: "Offenders are often partially prevented from reoffending by having a network, however loose, of persons in their life that reduce risk". This can either be psychological, such as "he wouldn't want to face his family if he did it again," or environmental, such as when a neighbor goes shopping with him on Saturdays so that he is not tempted.

- O1s and O2s: O1s include having an actual or perceived loss of relationship with someone who has been a positive influence on his life; being thrown out of positive social organizations; "blowing off" friends or engagements; increasing contact with someone who is a negative influence in his life. O2s include demonstrating appropriate enlistment of social supports when faced with emotionally taxing stressors.
- CRB1s and CRB2s: CRB1s include focusing on positive feelings about a negative peer influence; using verbal behavior that suggests that a source of social support may be collaborating with the offender to minimize or deny offence-related behaviors. CRB2s might include making appropriate requests for support from peers and therapists.

Substance abuse. The basic construct is: "The use of prohibited or inhibition-reducing substances. Urinalysis may be an additional source of evidence. This section may also involve the use of prescription drugs (pain killers)."

- O1s and O2s: O1s include receiving a violation or infraction for substance use; having a positive urinalysis. O2s could include making effective use of sobriety-supportive buttresses (e.g., AA, NA, and sponsor).
- CRB1s and CRB2s: CRB1s include presenting for session under the influence of drugs or alcohol; engaging in new prescription drug use suggesting abuse; requesting referral to prescriber. CRB2s include using breathalyzer as a regular pre-treatment assessment; appropriately including peers and therapist in commitment to sobriety.

What Does This Look Like in Practice?

Using FAP as an approach to treat sexual offense behavior is essentially similar to using FAP to treat any other behavioral problem. As with any behaviorally based approach, therapy begins with case conceptualization. Using FAP as an approach to treat sexual offense behavior has the added advantage of having research-identified risk factors to assist in the assessment and conceptualization of clinically relevant behaviors and functional classes. In practice, we look to see what the person gained by engaging in the harmful sexual practice (e.g., intimacy needs were met, aversive emotional state was avoided). Then the therapist notes which of these functional classes are consistent with identified risk factors, as well as for CRB1s and CRB2s related to the functional classes and class exemplars. Subsequently, the therapist observes the clients' behaviors and watches for CRBs, evokes CRBs, and contingently shapes CRBs in the context of a caring and supportive therapeutic relationship. Here are some examples of FAP questions that might occur in session

- How is the relationship with me similar or dissimilar to relationships you have with other people?
- What do you do well with me that you struggle to do well with others? What are some areas in which you struggle with me?
- Are there things you're afraid of telling me in session? What are you doing with those fears and worries?
- What is intimacy like with us? What are you doing to promote or quash it? What could I do?
- What would the conflicts you were having with your spouse right before you offended look like with us, if we were having similar conflicts?
- Are there times in session when you want to get up and leave? What are those times, what were we talking about when that happened? Can we talk about that again now?

• What do you do to handle yourself when you find yourself being aroused or having sexual thoughts in session? Is that helping in the short term or long term or both?

FAP with Women and Youth Convicted of Sexual Offenses

The dynamic risk-based approach presented above is derived from research that primarily has been conducted on adult male sexual offenders. Clinicians working with female offenders, however, could use an approach based on similar treatment principles, that is, collaboratively developing an ideographic treatment plan based on the client's specific dynamic risk-needs (c.f. Hart et al., 2003). Likewise, Newring, Parker, and Newring (Chapter 11, this volume) describe the use of FAP with adolescents. For those practitioners working with adolescent sexual offenders, several assessment instruments are available to help identify dynamic risk factors and treatment targets, including the Juvenile Sex Offender Assessment Protocol-II (J-SOAP-II; Prentky & Righthand, 2003), The Estimate of Risk of Adolescent Sexual Offense Recidivism (ERASOR; Worling, 2004), and the Youth Level of Service Inventory (Hoge, Andrews, & Leschied, 2002).

Therapist Features

The therapist behaviors associated with therapeutic change include being empathic, directive, respectful, flexible, attentive, confident, supportive, trustworthy, emotionally responsive, genuine, warm, rewarding, self-disclosing, encouraging participation, using humor, and instilling positive expectations (Marshall et al., 2003). These behaviors, consistent with FAP, facilitate change with general psychotherapy clients and with persons convicted of sexual offenses. Likewise, the therapist behaviors that reduce therapeutic change include being rejecting, nervous, dishonest, uninterested, unresponsive, rigid, judgmental, cold, critical, authoritarian, defensive, sarcastic, hostile and angry, manipulative, impatient, uncomfortable with silence, needing to be liked, and having boundary problems (Marshall et al., 2003, as cited in Page & Marshall, 2007). These behaviors interfere with effective FAP and effective sex offense treatment.

In FAP, the therapist's clinically relevant behaviors (Therapists 1s or T1s and Therapist 2s or T2s) impact the treatment process. For a therapist treating sexual offense behavior, there are likely to be a host of T1s and T2s. Depending upon the client, therapist, and relationship history, the balance of disclosure and guardedness might form a T1–T2 dyad. For another setting, a balance of directive and supportive might be a T1–T2 dyad. Just as case conceptualization is important for working with clients with sexual behavior problems, the therapist case conceptualization is important as well, as it will help clinicians monitor the impact of their behavior on clients (see Callaghan, 2006b).

When deciding to conduct treatment with persons who have exhibited sexual offense behaviors, it is important to ask yourself "why?" This therapy is often emotionally challenging, and offers limited short-term evidence of therapeutic success (particularly if the measure of "therapeutic success" is limited to whether or not an offender recidivates). Some providers may be motivated by a desire to prevent the offender from committing any future offenses. Accordingly, providers should be willing and able to employ the empirically based treatment approaches that are designed to facilitate therapeutic change (cited above). For some therapists, this may pose a challenge, particularly if they equate being supportive in a therapeutic setting with supporting or condoning the offense behavior. Of the many challenges therapists can face is being able to conceptualize the client's inappropriate sexual behavior as the best he could do at that time, given his history and contingencies of reinforcement.

When facing such a therapeutic challenge, it may be important for therapists to ask themselves which is more important: to *actually* facilitate prosocial change in an offender's behavior using empirically based therapeutic techniques, or to *feel* as though they have impacted the offender using other methods, such as communicating disapproval of sexual offense behavior, withholding support and understanding, or leveling further punishment. We argue that these types of behaviors are evidence of an important boundary violation, where the therapist is using the offender's treatment process to meet his or her own emotional needs (i.e., to express disapproval of sexual offense behavior and thus distinguish oneself as distinctly different from the client). More importantly, by approaching sex offense treatment from this perspective, therapists may be working in opposition to the more essential goal, which is reducing that offender's risk to re-offend. In other words, working effectively to treat sexual offense behavior demands that therapists set aside their personal opinions about what the offender has done in the past, so that they can facilitate therapeutic changes in the offender's behavior that will reduce his risk to re-offend in the future. In the words of Page (2007), "Treatment with this population is not an opportunity to work out your own issues" (p. 13).

Summary, Conclusions, and Recommendations

Much has changed in the 20 years since the first application of cognitive-behavioral techniques, including Relapse Prevention (RP), to the treatment of sexual offense behavior. RP quickly became a popular approach to sex offense treatment, and there is some evidence to support its effectiveness with some offenders (e.g., Marques, Weideranders, Day, Nelson, & van Ommeren, 2005; Nicholaichuk, Gordon, Gu, & Wong, 2000; Hanson et al., 2002). Nonetheless, RP has been subject to criticism for a number of reasons, including its utilization as a primary treatment strategy for sex offenses, rather than as a treatment adjunct as originally designed. Furthermore, increased emphasis has been placed on working collaboratively with persons convicted of sexual offenses to help address more positively oriented "approach goals," in addition to traditional avoidance-based treatment targets. Finally, there has been an explosion of research on sex offense risk assessment and risk-based treatment for offenders that have provided new directions for the field of sex offense evaluation and treatment.

FAP, at its core, is an intensely interpersonal psychotherapy in which the therapeutic relationship is both the context in which change occurs, and the meaningful agent that motivates and supports changes. As many of the dynamic risk factors for sexual offense recidivism are interpersonal in nature, FAP is ideally suited to direct treatment approaches when working collaboratively with persons convicted of sexual offending.

The challenges in working with clients convicted of sexual offenses are problems insofar as they impact the clinician's clinically relevant behavior. Can clinicians allow themselves to form a caring and therapeutic relationship with a person convicted of a sexual offense? Can they allow such a client to matter to them? How can they go about forging a meaningful relationship with the client? Can they forgo topography and instead focus on clinically relevant functions as they promote community safety?

There are no hard and fast rules to make your clients matter to you, and to allow you to matter to your clients. Instead, there are the guiding values of community safety, risk-based treatment principles, and the rules of FAP. Taken together, these have, can, and will continue to promote safe communities through the establishment and maintenance of healthy lives, free of sexual re-offending.

References

Callaghan, G. M. (2006a). The Functional Idiographic Assessment Template (FIAT) System: For use with interpersonally-based interventions including Functional Analytic Psychotherapy (FAP) and FAP-enhanced treatments. *The Behavior Analyst Today, 7*, 357–398.

Callaghan, G. M. (2006b). Functional Assessment of Skills for Interpersonal Therapists: The FASIT System: For the assessment of therapist behavior for interpersonally-based interventions including Functional Analytic Psychotherapy (FAP) or FAP-enhanced treatments. *The Behavior Analyst Today, 7*, 399–433.

Hanson, R. K., & Bussiere, M. T. (1998). Predicting relapse: A meta-analysis of sexual offender recidivism studies. *Journal of Consulting and Clinical Psychology, 66*, 348–362.

Hanson, R. K., Gordon, A., Harris, A. J., Marques, J. K., Murphy, W., Quinsey, V. L., & Seto, M. C. (2002). First report of the collaborative outcome data project on the effectiveness of psychological treatment for sex offenders. *Sexual abuse: A Journal of Research and Treatment, 14*, 169–194.

Hanson, R. K., & Harris, A. J. R. (2001). A structured approach to evaluating change among sexual offenders. *Sexual abuse: A Journal of Research and Treatment, 13*, 105–122.

Hanson, R. K., & Harris, A. (2002). *STABLE and ACUTE scoring guides: Developed for the dynamic supervision project: A collaborative initiative on the community supervision of sexual offenders.* Ottawa: Department of the Solicitor General of Canada. Available at www.psepc.gc.ca

Hanson, R. K., Harris, J. R., Scott, T., & Helmus, L. (2007). *Assessing the risk of sexual offenders on community supervision: The dynamic supervision project (User Report 2007–05).* Ottawa: Public Safety and Emergency Preparedness Canada. Available at www.psepc.gc.ca

Hanson, R. K., & Morton-Bourgon, K. (2004). *Predictors of sexual recidivism: An updated meta-analysis (User Report 2004–02)*. Ottawa: Public Safety and Emergency Preparedness Canada. Available at www.psepc.gc.ca

Hart, S. D., Kropp, R., Laws, D. R., Klaver, J., Logan, C., & Watt, K. A. (2003). *The Risk for Sexual Violence Protocol (RSVP) – Structured professional guidelines for assessing risk of sexual violence*. Vancouver, BC: Simon Fraser University, Mental Health, Law and Policy Institute.

Hoge, R. D., Andrews, D. A., & Leschied, A. W. (2002). *The youth level of service/case management inventory*. Toronto: Multi-Health Systems. Referenced in Schmidt, F., Hoge, R. D., & Gomes, L. (2005). Reliability and validity analyses of the youth level of service/case management inventory. *Criminal Justice and Behavior, 32*(3), 329–344.

Hudson, S. M., Wales, D. S., Bakker, L., & Ward, T. (2002). Dynamic risk factors: The Kia Marama evaluation. *Sexual Abuse: A Journal of Research and Treatment, 14*, 103–119.

Hudson, S. M., Ward, T., & Marshall, W. L. (1992). The abstinence violation effect in sex offenders: A reformulation. *Behavior Research and Therapy, 30*, 435–441.

Kohlenberg, R. (1974a). Directed masturbation and the treatment of primary orgasmic dysfunction. *Archives of Sexual Behavior, 3*, 349–356.

Kohlenberg, R. (1974b). In-vivo desensitization and aversive stimuli in the treatment of pedophilia. *Journal of Abnormal Psychology, 83*, 192–195.

Kohlenberg, R. J., & Tsai, M. (1991). *Functional analytic psychotherapy: Creating intense and curative therapeutic relationships*. New York: Plenum.

Laws, D. R., Hudson, S. M., & Ward, T. (Eds.). (2000). *Remaking relapse prevention with sex offenders: A sourcebook*. Thousand Oaks, CA: Sage.

Mann, R. E., Webster, S. D., Schofiled, C., & Marshall, W. L. (2004). Approach versus avoidance goals in relapse prevention with sexual offenders. *Sexual Abuse: A Journal of Research and Treatment, 16*(1), 65–75.

Marques, J. K., Weideranders, M., Day, D., Nelson, C., & van Ommeren, A. (2005). Effects of a relapse prevention program on sexual recidivism: Final results from California's Sex Offender Treatment and Evaluation Project (SOTEP). *Sexual Abuse: A Journal of Research and Treatment, 17*, 79–107.

Marshall, W. L., Serran, G. A., Fernandez, Y. M., Mulloy, R., Mann, R., & Thornton, D. (2003). Therapist characteristics in the treatment of sexual offenders: Tentative data on their relationship with indices of behaviour change. *Journal of Sexual Aggression, 9*(1) 25–30.

Marshall, W. L. (2005). Therapist style in sexual offender treatment: Influence on indices of change. *Sexual Abuse: A Journal of Research and Treatment, 17*(2), 109–116.

Marshall, W. L., Ward, T., Mann, R. E., Moulden, H., Fernandez, Y., Serran, G., & Marshall, L. E. (2005). Working positively with sexual offenders: Maximizing the effectiveness of treatment. *Journal of Interpersonal Violence, 20*(9), 1096–1114.

Newring, K. A. B., Loverich, T. M., Harris, C. D., & Wheeler, J. G. (2009). Relapse prevention. In W. O'Donohue & J. Fisher (Eds.), *Cognitive behavior therapy: Applying empirically supported techniques in your practice* (2nd ed.). New York: Wiley.

Nicholaichuk, T., Gordon, A., Gu, D., & Wong, S. (2000). Outcome of an institutional sexual offender treatment program: A comparison between treated and matched untreated offenders. *Sexual Abuse: Journal of Research and Treatment, 12*(2), 139–153.

Penix Sbraga, T., & Brunswig, K. A. (2003, May). *The functions of sexual coping responses: Taxonomic, research and treatment implications*. Paper presented at the 29th Annual Association for Behavior Analysis, San Francisco CA.

Prentky, R., & Righthand, S. (2003). *Juvenile Sex Offender Assessment Protocol-II (J-SOAP-II). Office of Juvenile Justice and Delinquency prevention*. Available at www.csom.org/pubs/JSOAP.pdf

Quinsey, V. L., Lalumiere, M. L., Rice, M. E., & Harris, G. T. (1995). Predicting sexual offenses. In J. C. Campbell (Ed.), *Assessing dangerousness: Violence by sexual offenders, batterers, and child abusers* (pp. 114–137). Thousand Oaks, CA: Sage.

Roberts, C. F., Doren, D. M., & Thornton, D. (2002). Dimensions associated with assessments of sex offender recidivism risk. *Criminal Justice and Behavior, 29*, 569–589.

Tsai, M., Kohlenberg, R. J., Kanter, J. W., Kohlenberg, B., Follette, W. C., & Callaghan, G. M. (2008). *A guide to functional analytic psychotherapy: Awareness, courage, love and behaviorism.* New York: Springer.

Ward, T., & Hudson, S. M. (2000). A self-regulation model of the relapse prevention process. In D. R. Laws, S. M. Hudson, & T. Ward (Eds.), *Remaking relapse prevention with sex offenders: A source book* (pp. 79–101). Thousand Oaks, CA: Sage.

Ward, T., Hudson, S. M., & Marshall, W. L. (1994). The abstinence violation effect in child molesters. *Behavior Research and Therapy, 32,* 431–437.

Ward, T., & Stewart, C. A. (2002). Good lives and the rehabilitation of sexual offenders. In T. Ward, D. R. Laws, & S. M. Hudson (Eds.), *Sexual deviance: Issues and controversies* (pp. 21–44). Thousand Oaks, CA: Sage.

Webster, S. D. (2005). Pathways to sexual offense recidivism following treatment: An examination of the Ward and Hudson Self-regulation model of relapse. *Journal of Interpersonal Violence, 20*(10), 1175–1196.

Wheeler, J. G. (2003). The abstinence violation effect in a sample of incarcerated sexual offenders: A reconsideration of the terms Lapse and Relapse. *Dissertation Abstracts International: Section B: The Sciences & Engineering, 63,* 3946.

Wheeler, J. G., & Covell, C. N. (2007). Stable dynamic risk-need rating manual for treatment planning, delivery, & progress evaluation. Unpublished manual. Available from the authors.

Wheeler, J. G., George, W. H., & Stephens, K. (2005). Assessment of sexual offenders: A model for integrating dynamic risk assessment and Relapse Prevention approaches. In D. M. Donavan & G. A. Marlatt (Eds.), *Assessment of addictive behaviors* (2nd ed., pp. 392–424). New York: Guilford Publications.

Wheeler, J. G., George, W. H., & Stoner, S. A. (2005). Enhancing the relapse prevention model for sex offenders: Adding recidivism risk reduction therapy (3RT) to target offenders' dynamic risk needs. In G. A. Marlatt & D. M. Donavan (Eds.), *Relapse prevention* (2nd ed.). New York: Guilford.

Worling, J. (2004). The Estimate of Risk of Adolescent Sexual Offense Recidivism (ERASOR). *Sexual Abuse: Journal of Research and Treatment, 16,* 235–254.

Chapter 14
FAP for Interpersonal Process Groups

Renee Hoekstra and Mavis Tsai

Functional Analytic Psychotherapy (FAP) (Kohlenberg & Tsai, 1991), with its behavioral focus on in vivo interactions and in-session equivalents of clients' daily life problems, offers a compelling conceptual framework from which to conduct interpersonal group psychotherapy (Gaynor & Lawrence, 2002; Vandenberghe, Ferro, & Furtado da Cruz, 2003). Although a wide variety of cognitive behavioral and behavioral approaches have been applied to group psychotherapy for issues such as skills training, coping deficits, and changes in thinking (Fisher, Masia-Warner, & Klein, 2004; James, Thorn, & Williams, 1993; Rittner & Smyth, 2000; Rhode, Jorgensen, Seeley, & Mace, 2004; Wilson, Bouffard, & Mackenzie, 2005), behaviorally oriented groups are generally characterized by the use of behavior modification techniques (Vinagrov, Co, & Yalom, 2003) and do not focus on interpersonal process. Behavioral and cognitive behavioral therapies for process-oriented groups that focus on interpersonal interactions as they occur in group do not appear to be very common. Only a few authors have addressed applied behaviorism in the context of interpersonal group psychotherapy (Rose, 1977; Upper & Flowers, 1994). Hollander and Kazaoka (1998) suggest that while behavioral approaches generally involve practical interventions, little or no attention has been paid to theoretical or conceptual issues. FAP enables treatment providers who work within a behavioral orientation to have a theoretical structure and format for interpersonally oriented groups.

The premise of FAP is that instances of clients' daily life problems will appear in session, and the contingent reactions of the therapist and other group members will naturally reinforce more adaptive behavior that can be generalized to clients' daily lives. This idea that group therapy can become a microcosm of clients' outside world has been a longstanding theme in psychodynamically oriented process groups:

> A freely interactive group, with few structural restrictions will, in time develop into a social microcosm of the participant members. Given enough time, group members will begin to be themselves; they will interact with the group members as they interact with others

R. Hoekstra (✉)
Private Practice, Boston, MA, USA
e-mail: renee_hoekstra@yahoo.com

J.W. Kanter et al. (eds.), *The Practice of Functional Analytic Psychotherapy*,
DOI 10.1007/978-1-4419-5830-3_14, © Springer Science+Business Media, LLC 2010

in their social sphere, will create in the group the same interpersonal universe they have always inhabited. In other words, clients will, over time, automatically and inevitable begin to display their maladaptive interpersonal behavior in the therapy group. (Yalom, 2005, pp. 31–32)

FAP differs from psychodynamic approaches, however, in (1) its focus on environmental events as the ultimate causes of behavior rather than mental entities such as drives and (2) its emphasis on the contextual meaning of behaviors – that the same behavior (e.g., an angry outburst) may be pathological or adaptive depending on the context in which it occurs. For a more detailed discussion of the differences between FAP and psychodynamic perspectives, see Kohlenberg and Tsai (1991, pp. 170–182).

The framework for FAP is based on five rules, or suggestions for therapist behavior. These rules, originally designed for individual psychotherapy, are effective in promoting cohesion, which is considered to be the key therapeutic factor in group psychotherapy. Burlingame, Fuhriman, and Johnson (2001) identified six empirically supported principles that maintain cohesion: pre-group preparation, early group structure, leader interaction, feedback, leader modeling, and member emotional expression. FAP's rules, consonant with these six principles, articulate more clearly the fundamental mechanisms of client change. Each rule and examples of its application to clients in group therapy is discussed in turn below.

Rule 1: Watch for Clinically Relevant Behaviors (CRBs)

Clients engage in three classes of clinically relevant behaviors (CRBs).

CRB1s are behavioral instances of the presenting problem occurring in session, CRB2s are in-session improvements and may be successive approximations of desired adaptive responses, and CRB3s are clients' observations and descriptions of their own behavior and what seems to cause it. CRB1s typically interfere with clients' abilities to make meaningful connections and to participate in intimate relationships. Intimacy promoting behaviors include being able to identify and express one's needs, give and receive feedback about interpersonal impact, deal with conflict, disclose feelings of closeness toward others, and express one's emotional experience (Callaghan, 2006).

For example, a client named Sally reports that her daily life problems include feeling lonely, having difficulty making friends, and being truly heard. In group, she talks in great detail about what she has done throughout the day. For Sally, her CRB1s can be identified as talking without pausing and not disclosing meaningful information. It would be difficult for other group members to engage in dialogue with her, and the result could be resentment by other members who believe she is unnecessarily taking up time. Sally's CRB2s or in-session improvements would include pausing to see if others are receiving what she is saying, giving others an opportunity to give feedback, and talking about topics that feel more vulnerable to her, such as her feelings of loneliness. CRB3s, the describing of functional connections, can help in obtaining reinforcement in daily life. An example of a CRB3 is Sally saying, "I think I may talk too much because I'm frightened no one really wants to hear what I have to say, so I don't say anything important."

The group setting offers far more opportunities than individual therapy for the occurrence of CRB1s and the natural reinforcement of CRB2s. A therapy group contains many potential built-in tensions: differences in social class, educational levels, income, and values; struggles for dominance and power; authority issues; distortions of others' verbalizations and actions; guardedness and distrust; envy; sexual attraction; judgment of others and fear of judgment from others; rivalry for therapist's attention and positive regard; fear of intimacy and vulnerability (punishment by group); fear of losing individuality; fear and wish to be known; desire for approval; and fear of rejection. Thus, group therapists, unlike individual therapists, can witness CRB1s evoked by a variety of individuals and can make use of the multitude of natural interpersonal reinforcers inherent in a group setting.

Rule 1 is the most important aspect of treatment. Attending to the many different ways that CRB1s and CRB2s can occur will enable a therapist to identify what to block, what to evoke, and what to reinforce naturally. This highlights the functional role of a therapist's response in reinforcing or extinguishing client behavior. The primary consequence of client behavior is the therapist's and other group members' reactions.

Getting Started: Rule 1 in Beginning Group Process

While the idea of screening and selecting clients for an ideally composed group is appealing, many contemporary therapists in public clinic and private practice settings have difficulty accumulating enough clients to form and maintain groups. Thus, they generally form groups by accepting the first seven or eight suitable group therapy participants (e.g., ruling out psychotic, dissociative, violent, and suicidal clients) using only the most basic principles of group composition, such as having an equal number of men and women, a range of age, professions, and interactional styles (such as active or passive) (Yalom, 2005).

Knowing what a client would like from joining group is a first step in identifying in vivo problematic behaviors. We ask potential group members these questions to assess their possible CRB1s:

1. What happens in group settings that prevent you from feeling connected to others? Please be as specific and clear as you can.
2. How do these behaviors serve to protect you, keep you sane, or keep you safe?
3. How might we observe these behaviors occurring in group?
4. Is there anything the group can do to help you observe when these behaviors occur in group? Please explain.
5. Are there things you do that keep you from making connections with other people that we would not be able to observe? Please elaborate.

6. Please describe anything you would like from other people in group that will help you to work on your concerns.
7. Please identify what you would like from the group leader that will help you to work on your concerns.
8. How will group members or the group leader know when what we ask is too much for you?
9. If you were upset with another group member, what would you do?
10. If you were thinking about leaving group, what would you do to let us know?
11. What is it that you would ideally like to gain from joining a group?

Ultimately, if each client's relevant history, presenting problems, daily life goals, in-session problems (CRB1s), and in-session improvements (CRB2s) are known to all group members, helping one another attain therapeutic goals becomes a clear joint undertaking.

Examples of Possible CRB1s

FAP views behavior based on its form and function. A behavior that has the same form (e.g., being warm and charming) may be a CRB1 or a CRB2 depending on its function (allows person to stay safe by focusing on others or invites others to become closer). With the caveat in mind that all behavior must be viewed contextually, below are examples of behaviors that tend to interfere with interpersonal effectiveness or intimacy:

1. Speaking in a way that is confusing or difficult for others to track: speaking in tangents; frequent shifts in topics; rambling, pressured or rapid speech; excessively loud talking; excessively quiet talking; inconsistent requests (asking and then withdrawing, changing one's mind, changing the subject).
2. Nonverbal issues: Excessive sighing, eye rolling, fidgeting, looking at the clock excessively, fixed facial expression or glare, unreadable or blank facial expression, closed posture (tightly crossed arms and legs), coming early or late, slouching, always sitting next to the leader.
3. Inability to give or receive positive feedback or validation.
4. Difficulty in reading other group members' emotions or attitudes, inability to hypothesize about the function of others' behaviors, lack of sensitivity to the affective tone of group (e.g., anger).
5. Insensitivity to group interaction: re-directing conversation toward oneself repeatedly, taking up all the group time with one's own difficulties without attending to the needs of others, difficulty recognizing one's impact on other group members.
6. Ineffective expression of affect: lack of affect; affect so intense it interferes with group communication; affect is expressed in a mixed/conflicting manner.

7. Rushed intimacy: insincere attempts to connect; over-disclosing by sharing intimate material too soon.
8. Assuming the group will make unanimous decisions prior to assessing the interests, wants, or desires of other group members.
9. Conflict avoidance: failure to identify one's own differences in regards to the group; inability to identify and describe disagreement or differences of opinion; inability to identify and describe conflict in regards to self and group; overly agreeable, acquiescent, or conciliatory; not acknowledging one's reaction to group conflict; inability to identify and describe emotional experiences and responses to group members' behavior.
10. Aggressive or attacking behavior: overly critical of group members' behavior, speaking in condescending tone, failure to observe the limits of others.
11. Avoiding contact: not talking, not sharing salient or meaningful material, withdrawing, tuning out or "going away in one's mind," not attending to what others are saying, making light of painful situations by joking, changing the subject when someone is discussing painful material, focusing on material that has no therapeutic benefit, keeping topics superficial and entertaining, storytelling.
12. Self-defeating/self-deprecatory behavior: self-derogatory comments, apologizing excessively, not accepting compliments, excessive expressions of hopelessness, persistent refusal to consider suggestions offered by group members.
13. Sub-grouping: whispering, casting "knowing" looks to another group member, banding or sharing with select group members but not the rest of the group, joining with group members outside of group, and failing to discuss these occurrences in group.
14. Thwarting/attacking group leader: excessive complaints about group leadership, consistently interrupting leader, taking over group leadership, and acting as if leading the group.

It is also important to attend not only to what is said, but what is omitted: the male member who offers feedback to female members but not to other men, the group that never confronts or questions the therapist, the topics that are never broached (e.g., sex, money, death), the member who never offers support or the one who never asks for it, or the member who does not ask questions of others. All these omissions may indicate CRB1s. A clear formulation of group members' CRBs will provide a structure for effective group interventions.

Rule 2: Evoke CRBs

The ideal therapeutic situation evokes CRB1s (so that clients can contact the controlling variables of their problematic behaviors) and provides for the development of CRB2s. The group setting, as previously stated, is a social microcosm that offers many therapeutic opportunities for clients: "The group . . . provides opportunities to evoke associations to current life relationships or to family of origin experiences" (Rutan & Stone, 2001, p. 72). When clients first come to therapy, however, they are not likely to have a comprehensive way of articulating their problems or observing occurrences of these problems in vivo. Data suggest that therapist and client disagreement over goals may play a role in therapeutic impasses (Hill, Nutt-Williams, Heaton, Rhodes, & Thompson, 1996), thus communicating fully with clients about therapeutic rationale and goals can serve to strengthen the therapeutic alliance with the group leader and prevent future misunderstandings. In addition, providing clients with group goals will make it more likely that everyone recognize their own and others' CRB1s and help one another develop intimacy facilitating repertoires that will generalize to daily life relationships.

Evoking CRBs involves both structuring the group environment to be evocative and focusing on relationships within the group.

Structuring the Group Environment to Be Evocative: Educating Clients About the FAP Rationale and Goals

In order for FAP to be most effective, it is important that clients understand its premise – that the therapist will be looking for ways that clients' outside life problems show up within the group setting because such an in vivo focus facilitates the most powerful change. This is a sample of an informed consent form we give to clients that describes the FAP rationale and goals:

What You May Expect in Functional Analytic Psychotherapy (FAP) Group

Clients come into group therapy with complex life stories of joy and anguish, dreams and hopes, passions and vulnerabilities, unique gifts and abilities. Your group therapy will be conducted in an atmosphere of caring, respect and commitment in which new ways of approaching life are learned. Embarking on a journey of exploration and growth with others is a privilege, and it is important to treat what others share with reverence and care. Validation of group members' feelings and experiences will create a safe environment in which to heal and to grow.

The type of therapy you are entering is called Functional Analytic Psychotherapy (FAP), a therapy that focuses on interpersonal effectiveness and intimacy. You will have the opportunity to explore how you are in relationships, to experiment with different ways of relating, and to learn how to express yourself more fully and to connect with others more deeply. You will be challenged to be more open, vulnerable, aware and present. Specifically, we'll be focusing on five classes of interpersonal skills: identifying and expressing needs, giving and receiving feedback about interpersonal impact, dealing with conflict, disclosing feelings of closeness towards others, and disclosing emotional experience and expression. These skills will increase the group's ability to work together so everyone can generate and benefit from compassion and closeness.

A primary principle in FAP is that your relationships within the group are a microcosm of your daily life relationships, and it is especially important for you to focus on issues (positive or negative) or difficulties that come up in group that also come up with other people in your life. You will identify your own problematic behaviors that interfere with closeness, learn to understand their protective functions, practice more intimacy-promoting behaviors, and rely on the other group members to provide helpful feedback. So we will be exploring how you interact in group in a way that is similar to how you interact with other people, what problems come up in group that also come up with other people, and what positive behaviors you can develop in group that you can translate into your relationships with others.

Therapy has a greater impact when you talk about your experience in the present moment rather than reporting about things felt during the week. For example, sharing what you are thinking, feeling, or needing, or your experience of another group member, is encouraged even if it feels scary or risky. When we look at something that is happening in the moment, we can get immediate feedback from other group members, we can experience and understand it more fully, and therapeutic change is faster and stronger. There is an optimal level of risk-taking in any situation, however, and it's important that you monitor how much outside your comfort zone to be is best for you at any given time.

Overall, FAP group will focus on bringing forth your best self. The most fulfilled people are in touch with themselves, are able to speak and act compassionately on their truths and gifts, and are able to fully give and receive love. When one feels the power in expressing one's thoughts, feelings, and desires in an authentic, caring and assertive way, one is more connected to others and has a greater sense of mastery in life. This group will be an ideal place for you to practice sharing your inner voice in an environment that is able to receive and respond.

I accept the above statement, and have been given a copy for myself. I have had the opportunity to ask questions and to voice my reactions. I am committed to doing my best in this group therapy.

Focus on Relationships Within the Group

It is important to guide group members away from talking about daily life issues and focus instead on their relationships with one another, because the more spontaneously they interact with one another, the more rapidly and authentically their social microcosm will develop that will evoke their CRB1s.

Begin by focusing on positive interactions – "Who do you feel the most warmly towards here?" "Who is easiest person in the group for you to trust?" "Who is the most similar to you – what do you most like or admire about him/her?"

As trust builds within the group, the therapist can pull for more difficult disclosures: "I wonder if we can share some thoughts that we've been having but are a little reluctant to share with the group," or "I'm wondering if you're sizing each other up, arriving at impressions about the group, wondering how you'll fit in. Can we spend some time discussing what each of us has come up with so far?" or "Is there anything that disappointed you about our meeting today?"

Table 14.1 provides examples of reasons clients give for wanting treatment, how their CRB1s may show up in group (Rule 1), and what the therapist might say to evoke CRB (Rule 2) – to help the client get in touch with how his/her in-session behavior may be a reflection of daily life problems, to provide an opportunity for the

Table 14.1 Client presenting problems, corresponding CRB1s, and possible therapist statements

Presenting problem	CRB1	Possible therapist statement
I have low self-esteem	Client makes self-deprecating remark when complimented by another group member	What happened when you were complimented? Did anyone in this group notice what she did just now with that compliment? What did she do to block it? (To member) What would happen if you really let yourself take in the compliment and feel the positive regard behind it?
I tend to take on everyone else's problems and worry about them	Client refrains from talking about personal problems and is overly accommodating to other group members	You've been pretty quiet. Are you taking on everyone else's problems? Anyone else in the group have a hypothesis of what's happening based on the reasons why X came into treatment?
I can't hold down a job	Client fails to inform leader of missing sessions and comes to group irregularly	You say you have a hard time holding down a job because your work attendance is spotty. Twice you've failed to attend group and didn't inform me you were going to miss group. Is this the kind of thing that happens with new jobs?
It is hard for me to make friends	Client talks about office dynamics at length	It may be hard for the group to respond to what you're saying because it's somewhat abstract and impersonal. I'd be more interested in how you've been feeling about group the last couple of meetings. Are there some interactions you've been especially tuned into? Or, what reactions have you had to other members here?

Table 14.1 (continued)

Presenting problem	CRB1	Possible therapist statement
I'm angry at my partner a lot	Client makes critical statements about how group is going	Are you unhappy with the way group is going? Is there anyone in group who you can foresee getting into a similar type of struggle as you do with your partner?
I'm too passive and too easily influenced by others	Is very agreeable in group	Who in the group could influence you the most?
Other people don't like me, and I think they make fun of my feelings	Doesn't talk in group	Are you thinking that we'll make fun of your feelings if you disclose them? Who do you imagine will be most likely to ridicule you? Least likely?

development of CRB2s, and to increase the group members' capacity to help each other with CRBs. In each of these instances, the therapist can deepen interaction by encouraging further responses from other group members: "How do you feel about his fear that you would ridicule him? Can you imagine doing that?" or "What can she say or do right now that would help you feel more connected?"

Rule 3: Reinforce CRB2s

If a therapist responds immediately to client improvements, however small, the likelihood is increased that the new behavior will be strengthened. A group leader who responds positively to a client in a warm and genuine manner when the client tries different behaviors may naturally increase the likelihood that the new behaviors will continue to occur. This type of response, however, needs to be reinforcing for the client. Something becomes a reinforcer only in the context of the process and cannot be identified independent of it. Therapist statements that are intended to reinforce client behavior must actually be reinforcing to the client; thus a group leader's use of Rule 3 must be flexible and contingent on client improvement. From a behavioral perspective, group behavior is always reinforcing if a client returns to group. Clients who are deprived of meaningful social contact naturally will be reinforced by a group that expresses a genuine interest in the client.

Group leadership demands flexibility, genuineness, and the ability to shift with the group process. A therapist can make a hypothesis about what is reinforcing based on the identification of CRBs, and can employ an array of natural responses that could be reinforcing to the client. Here are some examples of what a therapist might say to the clients: "I like it when you pause and let the rest of the group catch up. It feels nice to be able to respond to what you're talking about." "I feel like now we are getting to know the real you, the one behind the words, and you have a lot of depth." "Your self-disclosure took the group a lot deeper, and brought forth a lot of positive and caring responses from other group members." In the third example, the therapist is increasing the client's contact with controlling contingencies (the interest and caring of other group members).

A leader fosters relationships among group members and between them and himself/herself in order to promote the natural reinforcement of CRB2s. Essential to the process of reinforcement is the concept of shaping successive approximations to a target behavior. If we are hooked by the interpersonal behavior of a group member, therapeutic value follows if we do not engage in the typical behavior the client elicits from others, which only reinforces the usual cycles. For example, if a client talks at length about tangential issues, a typical response would be to ignore this client and not get to know him or her better. In FAP group, the responsibility of the therapist would be to help this client: (1) recognize the CRB1 when it's occurring, (2) understand the function of the CRB1 (e.g., protecting the client from making connections with others and the eventual disappointment and hurt that has occurred in past relationships), (3) make successive approximations to more adaptive behavior (talking more briefly; talking about feelings first about outside issues; then about feelings toward others in the group), and (4) be naturally reinforced for these improvements or CRB2s by the therapist as well as by other group members. If the therapist makes his or her response contingent upon client improvement, the therapist will have a powerful tool to facilitate and positively influence the outcome of treatment.

Rule 4: Observe the Potentially Reinforcing Effects of Therapist (and Group) Behavior in Relation to Client CRBs

As stated in Rule 3, a therapist thinking his or her response is reinforcing may not make it so. The way to tell if a client truly is being reinforced is if the target behavior in question increases in strength over time. The therapist must be aware of how his or her interventions impact the client, both immediately and in the long term.

Rule 4 encourages the therapist not only to be aware of the impact of his or her interventions, but to attend to private experiences that can be a useful resource in identifying CRBs. This can enable the therapist to observe functional connections between the therapist's private experience (e.g., frustration), the client's presenting concern (e.g., loneliness), and the client's CRB1 (e.g., not saying anything meaningful in group).

In addition, if a therapist is aware of his or her own in vivo problems (T1s) that may negatively influence treatment, he or she needs to work on T2s (therapist target behaviors) that will facilitate progress. For example, a therapist may come from a background in which interrupting someone is disrespectful. For a client whose long-windedness is a CRB1, however, the therapist's unwillingness to interrupt could interfere with his or her ability to intervene effectively. In a group setting, this can be a unique challenge in the sense that the therapist cannot hide from a group: group leader behaviors become the public domain of the group. A failure to identify and work on T2s in a group setting can increase a leader's vulnerability to engaging the group in an anti-therapeutic manner, thus risking the loss of emotional valence and group interest.

In the above scenario, the remaining group members will likely become bored, frustrated, and agitated. These private experiences of other group members are naturally occurring consequences of the client's loquaciousness, and offer the group leader an excellent opportunity to extrapolate Rule 4 to a group setting. The idea here is to teach the group how to use each other by augmenting and enhancing the private experience of group members when the person in question is rambling on in a tangential manner. For instance, the group leader can ask the remaining members questions such as: "What are you noticing or experiencing as X is talking? What is it like to sit here in this group right now and listen to X talk about her laundry? Who got lost a few paragraphs ago? Why isn't anyone in this group asking questions about X's personal life? Is there anyone that wants to ask questions but feels as if X can't be interrupted?" Getting the group to talk about what is occurring in group without ignoring or negating the talkative member can serve to increase authenticity of group members and to reinforce the client for being more real to the group.

Rule 5: Give Interpretations of Variables That Affect Client Behavior

This rule involves describing observed behavior and its possible functions, and corresponds to CRB3s, the reasons clients give for their behavior. Understanding the historical functions of client CRB1s can help both the client and the group work with these behaviors in a non-punitive fashion. Clients who understand the functions of their problematic behaviors are better positioned to take risks in the future as a means to remedy the problem. Consider the example of the client who talks incessantly. It would help for everyone to understand that she had many siblings who talked over her, inhibited her from speaking, or ignored her. Because her current group experience is similar to being around many siblings, she becomes anxious that she will not get an opportunity to speak. Furthermore, by talking non-stop, she will not have to observe that others are not listening. In this situation, the therapist can first describe the observed behavior or CRB1: "I notice that you have been talking a lot about the details of your day, such as your laundry and your dishes." Second, the therapist hypothesizes about the function of the client's behavior: "Perhaps talking about non-important things is one way to avoid talking about the things that matter. When you don't tell people how you really feel about what's going on, you don't have to make yourself vulnerable. Then you don't risk finding out if people really do care about what you have to say. What do you think?" Third, the therapist encourages new behavior (Rule 2): "I don't hear anybody here in group treating you like your siblings used to treat you. What if you talk about something that feels a little risky for you to talk about?" Fourth, the therapist helps evoke naturally reinforcing responses from other group members (Rule 3) in response to this client's CRB2 of talking about something more potent in a brief manner. Once the client is exposed to new responses contingent on her behavior, such as having positive input from others, change can occur.

In sum, reasons generated for behavior provide motivation for understanding, identifying, and controlling the unknown, and result in a sense of mastery and freedom. Reason-giving is an essential aspect of the change process because it moves people from a "passive, reactive posture to an active, acting, changing posture" (Yalom, 1995, p. 171). If clients are able to articulate how their behavior functions in their life they can find solutions and generalize progress in therapy to daily life.

Future Directions and Precautions

As current publications in support of FAP application to groups (Hoekstra, 2008; Vandenberghe et al., 2003) are theoretical in nature, future directions for FAP groups could include empirical data collection. The FAP Session Bridging Form and the FAP Experience of Closeness in the Therapeutic Relationship (Tsai et al., 2008) could easily be modified to collect information about groups between sessions. Additionally, measures of cohesion, loneliness, social phobia, depression, and intimacy could provide baseline data about symptoms and functioning. One suggestion for collecting data on FAP groups includes soliciting clients who utilize healthcare services for physical symptoms exacerbated by stress (e.g., headaches). This would enable the researcher to identify additional health-related symptom measures to include in the study.

Clinicians should also inform their clients of the potential risks associated with groups. While the group leader can foster certain norms and have a strong influence in structuring the group, there are no guarantees about how the group will unfold and what content may come up. Information is not guaranteed to be confidential, and feedback may be painful to hear. Clients may discontinue treatment if it is not beneficial for them, as long as there is exploration that this is not part of a CRB1 pattern of avoidance. Seeking individual therapy or meeting with the group leader individually may be an additional option if the group experience becomes too intense.

Conclusion

Burlingame et al. (2001) identified that two out of six empirically supported principles of group psychotherapy include pre-group preparation and early group structure. Therefore, providing an informed consent, conducting a screening interview, and accurately reiterating the client's functional patterns prior to the group process will be critical components of starting a group effectively. The FAP approach to group psychotherapy enables therapists to (1) elicit statements about CRB1s in the screening interview ("Yes, I talk a lot in groups, especially when I am anxious"), (2) elicit client agreement to work on presenting concerns in group ("Yes, I agree to attend to times during group in which I talk a lot"), (3) encourage client disclosure of CRB1s to the group ("If I'm talking a lot in group, I am probably getting anxious and need help"), and (4) remind clients of their commitment when the CRB1 shows up in group ("You are talking a lot. This is what you agreed to work on in group. How could we help you right now?"). As the group therapist allows the group to develop, he/she can enhance and augment the private experiences and reactions of group members, offer statements of functional relationships, and teach the group as a whole to watch for the CRBs of its members. Thus, the FAP application to group provides therapists not only a foundational structure for the group, but a clear focus on both the group agenda and the goals of the clients throughout the life of the group.

References

Burlingame, G. M., Fuhriman, A., & Johnson, J. (2001). Cohesion in group psychotherapy. *Psychotherapy: Theory, Research, Practice, Training, 38*(4), 373–379.

Callaghan, G. M. (2006). The Functional Idiographic Assessment Template (FIAT) System: For use with interpersonally-based interventions including Functional Analytic Psychotherapy (FAP) and FAP-enhanced treatments. *The Behavior Analyst Today, 7,* 357–398.

Fisher, P., Masia-Wartner, C., & Klein, R. G. (2004). Skills for social and academic success: A school-based intervention for social anxiety disorder in adolescents. *Clinical Child and Family Psychology Review*, *7*, 241–249.

Gaynor, S. T., & Lawrence, P. (2002). Complementing CBT for depressed adolescents with Learning through In Vivo Experience (LIVE): Conceptual analysis, treatment description, and feasibility study. *Behavioural & Cognitive Psychotherapy*, *30*(1), 79–101.

Hill, C. E., Nutt-Williams, E., Heaton, K., Rhodes, R. H., & Thompson, B. J. (1996). Therapist retrospective recall of impasses in long-term psychotherapy: A qualitative analysis. *Journal of Counseling Psychology*, *43*, 207–217.

Hoekstra, R. (2008). Interpersonal process groups redefined: A behavioral conceptualization. *International Journal of Behavioral Consultation and Therapy*, *4*, 188–198.

Hollander, M., & Kazaoka, K. (1998). Behavior therapy groups. In Long, S. (Ed.), *Six group therapies* (pp. 257–342). New York: Plenum Press.

James, L. D., Thorn, B. E., & Williams, D. A. (1993). Goal specification in cognitive-behavioral therapy for chronic headache pain. *Behavior Therapy*, *24*, 305–320.

Kohlenberg, R. J., & Tsai., M. (1991). *Functional analytic psychotherapy: Creating intense and curative therapeutic relationships*. New York: Plenum Press.

Rhode, P., Jorgensen, J. S., Seeley, J. R., & Mace, D. E. (2004). A cognitive-behavioral intervention to enhance coping skills in incarcerated youth. *Journal of the American Academy of Child and Adolescent Psychiatry*, *43*, 669–676.

Rittner, B., & Smyth, N. J. (2000). Time-limited cognitive-behavioral group interventions with suicidal adolescents. *Social Work with Groups*, *22*, 55–75.

Rose, S. (1977). *Group therapy: A behavioral approach*. Englewood Cliffs, NJ: Prentice-Hall.

Rutan, J. S., & Stone, W. N. (2001). *Psychodynamic group psychotherapy*. New York: Guilford Press.

Tsai, M., Kohlenberg, R. J., Kanter, J. W., Kohlenberg, B., Follette, W. C., & Callaghan, G. M. (2008). *A guide to functional analytic psychotherapy: Awareness, courage, love, and behaviorism*. New York: Springer.

Upper, D., & Flowers, J. (1994). Behavioral group therapy in rehabilitation settings. In Bedell, J. R. (Ed.), *Psychological assessment and treatment of persons with severe mental disorders* (pp. 191–214). Washington, DC: Taylor and Francis.

Vandenberghe, L., Ferro, C. B. L., & Furtado da Cruz, A. C. (2003). FAP-enhanced group therapy for chronic pain. *The Behavior Analyst Today*, *4*, 369–375.

Vinagrov, S., Co, P., & Yalom, I. (2003). Group therapy. In Hales, R. E. & Yudofsky, S. C. (Eds.), *Textbook of clinical psychiatry* (4th ed., pp. 1333–1371). Washington, DC: American Psychiatric Publishing.

Wilson, D. B., Bouffard, L. A., & Mackenzie, D. L. (2005). A quantitative review of structured, group-oriented, cognitive-behavioral programs for offenders. *Criminal Justice and Behavior*, *32*, 172–204.

Yalom, I. (1995). *The theory and practice of group psychotherapy*. New York: Basic Books.

Yalom, I., & Leszcz, M. (2005). *The theory and practice of group psychotherapy* (5th ed.). New York: Basic Books.

Index

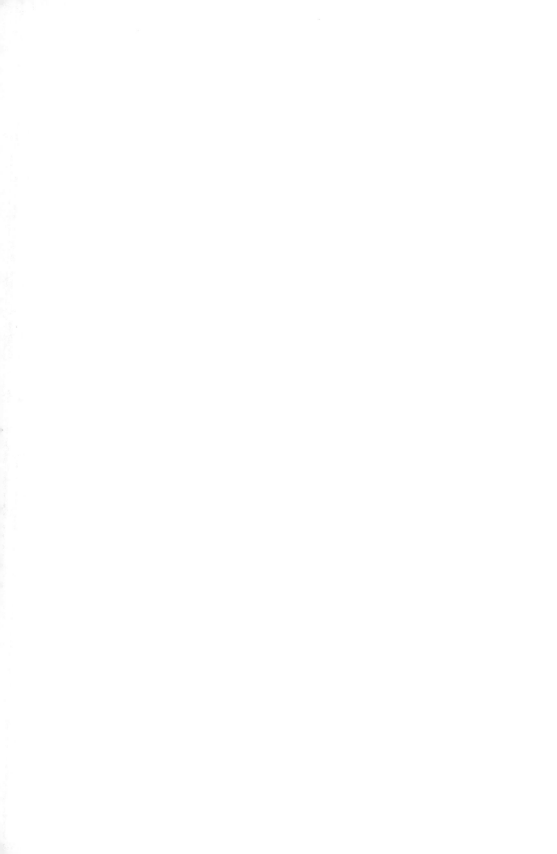

LaVergne, TN USA
11 June 2010
185788LV00001B/11/P